THE COMPLETE ILLUSTRATED GUIDE TO
NATURAL
HOME REMEDIES

Safe and Effective Treatments for Common Ailments

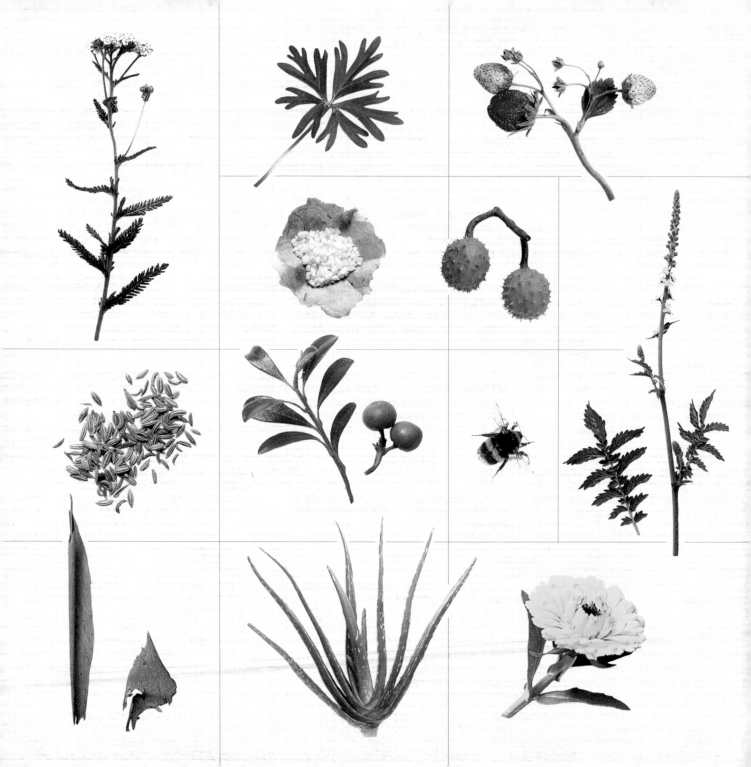

THE COMPLETE ILLUSTRATED GUIDE TO
NATURAL
HOME REMEDIES

Safe and Effective Treatments for Common Ailments

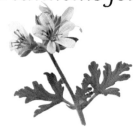

GENERAL EDITOR: KAREN SULLIVAN
CONSULTANT EDITOR: C. NORMAN SHEALY, M.D., PH.D.

Harper
Collins

HarperCollins*Publishers*
77–85 Fulham Palace Road,
Hammersmith, London W6 8JB

© 1997 by Element Books Limited

www.harpercollins.co.uk

First published in the USA, the UK and Australia in 1997 by Element Books Inc.

1 3 5 7 9 10 8 6 4 2

Cover illustration © Rebekah Nichols/illoreps.com

Designed by **quadrum**
Quadrum Solutions, Mumbai, India
www.quadrumltd.com Tel: 91-22-24968210

A complete listing or picture credits can be found at the back of this book.

A catalogue record of this book is available from the British Library

ISBN 978-0-00-788539-8

Printed and bound in China by South China Printing Company Ltd

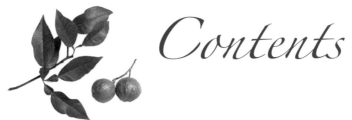

Contents

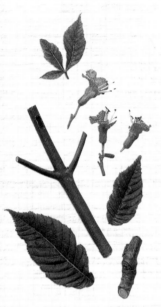

Foreword

Folk medicine has been the standard throughout the world and throughout history. Indeed, even today a majority of individuals living on the planet Earth have little or no access to physicians. It is estimated in the United States alone that at least 80 percent of ailments are treated in the "folk" domain.

Obviously there is a place for physicians in treating many acute illnesses and conditions such as seizures, fractured bones, serious infections and abscesses, congestive heart failure, strokes, etc. For less serious problems, and for a majority of chronic difficulties, home remedies and using common sense may often offer the best approach.

The Complete Illustrated Guide to Natural Home Remedies is an encyclopedic treasure providing the most comprehensive approach to date. For esthetic reading, browsing, or a quick reference, you have here my recommendation of the best guide to assist you in taking responsibility for your well-being.

C. NORMAN SHEALY, M.D., Ph. D.
Founder, *Shealy Institute for Comprehensive Health Care*
Founding President, *American Holistic Medical Association*
Research and Clinical Professor of Psychology,
Forest Institute of Professional Psychology

Introduction

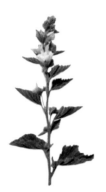

ABOVE
Marshmallow
(Althaea officinalis)
*is a traditional
herbal remedy with
many uses. Its leaves
make a soothing
tea for coughs and
its root is useful for
digestive problems.*

From the very earliest days of civilization we have turned to plants for healing, a tradition that has survived the arrival of conventional medicine and found new strength at the end of the twentieth century. Until fairly recently, every family had a cornucopia of favorite home remedies—plants and household items that could be prepared to treat minor medical emergencies, or to prevent a common ailment becoming something much more serious. Most households had someone with a little understanding of home cures, and when knowledge fell short, or more serious illness took hold, the family physician or village healer would be called in for a consultation, and a treatment would be agreed upon. In those days we took personal responsibility for our health—we took steps to prevent illness and were more aware of our bodies and of changes in them. And when illness struck, we frequently had the personal means to remedy it. More often than not, the treatment could be found in the garden or the larder.

Modern Miracles?

In the middle of the twentieth century we began to change our outlook. The advent of modern medicine, together with its many miracles, also led to a much greater dependency on our physicians and to an increasingly stretched healthcare system.

The growth of the pharmaceutical industry has meant that there are indeed "cures" for most symptoms, and we have become accustomed to putting our health in the hands of someone else, and to purchasing products that make us feel good. Somewhere along the line we began to believe that technology was in some way superior to what was natural, and so we willingly gave up control of even minor health problems.

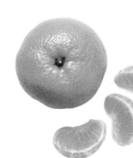

We are no longer in touch with our bodies, and when we become ill we expect someone else to treat us and to make us well again. Studies show that we are not really satisfied unless we leave our physician's surgery with a prescription. We are more dependent, and less self-sufficient, than we once were.

Increasingly, however, we are learning that the conventional medical system is not infallible. Its "miracle cures" may make us feel better, but they do so by suppressing the symptoms, not by curing their cause. For example, hydro-cortisone cream may ease the itching of eczema, but it does nothing to treat whatever is causing it. Cough suppressants will ease a cough, but the natural reflex of the body to expel mucus from the lungs has also been suppressed, which means that in the long run our bodies are unable to fight off illness and infection.

Many members of the medical community consider natural remedies to be old-fashioned and outdated, although some of the most effective drugs on the market are derived from plants. Foxglove provided digitalis, which has saved the lives of hundreds of heart patients, and the active ingredient in the bark of the white willow tree is none other than aspirin, one of the most important discoveries of modern medicine. There are plenty of other herbal remedies already in use within orthodox medicine; components of the yew tree, for example, have been successfully used to halt cancer, and the rosy periwinkle is used to control leukemia, especially in children. Plants are effective medicine, and when used prudently they can provide us with good health—free of side effects.

In the West, we are accustomed to taking medicine when we are ill, and it is difficult to teach ourselves that good health means taking a holistic approach. Natural remedies are designed to be holistic—taking into consideration the mind, body, and spirit as equally important elements of good health. When all three elements are successfully balanced, when we have optimum energy levels and a good sense of well-being, our bodies have the ability to cure themselves.

Remedies from the Home and Garden

Many of the remedies suggested in this book comprise natural items that you will find in your larder or growing in the garden. For others you may have to look a little further afield. There are detailed descriptions of each home remedy—for example, the variety of uses for the marigold plant, vinegar, wild cherry, arnica, and apples. You will also find a useful discussion of the forms in which each remedy can be taken. Some plants can be infused and drunk as a tea; some can be used as a poultice on an injured limb; others can be taken in homeopathic dilutions to treat specific conditions and ensure that our bodies are balanced. Certain plants have their "essences" extracted and distilled in alcohol (flower essences or tinctures), and we use the "essential oils" of many plants in aromatherapy, which is the fastest-growing complementary therapy in the Western world.

ABOVE *Natrum mur is a very useful homeopathic remedy which suits many symptoms; its source is common salt.*

More and more of us are developing a sense of personal responsibility, and taking our health back into our own hands. Today, with the benefit of knowledge of plants and traditional remedies from around the world, we have a vast and exciting pharmacy from which to choose our remedies, and an equally wide array of forms in which to prepare and purchase them. Our bodies are miraculous things and, by using natural remedies, we can encourage them to heal themselves.

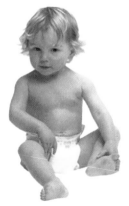

LEFT *Babies and children respond particularly well to home remedies; home remedies can be safely used to treat everyday complaints such as diaper rash.*

How to Use This Book

The aim of The Complete Illustrated Guide to Natural Home Remedies *is to introduce the reader to simple, natural remedies that can safely be used at home for the common ailments and everyday mishaps that every household experiences at some point. It is divided into four parts.*

PART ONE, **Home Therapies**, covers herbalism, homeopathy, flower essences, and aromatherapy, the therapies you are most likely to use at home, employing remedies that you can obtain easily or make yourself. There is also an essay entitled "From the Larder," which shows you the healing properties of everyday kitchen ingredients.

PART TWO, **The Ailments**, lists common ailments and the injuries that are most likely to occur at home, grouped under the body system they affect, beginning with the immune system, then working from the head downward. Children's problems and childhood diseases are covered in a self-contained section. Remedies from each of the five home therapies are suggested, as well as self-help tips.

PART THREE, **The Remedy Sources**, introduces the vegetable, animal, and mineral sources that provide the most familiar remedies used in the therapies outlined in Part One. It is interesting to note how many sources provide more than one therapeutic remedy.

PART FOUR, **Practical Matters and Useful Information**, contains a first-aid section and suggestions for the contents of a home medicine chest. These are followed by a table of vitamin and mineral data covering recommended daily intake, a glossary of terms, a directory of healing plants, suggestions for further reading, some useful addresses, and a general index.

THE ICON SYSTEM

Icons are used throughout the book to help you see at a glance which therapy is under discussion or recommended. There is also a special symbol to lead you to the most suitable remedies for children. A key is given to the right.

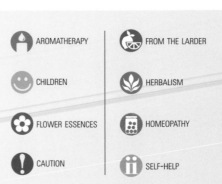

AROMATHERAPY

CHILDREN

FLOWER ESSENCES

CAUTION

FROM THE LARDER

HERBALISM

HOMEOPATHY

SELF-HELP

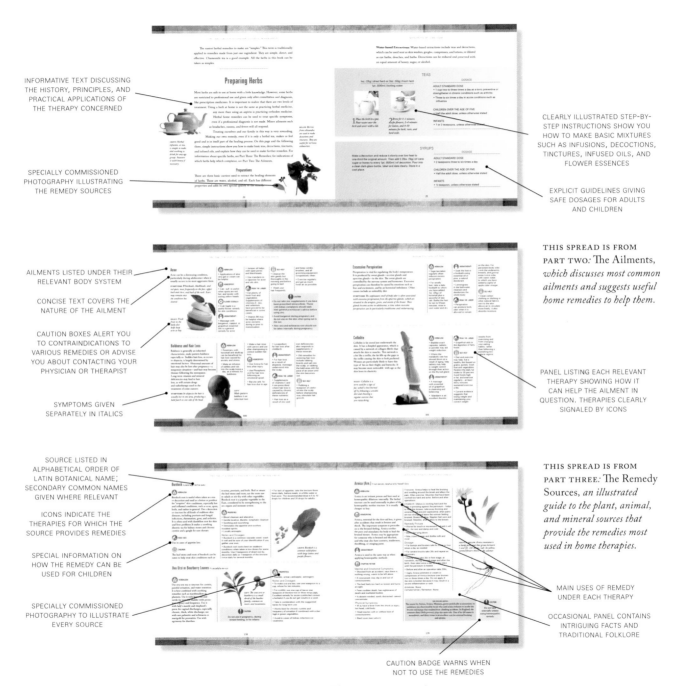

INFORMATIVE TEXT DISCUSSING THE HISTORY, PRINCIPLES, AND PRACTICAL APPLICATIONS OF THE THERAPY CONCERNED

SPECIALLY COMMISSIONED PHOTOGRAPHY ILLUSTRATING THE REMEDY SOURCES

CLEARLY ILLUSTRATED STEP-BY-STEP INSTRUCTIONS SHOW YOU HOW TO MAKE BASIC MIXTURES SUCH AS INFUSIONS, DECOCTIONS, TINCTURES, INFUSED OILS, AND FLOWER ESSENCES

EXPLICIT GUIDELINES GIVING SAFE DOSAGES FOR ADULTS AND CHILDREN

AILMENTS LISTED UNDER THEIR RELEVANT BODY SYSTEM

CONCISE TEXT COVERS THE NATURE OF THE AILMENT

CAUTION BOXES ALERT YOU TO CONTRAINDICATIONS TO VARIOUS REMEDIES OR ADVISE YOU ABOUT CONTACTING YOUR PHYSICIAN OR THERAPIST

SYMPTOMS GIVEN SEPARATELY IN ITALICS

THIS SPREAD IS FROM PART TWO: The Ailments, *which discusses most common ailments and suggests useful home remedies to help them.*

PANEL LISTING EACH RELEVANT THERAPY SHOWING HOW IT CAN HELP THE AILMENT IN QUESTION. THERAPIES CLEARLY SIGNALED BY ICONS

SOURCE LISTED IN ALPHABETICAL ORDER OF LATIN BOTANICAL NAME; SECONDARY COMMON NAMES GIVEN WHERE RELEVANT

ICONS INDICATE THE THERAPIES FOR WHICH THE SOURCE PROVIDES REMEDIES

SPECIAL INFORMATION ON HOW THE REMEDY CAN BE USED FOR CHILDREN

SPECIALLY COMMISSIONED PHOTOGRAPHY TO ILLUSTRATE EVERY SOURCE

THIS SPREAD IS FROM PART THREE: The Remedy Sources, *an illustrated guide to the plant, animal, and mineral sources that provide the remedies most used in home therapies.*

MAIN USES OF REMEDY UNDER EACH THERAPY

OCCASIONAL PANEL CONTAINS INTRIGUING FACTS AND TRADITIONAL FOLKLORE

CAUTION BADGE WARNS WHEN NOT TO USE THE REMEDIES

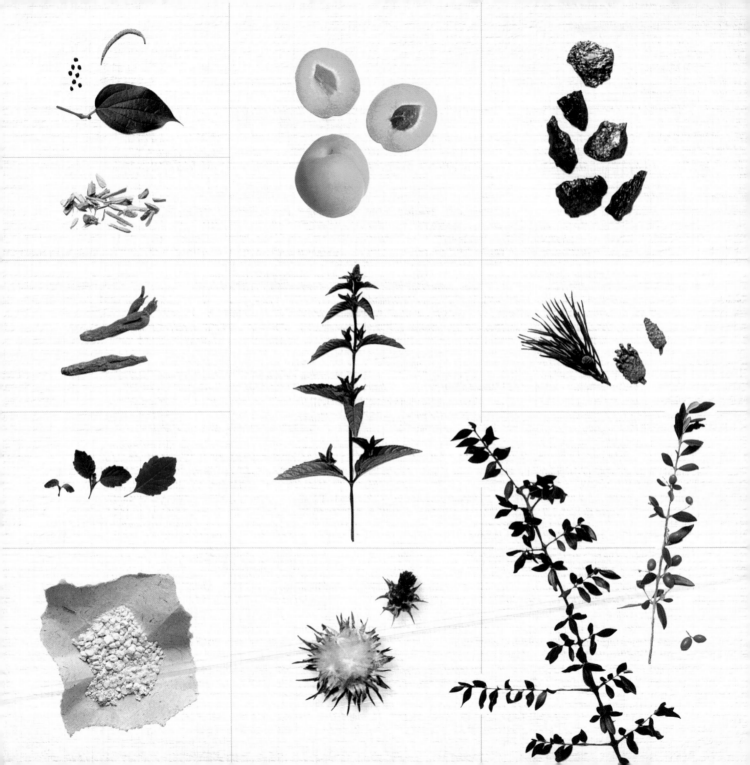

PART ONE

Home Therapies

Many natural healing therapies can be usefully applied at home. This part of the book offers a brief introduction to major therapies sympathetic to the natural approach: herbalism, homeopathy, flower essence therapy, and aromatherapy. There is also a section on food, covering basic nutrition and discussing foods that can heal and those that can do damage.

Each section gives a brief history of the therapy, its major principles and personalities, and practical advice and useful tips on how and when to use it in the home. Step-by-step illustrated instructions show you how to make your own basic herbal and flower essence remedies.

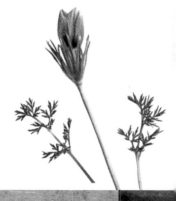

Herbalism

*H*erbalism is the oldest form of medicine known to humankind, and our knowledge of the healing power of herbs has accumulated over thousands of years. People from every culture explored the natural world around them and used it to furnish sustenance, shelter, and medications. Often the differentiation between food and medicine was slight, but medicine people discovered through trance, journeying, observation, and experimentation what was good or bad for the human body. The Ebers papyrus of ancient Egypt names eighty-five herbs including dill, lettuce, mint, and poppies. The Greek herbalist Dioscorides, who lived in the first century B.C., lists about 400 herbs, most of which are still used today.

The golden age of English herbalism was the sixteenth and seventeenth centuries. Culpeper wrote his *Complete Herbal* in 1653 as an aid to the "common man" to treat himself. It has been in print ever since. Culpeper's language is archaic but poetic. He recommends rose petal syrup "as an excellent purge for small children and grown people of a costive habit" and sloe berries for "the lax of the belly or stomach [diarrhea] or too much abounding of women's courses."

The tradition of self-help herbals was continued into the eighteenth century by John Wesley, a traveling preacher and founder of the Methodist Church, who collected many folk remedies on his journeys.

During the last century, as people moved into the new industrial cities, they lost touch with

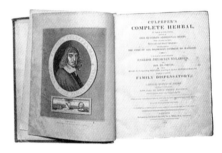

ABOVE *The title page from a nineteenth-century facsimile of Nicholas Culpeper's famous* Complete Herbal, *completed in 1653. Interest in Culpeper's art is still strong more than 300 years after his death.*

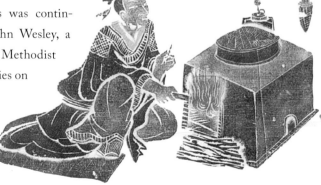

BELOW *Herbal remedies are central to traditional Chinese medicine. This stone rubbing shows a herbalist at work preparing his medicines.*

the herbal traditions of the countryside. However, herbal medicine was reintroduced by people such as Dr. Albert Coffin who learned his herbalism in America from the native people. He set up practice in England and was influential in founding the National Association of Herbalists, a key body in bringing herbal medicine up-to-date.

Today there is a revived interest in herbalism. It is being embraced by people seeking an alternative to drug therapy, and by the medical and pharmaceutical professions who use the active ingredients of plants to formulate new medicines. In most parts of the world herbalism is the main source of medicine, and in recent years interest in Western countries has been boosted by a greater understanding of the ancient traditions of China, India, and South America. Herbalists trained in the West use herbs grown mainly in the West, but they are developing uses for herbs from some of the Eastern disciplines.

What is a Herb?

In botany a herb is a green plant without a woody stem. In medicine the term is extended to include any plant, and any part of a plant, that can be used to make a remedy. This term "herb" embraces seaweeds, ferns, flowers, roots, bulbs, barks, seeds, and leaves and includes cooking herbs, spices, and many fruits and vegetables.

How Herbs Work

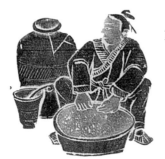

Herbal medicine occupies the middle ground between drugs and food. At one end of the herbal spectrum are strong remedies that have been used as the source of modern drugs; these include poppies and deadly nightshade, which are used to produce opium and atropine. At the other end are nourishing remedies such as bladderwrack and horsetail, which are rich sources of vitamins and essential trace nutrients.

The aim of the pharmaceutical industry is to find one "active" ingredient in a plant and extract it to make a more "powerful" medicine. Herbalists say that a plant is made up of many different ingredients that act together to make a safer and more effective medicine. Modern research tends to support this point of view.

Herbs are usually chosen to work with the inherent healing powers of the body. For example, fevers are treated with herbs, such as elderflower, that bring down the temperature by encouraging the body to sweat, which is its natural response. Recurrent infections are treated with herbs, such as echinacea, that stimulate the immune system to help the body fight off infection.

Many herbs are especially strengthening to particular organs and parts of the body. For example, hawthorn strengthens the heart and dandelion strengthens the liver. These herbs can be used for most diseases affecting those organs. Bitter tonics such as rosemary strengthen digestion and encourage the absorption of foods and are therefore applicable to most chronic illnesses, by helping to build up the whole body.

Herbalists consider that orthodox drugs suppress the body's healing powers. They have obvious advantages in crisis situations and for serious diseases, but they often leave the body in a partially healed state, setting up more health problems for the future.

For example, cortisone cream used in eczema quickly stops the inflammation but eventually thins the skin making it even more sensitive. Bronchial dilators used in asthma quickly stop an attack but lead to dependence, which discourages long-term healing. In both these conditions, the root cause of the illness is not addressed. The symptoms are eased, which is the form that all orthodox treatment takes. In contrast, the proper use of herbs strengthens rather than weakens the body.

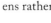

ABOVE *Bearberry* Arctostaphylos uva ursi *is a powerful astringent and antiseptic. It is useful for infections of the kidney and urinary tract.*

BELOW *Elder* Sambucus nigra *has many healing uses; its berries are useful for rheumatism, its flowers for catarrh complaints, colds, and influenza, and its leaves for wounds, sprains, and bruising.*

Herbalism in Action

*H*erbs are ideal medicines for home treatment of minor ailments and chronic, non-life-threatening diseases. Herbs used for chronic complaints are slow and sure and need to be taken for many months for maximum effect.

Children respond very well to herbal medicine, but remember that children's illnesses can develop very quickly. Seek a diagnosis from your medical practitioner or professional herbalist before beginning a herbal treatment.

Pregnant women like herbs for their relative safety and lack of side effects, but no herbal remedy should be started while pregnant without first consulting a herbal expert. Some herbs are contraindicated in pregnancy. These include angelica, Chinese angelica, comfrey, dang gui, devil's claw, ginseng, Siberian ginseng, lady's mantle, licorice, motherwort (except in the last three weeks), peppermint, sage, thyme, uva ursi, vervain, wild yam, and yarrow.

Some herbs are best avoided in early pregnancy. These include artemesia, Roman chamomile, burdock root, fennel seed, penny royal, raspberry leaves (best when taken in the last four to six weeks), and rue. A pregnant woman should not use any laxative except dandelion and yellow dock or any worming herbs except garlic.

When breast-feeding, women should avoid herbs that are contraindicated for infants. They should also avoid sage, which tends to dry up the milk.

Professional herbalists often use their remedies to complement orthodox therapies, and there has been much research validating this approach. This should not, however, be done at home, except in the specific instances mentioned under the appropriate herbs. If you are using herbs at the same time as orthodox treatment be sure to tell your medical practitioner, or ask your herbalist to contact your practitioner.

ABOVE *Use herbs gathered in the wild as quickly as you can after picking them to enjoy their maximum power.*

Where to Find Herbs

Herbs can be obtained from many different sources:

• Culinary herbs, fresh and dried, can be bought from most supermarkets, fruit and vegetable shops, and markets.

• Other herbs can be bought from specialist shops and mail-order suppliers.

• Chinese herb shops.

• Some herbs and a selection of herbal tablets and remedies are usually available at healthfood stores.

• Over-the-counter herbal remedies sold in most countries have to conform to strict rules governing their quality and safety.

• A range of herbal tablets may be found at pharmacies.

• Many herbs can be bought from garden nurseries.

• Seeds can be bought and the herbs grown in window boxes or gardens.

• Herbs can be gathered from the wild (wild crafted).

Purchase from a retailer with a fast turnover to ensure that herbs are as fresh as possible. To avoid confusion always specify the exact part of the plant you want: the leaf, flower, bark, or whole herb, etc. Botanical names are also useful. Although powders are convenient, it is best to buy whole herbs and spices and grind them when you need them—this way they retain their strength and flavor longer. Buy sufficient for your immediate needs and restock regularly. Store in jars in a cool dark place.

ABOVE *Growing herbs from seed can be very satisfying. Buy seeds from a reputable source, or better still take them from growing plants if you can.*

ARE HERBS SAFE?

Herbs have fewer side effects than orthodox medicines, and they are safer to use provided the following simple guidelines are used:

• Always follow the advice given. The dosages represent the most effective herb use. Double dosages do not work more quickly; they merely give the body too much work to do at once.

• Never pick your own herbs without being sure of identification. There are many strong and powerful herbs such as lily of the valley and gelsemium that need to be taken under professional guidance.

• Be sure you have your diagnosis correct. If the symptoms do not improve consult your medical practitioner or professional herbalist.

Wild crafting—gathering herbs from the wild—is becoming increasingly popular, but it is important to have an accurate identification and to pick with due regard to conservation. Many plants are protected by law. In some areas wild crafting is prohibited. Consider the rules of the countryside and treat all growing things with respect. Plants cannot be dug or roots gathered without the consent of the landowner. Gather well away from main roads and recently sprayed fields.

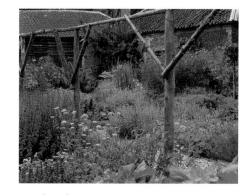

Growing herbs is rewarding and worthwhile. There is also the assurance, with homegrown produce, that it is free from sprays, chemical residues, and pollution. Follow the instructions on the seed package or buy a specialist herb gardening book. Each individual herb has an optimum harvesting time. Flowers are best when they have just opened. Leaves are most potent just before the plant has flowered. Gather roots in the fall and barks in the spring.

Fresh Herbs

Fresh herbs can be prepared in many different ways. They can be eaten in salads and sandwiches or added to soups and stews. They can be infused to make a tea or boiled to make a decoction. Fresh herbs are seasonal, but their healing virtues can be preserved in an alcoholic tincture for year-round use or they can be made into other preparations such as syrups and creams for convenience.

Dried Herbs

Most herbs will be purchased in their dried form, which is available all year round. They can be used in the same way as fresh herbs although the amounts differ slightly since dried herbs are a little more powerful. For example, when using dried herbs the standard recipe for a herbal tea is 1oz. to 1pt. (25g. to 500ml.) of water; when using fresh herbs it is 2oz. to 1pt. (50g. to 500ml.) of water.

The easiest herbal remedies to make are "simples." This term is traditionally applied to remedies made from just one ingredient. They are simple, direct, and effective. Chamomile tea is a good example. All the herbs in this book can be taken as simples.

Preparing Herbs

Most herbs are safe to use at home with a little knowledge. However, some herbs are restricted to professional use and given only after consultation and diagnosis, like prescription medicines. It is important to realize that there are two levels of treatment. Using a herb at home is not the same as practicing herbal medicine, any more than using an aspirin is practicing orthodox medicine. Herbal home remedies can be used to treat specific symptoms, even if a professional diagnosis is not made. Minor ailments such as headaches, nausea, and fevers will all respond.

Treating ourselves and our family in this way is very rewarding. Making our own remedy, even if it is only a herbal tea, makes us feel good and is in itself part of the healing process. On this page and the following three, simple instructions show you how to make basic teas, decoctions, tinctures, and infused oils, and explain how they can be used to make further remedies. For information about specific herbs, see Part Three: The Remedies; for indications of which herbs help which complaint, see Part Two: The Ailments.

ABOVE *Herbal infusion, or tea, is simple to make and soothing to drink for any age group. Sweeten it with honey if necessary.*

BELOW *Berries from schisandra are used to make decoctions and tinctures. They are useful for nervous exhaustion.*

Preparations

There are three basic carriers used to extract the healing elements of herbs. These are water, alcohol, and oil. Each has different properties and adds its own special quality to the remedy.

Water-based Extractions: Water-based extractions include teas and decoctions, which can be used neat as skin washes, gargles, compresses, and lotions, or diluted as eye baths, douches, and baths. Decoctions can be reduced and preserved with an equal amount of honey, sugar, or alcohol.

TEAS

1oz. (25g.) *dried herb* or 2oz. (50g.) *fresh herb*

1pt. (500ml.) boiling water

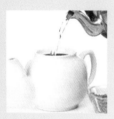

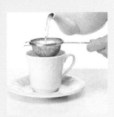

1 *Place the herb in a pot. Pour water over the herb and cover with a lid.*

2 *Brew for 1–3 minutes for flowers, 2–4 minutes for leaves, and 4–10 minutes for bark, roots, and hard seeds.*

DOSAGE

ADULT STANDARD DOSE
- 1 cup two to three times a day as a tonic preventive or strengthener in chronic conditions such as arthritis
- Three to six times a day in acute conditions such as influenza

CHILDREN OVER THE AGE OF FIVE
- Half the adult dose, unless otherwise stated

INFANTS
- 1 or 2 teaspoons, unless otherwise stated

SYRUPS

Make a decoction and reduce it slowly over low heat to one-third the original amount. Then add 2.2lbs. (1kg.) of cane sugar or honey to every 1pt. (500ml.) of decoction. Pour into a clean dark-glass bottle, label and date clearly. Store in a cool place.

DOSAGE

ADULT STANDARD DOSE
- 2 teaspoons three to six times a day

CHILDREN OVER THE AGE OF FIVE
- Half the adult dose, unless otherwise stated

INFANTS
- ½ teaspoon, unless otherwise stated

1oz. (25g.) *dried herb* or 2oz. (50g.) *fresh herb*

1pt. (500ml.) water

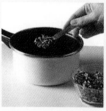

1 *Put herb into a pan.*

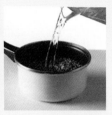

2 *Cover with water, and put on a tight lid.*

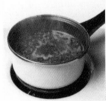

3 *Bring to a boil and simmer gently for twenty minutes.*

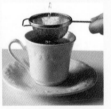

4 *Strain and make back up to 1pt. (500ml.) by adding fresh water.*

DECOCTIONS

Decoctions are made from seeds, barks, and roots. Decoctions will keep for three or four days.

DOSAGE

ADULT STANDARD DOSE
- ½ cup two to three times a day as a tonic
- ½ cup three to six times a day for acute conditions

CHILDREN OVER THE AGE OF FIVE
- Half the adult dose, unless otherwise stated

INFANTS
- ½ or 1 teaspoon, unless otherwise stated

COMPRESS: Use a standard tea at the required temperature: cold for inflammations, hot for joints and swellings, and warm for spasm, cramp, and muscle tension. Use hot alternating with cold for drawing abscesses. To make a compress, soak a bandage in the tea, wrap it around the affected part, cover, and leave on for ten to twenty minutes. Repeat as necessary. Use the same method for children and infants.

GARGLE: Add a pinch of salt to a standard tea or decoction and gargle three to six times a day. Use the same methods for children, although children under six are generally unable to gargle.

EYE BATH: Make sure that all utensils are scrupulously clean. Add a pinch of salt to a standard-strength tea and then strain carefully through unbleached filter paper. This may take some time. Make the tea fresh each time.

Use the eye bath to wash the eyes twice a day. Wash out the eye bath between bathing each eye.

Use the same method for children, although it may be more practical to use as eye drops by dropping the mixture directly into the eye.

TINCTURES

7oz. (200g.) *dried herb* or 14oz. (400g.) *fresh herb*

2pt. (1l.) liquid made up of 3 parts vodka to 2 parts water

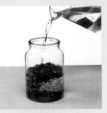

1 *Put herbs in a large, clean glass jar and pour the liquid mixture over them.*

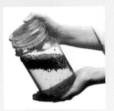

2 *Seal and store in a cool, dark place for two weeks, shaking occasionally.*

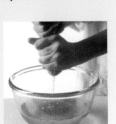

3 *Strain the mixture through a cloth and carefully wring out all the liquid.*

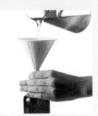

4 *Bottle and label with name and date.*

Herbal tinctures can be used internally and externally, in gargles, douches, compresses, liniments, mouthwashes, and baths.

Dilute 1 part tincture with 4 parts water for gargles, douches, and compresses.

Add 1 cup of tincture to a bath.

DOSAGE

ADULT STANDARD DOSE
• 1 teaspoon three times a day for chronic conditions
• 1 teaspoon six times a day for acute conditions

CHILDREN OVER THE AGE OF FIVE
• ½ teaspoon three times a day, or mix well with equal amounts of honey and give 1 teaspoon of the mixture

INFANTS
• 5-10 drops in a little fruit juice

BATH: 1 to 2 quarts (1-2 l.) of standard tea may be added to a bath, or one to two pints (½-1 l.) to an infant's bath or hand bath.

Adults should soak for twenty minutes. Children and infants should soak for ten minutes.

Alcohol-based extractions: Alcohol is used to make herbal tinctures, which are stronger than infusions or decoctions.

CREAMS: The simplest way to make a cream is to add tincture to a base cream. Base cream or emulsifying creams are available from pharmacists or specialist shops. As a last resort use an unscented hand cream. Creams soak into the skin and nourish it.

Add 1 part tincture, drop by drop, to 3 parts base cream, stirring all the time.

VINEGARS

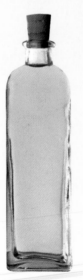

Vinegars are regarded as the "poor man's" tincture and are useful when you do not wish to use alcohol, or if it is contraindicated.

Make as for tinctures (*see page 25*) using 2pt. (1 l.) cider vinegar instead of the alcoholic liquid.

Use diluted with water as douches, washes, baths, disinfectants, and cooling drinks.

DOSAGE

ADULT STANDARD DOSE
• 1 tablespoon to 1 cup of water

CHILDREN OVER THE AGE OF FIVE
• 1 or 2 teaspoons mixed with water

INFANTS
• ½ or 1 teaspoon mixed with honey, if they will take it, up to six months

LEFT *Herbal vinegar, a nonalcoholic tincture.*

For infants and people with sensitive skin, use only marigold or chamomile, or test first on a small patch of skin.

Oil infusions: Traditionally bear or goose grease, butter, suet, or lard were used for infusions, but today we use vegetable oils.

INFUSED OILS

Use fresh or dried herbs (between 4 to 8oz. [100-200g.]) and pure unblended vegetable oil. A light oil such as sunflower or grapeseed is preferable to olive oil, which may overwhelm the natural fragrance of the herbs.

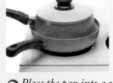

1 *Use a pan with a light lid. Put half the herbs into the pan and cover completely with oil.*

2 *Place the pan into a water bath or steamer and simmer gently for two hours. Do not use direct heat.*

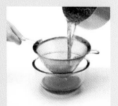

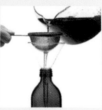

3 *After two hours strain well. The oil will change color, picking up some of the qualities of the herbs. Discard the spent herbs. Repeat the whole process. Put the remaining half of the original herbs in the pan and cover with the strained oil.*

4 *Return to the water bath and simmer for two hours. Strain. The oil will now have a rich herbal color. Pour into clean dark-glass bottles. Label and date. The infused oil will keep longer if you add 10 percent wheatgerm or vitamin E oil.*

DOSAGE

ADULT STANDARD DOSE
- ½ cup two to three times a day as a tonic
- Three to six times a day for acute conditions

CHILDREN OVER THE AGE OF FIVE
- Half the adult dose, unless otherwise stated

INFANTS
- ½ or 1 teaspoon, unless otherwise stated

Homeopathy

*H*omeopathy is a medical system whereby an ill person is treated with a remedy that would produce the symptoms of that illness in a healthy person. Although considered controversial by orthodox medical science, it is not a new idea. In *c.*450, Hippocrates—a Greek physician considered to be the father of medicine— noted that things that caused illness, such as poisons, could be used to treat illnesses they caused. Throughout history this principle was expounded and reconsidered, but it was not until Dr. Samuel Hahnemann (1755-1843) made it his life's work that the principle was formalized into a medical system.

The History of Homeopathy

Dr. Hahnemann was a German doctor who was fluent in many languages; by translating scientific papers he paid his way through university, qualifying in medicine and chemistry. He had a successful practice as a doctor but became disillusioned with the barbaric medical treatments of the day, which included bleeding, purging, and the use of unsafe, occasionally poisonous medicines. He returned once again to translation, whereupon the beginning of his theory was developed.

Hahnemann received a paper attributing the curative effect of cinchona bark (China) on malaria to its astringent and bitter properties. He found this difficult to believe and decided to take some China himself. He found that he suffered the symptoms of malaria, which disappeared within a few hours and did not reappear unless he repeated the dose.

He repeated the experiment on healthy friends and family, carefully noting the drug's effect, and he found that the same thing happened but the variety and strength of symptoms and the speed of recovery was different from person to person.

Hahnemann felt that he had now proved the action of the drug and called the list of symptoms "the proving." The healthy people who had taken the drug were "the provers." He then graded the symptoms into first (keynote), second, and third line, according to the frequency and strength of their appearance. Fired with enthusiasm he went on to prove other common drugs of the day including belladonna, arsenic, and mercury.

The Single Remedy

Hahnemann prescribed single remedies because they had been proven individually. He believed that if more than one remedy was given at a time, the combination might have a different effect on the body and it would be more difficult to pinpoint which remedy was having which effect. Other homeopaths have since gone on to develop combination remedies, but these should only be taken under the guidance of a professional practitioner.

THE FIRST LAW OF HOMEOPATHY

In 1796 Hahnemann wrote that there are three systems of medicine:

1. Prevention, where you remove the causes, such as poor hygiene, and so prevent illness.
2. *Contraria contraris*, which is healing by opposites (allopathy). An example of allopathic medicine is giving a laxative drug that will cause diarrhea to cure constipation.
3. *Similia similibus curentur*, which means "like cures like," or a substance that causes symptoms in a healthy person will cure similar symptoms in an ill person. He named this system homeopathy from the Greek meaning "similar suffering or disease." Similia similibus curentur became the first law on which homeopathy is based (the Law of Similars). Hahnemann then set up in medical practice but this time he closely questioned his patients as to the effect their illness had on them: were they hot or cold? Thirsty or thirstless? What did the pain feel like? When he had their answers, he prescribed a single remedy accordingly.

RIGHT Kali bichromium, *or* Kali bich., *is an excellent remedy for complaints characterized by excessive, thick mucus.*

REMEDY DILUTION, POTENTIZATION, AND THE MINIMUM DOSE

In homeopathy, the smallest dose (the minimum dose) is given to stimulate the body's natural defenses. During his early studies, Dr. Hahnemann found that people often suffered an initial severe aggravation of their complaint when taking a homeopathic remedy. He deduced from this that the dose must be too large, and so he devised a method of reducing it by progressive dilution *(see below)*. The more he diluted the remedy, the more powerful it became, and so he called the degrees of dilution "potencies," and the process "potentization." Most homeopathic remedies are diluted in a ratio of 1:100, the centesimal scale (c). Once the remedy is higher than 12c potency, there is little or none of the original substance left and yet the curative action is enhanced, not diminished. Remedies can also be potentized along the decimal scale.

The mother tincture is made directly from the source material.

One drop of the tincture is mixed with 99 drops of water or alcohol to make the first potency, 1c.

The tube is vigorously shaken over 100 times. This process is called succussion.

One drop is mixed with 99 drops of alcohol or water and the sequence is repeated.

Polentized remedies are used to make pills or creams, or taken as a tincture.

The Homeopathic Remedy

Many people mistakenly believe that because homeopathic remedies are sold over the counter in minute doses, it is the tiny size of the dose that makes it homeopathic. This is not so. For a remedy to be homeopathic it has to be chosen or prescribed according to the First Law of Homeopathy—*similia similibus curentur* or "like cures like"—and the symptoms of the person taking it must fit the remedy picture as given by the healthy provers.

Materia Medica and Remedy Pictures

A collection of remedy descriptions is known as a *materia medica*. An easy way to learn remedies is by getting to know them as people—think of the symptoms as making up a picture of a person. For example, a thin, hardworking, and irritable person who is prone to hangovers and indigestion would represent *Nux vomica*. Homeopaths call these "remedy pictures."

The Advance of Homeopathy

Despite being dismissed by the orthodox medical profession as unscientific, Dr. Hahnemann's practice flourished and gradually other doctors converted to homeopathy, and so it spread throughout the world. It was an ideal form of medicine for missionaries, explorers, and adventurers since the remedies were not bulky and each remedy often covers a wide list of ailments.

Hahnemann wrote many books in which he explained the philosophies on which homeopathy is based, the drugs he had proved with the symptoms elicited, and the use of such remedies up to the 30c potency.

Vital Force

The vital force is the energy that sustains life and gives strength to our constitution. Our minds, will, and intentions inspire and drive us to keep going, but whether or not we can depends on our vitality. Someone with a strong vitality will be full of energy and vigor, be able to work hard and sleep well. Because such people are strong, illnesses tend to have a violent sudden onset.

Other people have a reasonable vitality, so illnesses may come on suddenly, but once laid low these people do not have the reserve to bounce back and illnesses tend to linger. Yet others have a low vitality—illnesses creep up on them slowly, with symptoms gradually increasing in severity and then lingering a long time. People with low vitality are slow to recover.

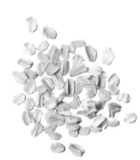

RIGHT *Grain cereals such as oats are rich in magnesium phosphate, the source of the remedy Mag. phos.*

Our vitality is part of our inherited constitution and is very much affected by our lifestyle: adequate sleep, a nutritious diet, regular moderate exercise, and good hygiene all maintain and improve our vitality. Likewise, inadequate sleep, a poor diet, excessive or insufficient stimulation, and bad hygiene will deplete it and make us susceptible to ill-health.

HERING'S LAW OF CURE

Dr. Constantine Hering (1800-80) formulated principles that govern the direction of cure. He stated:

• Cure takes place from within outwards, meaning the most vital organs will get better first. So the brain, lungs, heart, liver, and kidneys would improve before the gut, muscles, joints, or skin.

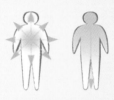

• Cure takes place from above to below; for example, psoriasis should clear up first on the head followed by the hands.

• Cure takes place in reverse order to the onset of symptoms. If a child has a history of eczema but presents with asthma, as the asthma is cured the eczema should return before healing for good.

Susceptibility to Disease

BELOW *Susceptibility varies from person to person. In a crowd of people exposed to the same conditions only a certain percentage will catch a contagious disease.*

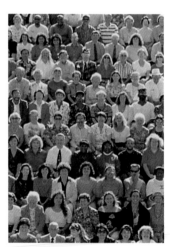

We will not catch a disease if we are healthy. During an epidemic not everyone will succumb to the disease; we have to be susceptible in order to suffer from disease. This is attributable not only to our inherited constitution and our lifestyle but also to our state of mind. Traditionally, doctors and nurses rarely succumbed to the infectious diseases that they treated. This is thought to be because their work was their vocation and they were happy and fulfilled. They were mentally and emotionally healthy and their bodies were too.

Homeopathy states that the most important key to good health is the mind—the intellect and will—and the emotions, and it is well recognized that depressions and neuroses are linked to physical diseases such as rheumatism, asthma, heart disease, and cancers. A depressed person has suppressed immunity, which makes him or her more susceptible to illness. Any physical, mental, or emotional stress depletes the vital force.

Homeopaths believe that the body instinctively seeks to be well and symptoms are a sign that the body is trying to maintain an equilibrium; for that reason, symptoms should never be suppressed, which simply drives the ailment inward. For example, suppressing eczema can lead to asthma, as the body tries to rid itself of disease through another route.

BIOCHEMIC TISSUE SALTS

Dr. W. H. Schuessler, a homeopath and chemist in the nineteenth century, noted that there are twelve mineral salts within the body that are vital for the healthy functioning of all the cells. He called them biochemic tissue salts and recorded their action on various bodily tissues and the symptoms caused by a lack or imbalance of each. He maintained that disease will not occur if cells receive adequate nutrition—the mineral salts are vital for this—so he decided that tissue salts singly or in combination were the only form of medicine the body needed. Because they are minerals, an ill body may not be able to assimilate them. So Schuessler used the homeopathic method of pharmacy and triturated (ground) the salts until they were soluble, in a 6x potency, and thus could be easily utilized by the body.

He maintained that his remedies are not homeopathic because they do not follow the like cures like rule; they supply the body with a substance it lacks to cure symptoms that have been produced because of the deficiency.

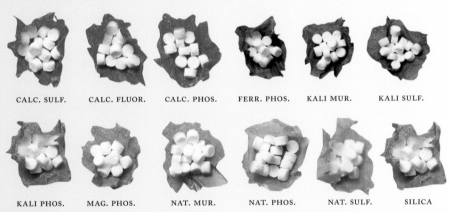

| CALC. SULF. | CALC. FLUOR. | CALC. PHOS. | FERR. PHOS. | KALI MUR. | KALI SULF. |

| KALI PHOS. | MAG. PHOS. | NAT. MUR. | NAT. PHOS. | NAT. SULF. | SILICA |

DOSAGES

Dr. Schuessler recommended prescribing tissue salts in the 6x potency:

• Acute cases: every half hour until better

• Chronic cases: three times a day until better

Homeopaths will always use the same remedy to fit a symptom picture, but the potency may differ as will the frequency of the dosage, according to the Law of Similars. The twelve biochemic tissue salts are:

CALC. FLUOR. *Calcium flouride*
CALC. PHOS. *Calcium phosphate*
CALC. SULF. *Calcium sulfate*
FERR. PHOS. *Iron phosphate*

KALI MUR. *Potassium chloride*
KALI PHOS. *Potassium phosphate*
KALI. SULF. *Potassium sulfate*
MAG. PHOS. *Magnesium phosphate*

NAT. MUR. *Sodium chloride*
NAT. PHOS. *Sodium phosphate*
NAT. SULF. *Sodium sulfate*
SILICA *Silicon dioxide*

Homeopathy in Action

$\mathcal{R}$emedies are made from any substance that can be proven to have an effect on humankind. They are derived mostly from plants and minerals but are also taken from the animal kingdom—mostly in the form of secretions, such as snake venom and bee sting. Remedies are also made from disease products, such as pus, and also from sunshine, electricity, and sea water.

As previously mentioned, remedies are made according to two potency scales—decimal and centesimal. If a substance is easily soluble it is dissolved in alcohol for eight to fourteen days, then strained and the liquor is called the Mother tincture (Q) from which all other potencies are derived. If the substance is not easily soluble it is triturated (ground) with lactose and after the sixth potency it will be soluble in alcohol.

Remedies are dispensed as hard or soft tablets, powders, granules, or globules made from lactose. These may be sucked until they dissolve away, or be dissolved in a glass of water first and then taken by the spoonful. Remedies may also be dispensed as tinctures (liquids) and taken as drops directly on the tongue or diluted in water.

Remedies should be stored in cool, dry conditions, out of direct sunlight and away from strong smells; they should be handled minimally.

Do not eat, drink, or clean your teeth for fifteen minutes before and after taking a remedy so that your mouth is relatively free of tastes and odors. While being treated homeopathically, it is best to avoid coffee and other caffeine-containing foods and drinks because some remedies may be antidoted.

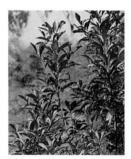

ABOVE *The quinine tree* Cinchona officinalis, *source of the homeopathic remedy Cinchona or China. This was the remedy that inspired Hahnemann's theory.*

Case-taking

A professional homeopath will make a very detailed study of patients—not just their presenting complaint and its causes, but a full medical history noting their constitution and appearance, mental and emotional symptoms, physical symptoms, general symptoms and any peculiar symptoms that accompany them.

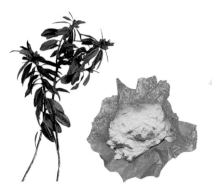

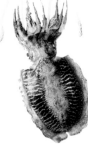

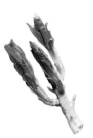

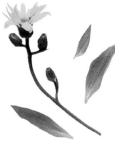

Ledum palustre
LEDUM

Flowers of Sulfur
HEPAR SULF.

Sepia officinalis
SEPIA

Atropa belladonna
BELLADONNA

Arnica montan
ARNICA

LEFT AND BELOW
*Homeopathic
remedies come from
a wide variety of
sources from the
animal, vegetable,
and mineral
kingdoms.*

Then they prescribe the similar remedy and required potency.

When taking a case yourself, jot down everything you notice about your patient, whether it is a friend or your child. Be observant, note their skin color and texture, whether they sweat or have a particular odor. What mood do they appear to be in, have they noticed a mood change themselves? Find out what they are complaining of—how severe it is, what the pain is like, whether it radiates anywhere, what things make them better or worse, and so on—until you have a picture of how their complaint affects them.

Compare your picture to the remedies in this book—it is not necessary to have all the symptoms listed under the remedy, just the main ones for the complaint. It is best to start by prescribing remedies for minor ailments that are not too severe and are of limited duration such as coughs and colds, conjunctivitis, cuts and bruises, and teething.

Acute complaints are usually of a sudden onset and, by their nature, have a limited duration. Recovery is usually quick and uneventful. A chronic complaint is a recurring, long-term condition and may have a much slower recovery. Chronic complaints gradually increase in severity; acute attacks may occur on top of the chronic symptoms—for example, in asthma or arthritis. Chronic conditions usually weaken the system making it susceptible to further chronic and acute illnesses.

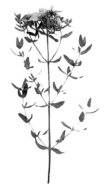

*Hypericum
perforatum*
HYPERICUM

WHAT TO EXPECT

• The condition improves according to Hering's Law and the person feels well in themselves: the correct remedy has been given.

• There is an initial aggravation of symptoms but then the person improves: the correct remedy has been given.

• The condition improves at first, then stops: review the case, either repeat the remedy in the same or higher potency, or change the remedy.

• The condition remains unchanged: review the case. If the remedy still appears to be correct review the potency given. Or change the remedy. Or consult a professional homeopath.

• New symptoms appear that the person has never experienced before: they could be "proving" the remedy. Stop taking the remedy, and the symptoms should clear up. If they do not, try drinking a cup of very strong black coffee—it will often antidote the actions of remedies. Or consult a professional homeopath.

Prescribing the Remedy

Having decided on the appropriate remedy you have to decide on the potency and the frequency of the dose to be given.

As a general rule, never repeat the remedy while improvement continues.

• For acute physical ailments where the physical symptoms predominate: 6x or 6c potency every fifteen to thirty minutes.

• Then, as symptoms settle down, stretch the dose to every couple of hours.

• Finally, reduce the dose to three times a day if required.

Once improvement is seen do not repeat the remedy until the action appears to stop and improvement does not continue.

• For acute physical or emotional ailments where the mental or emotional symptoms predominate, take one 30c dose and do not repeat unless needed.

• For chronic physical complaints, give a 6x or 6c potency three times a day for a week, or longer if you feel this is necessary.

Flower Remedies

*F*lower remedies use the vibrationary essence of flowers to balance the negative emotions that lead to and are symptoms of disease. They are a simple natural method of establishing personal equilibrium and harmony. Flower remedies are simple to make and use; they can be safely taken by people of all ages and levels of health; and they will not interfere with any other medication.

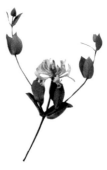

ABOVE
Honeysuckle is the Bach remedy for grief and excessive nostalgia.

The History of Flower Remedies

Until recent years the term "flower remedies" was synonymous with Dr. Edward Bach. Dr. Bach was born in Warwickshire, England, in 1886. He trained at University College Hospital in London where he worked as a bacteriologist during World War One. His work with F. H. Teale on intestinal bacteria was an important contribution to modern medicine, and in March 1919, he went on to the London Homeopathic Hospital. It was here that he began to study and develop the concept and application of flower remedies. He believed that diseases

DR. BACH'S FIVE PRINCIPLES

Dr. Bach realized during the clinical trials that the remedies would be ideal for home use. Medical knowledge could lead to restrictive thinking and practices, but the use of flower remedies was available to everyone because it was based on five simple principles:

1. *No medical knowledge whatsoever is required.*
2. *The disease itself is of no consequence whatsoever.*
3. *The mind is the most sensitive part of our bodies, and the best guide to tell us what remedy is required.*
4. *The manner in which a patient reacts to an illness is alone taken into account, not the illness itself.*

5. *Conditions such as fear, depression, doubt, hopelessness, irritability, desire for company or desire to be alone, and indecision are the true guides to the way in which a patient is being affected by his or her malady, and to the remedy he or she needs.*

The same disease may have different effects on different people. It is these individual effects that require treatment. In illness there is a change of mood from that of ordinary life. It is possible to notice and treat the changes long before signs of the disease itself appear. Flower remedies affect on every level—spiritual, psychological, and physical. In this way, flower remedies are truly holistic.

THE BACH FLOWER REMEDIES

AGRIMONY*: For those who hide their feelings behind a cheerful face. They claim that all is well even when it is not.

ASPEN: This "trembling tree" remedy is for fear of unknown things.

BEECH*: For the perfectionist who finds it hard to tolerate or understand the shortcomings of those they believe to be foolish, shortsighted, or ignorant.

CENTAURY*: For those who are kind, gentle, and eager to please, but so unwilling to let anyone down that they find it impossible to say no.

CERATO*: For those who seek the reassurance of others because they do not trust their own judgment or intuition. Dithering means that they miss out on opportunities.

CHERRY PLUM: For irrational thoughts and those who fear losing their sanity. They often feel anxious and overwhelmingly depressed.

CHESTNUT BUD: For those who keep making the same mistakes, never seeming to learn from past experiences.

CHICORY*: For the mothering type who is loving but overprotective and possessive. They demand love, sympathy, and appreciation.

CLEMATIS*: For the artistic dreamer, who may become absent minded, inattentive, easily bored, and lacking in concentration.

CRAB APPLE: For those who feel infected or unclean, revolted by eating or sex, or who have a hygiene fixation.

ELM: For those who are overwhelmed and made to feel inadequate by pressure from work, family, and other commitments.

GENTIAN*: For the eternal pessimist, who is easily discouraged.

GORSE: For those who believe that they were born to suffer and are pessimistic about everything.

HEATHER: For those who are always talking about themselves, so nobody else can get a word in.

HOLLY: For those who develop the victim mentality, overcome with hatred, jealousy, envy, or suspicion.

HONEYSUCKLE: For those who dwell on the past to the extent that they lose interest in the present. Can help with bereavement.

HORNBEAM: For those who are mentally exhausted at the thought of work so what used to be a pleasure becomes a chore.

IMPATIENS: For those who do everything in a hurry. They are brusque, finish sentences for people, fidget, look at their watches, and edge toward the door when others are still talking.

LARCH: For those with ability but no confidence.

MIMULUS*: For those who are shy, nervous, and blush easily. This is also the remedy for the fear of known things.

MUSTARD: For those who are gloomy for no apparent reason.

OAK: For the fighter who never gives in.

OLIVE: For those who are exhausted through overwork or overexhaustion.

PINE: For those who feel guilty, even when things are not their fault. They are always apologizing.

RED CHESTNUT: For those who are overanxious for family and friends and afraid of impending disasters.

ROCK ROSE*: For terror and panic, which may not be rational but is still real.

ROCK WATER: For those who are strict with themselves and who demand perfection.

SCLERANTHUS*: For emotional distress due to indecision.

STAR OF BETHLEHEM: For the inconsolable after shock, bereavement, bad news, or trauma.

SWEET CHESTNUT: For those in utter despair, when they can see no way out of the darkness and wish they could die.

VERVAIN*: For the enthusiastic, principled perfectionist who is incensed by injustice and fights for the underdog.

VINE: For the leader—the strong, dominant, ambitious, and determined but sometimes tyrannical.

WALNUT: This is the remedy for change. It settles one into a new environment and helps to cope with life changes.

WATER VIOLET*: For the reserved, self-contained, and dignified.

WHITE CHESTNUT: For those who are tormented by persistent worries and unwanted thoughts.

WILD OAT: For those dithering at a crossroads in life.

WILD ROSE: For those who drift and do not have the enthusiasm or ambition to change any aspect of their life.

WILLOW: For the grouchy, introspective pessimist who dwells on misfortune and wallows in self-pity.

One of Dr. Bach's original "Twelve Healers."

were not primarily due to physical causes but some deeper disharmony, which would lower the individual's vitality and resistance. In 1930, Dr. Bach decided to devote his life to a search for simple remedies from the countryside.

Between 1928 and 1932, Dr. Bach discovered the "twelve healers," Agrimony, Beech, Centaury, Cerato, Chicory, Clematis, Gentian, Mimulus, Rock Rose, Scleranthus, Vervain, and Water Violet. Dr. Bach based the remedies on his observation that all people could be categorized into one of twelve easily recognizable types. He knew intuitively that there were more states to explore but he published the "Twelve Healers" saying, "The relief of suffering was so certain and beneficial, even when there were only twelve remedies, that it was deemed necessary to bring these before the public at the time, without waiting for the discovery of the remaining twenty-six."

Dr. Bach was very religious; he believed that health and harmony is our natural state and that we can achieve it if we listen to our true souls. Problems developed when an individual had difficulty learning one of the fundamentals of life, which according to Dr. Bach, are:

- Power
- Balance
- Wisdom
- Intellectual knowledge
- Service
- Spiritual perfection
- Love

Disease indicates that the personality is in conflict. He believed that qualities and virtues are relative and that a virtue in one person may be perceived as a fault in another. Dr. Bach said that the primary diseases are caused by the lessons of:

- Cruelty
- Self-love
- Instability
- Hate
- Ignorance
- Greed
- Pride

Negative states could be broken down into groups:

- Fear
- Insufficient interest in present circumstances
- Uncertainty
- Loneliness

The thirty-eight remedies developed by Dr. Bach are all rooted in one of these seven states and they respond to the seven steps of healing, generated by peace, hope, joy, faith, certainty, wisdom, and love.

The flower essences work with these positive emotions, so that the emotions may flow freely. Dr. Bach believed that flower remedies worked by "like repelling like." In his book *Heal Thyself*, he advises those who suffer to seek within themselves for the real origin of their maladies, so they may assist themselves in their own healing.

Flower Remedies in Action

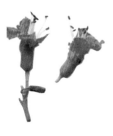

ABOVE *Red Chestnut is used to soothe the overanxious, those distressed by news of distant disaster.*

*W*hen buying flower essences you purchase a stock bottle of remedy, which is a stock of the concentrated remedy from which personal remedies and medicines can be made. Do not use this in its undiluted state.

A personal remedy may contain one to six remedies. It depends on the areas being addressed. Decide on the remedies needed, put 4 drops of each into a clean 1fl. oz. (30ml.) bottle, add water and 1 teaspoon of brandy to act as a preservative. Shake well and label with your name and the date. The remedy is now ready to use. All stock remedies should be diluted in this way before use.

The standard dose is 4 drops four times a day under the tongue. Remedies can be taken every half hour during extreme crisis.

There is some debate as to whether the remedies should be taken before or after meals, or if coffee and strong herbs and spices should be avoided. There is little evidence that anything affects the efficiency of the remedies, but it is useful to space them carefully across the day so that the remedy may take advantage of your personal rhythms.

Remedies are about growth and change, so it is worth looking for the periods of the day when you have some mental space. Some people find this time in the

RESCUE REMEDY

The most frequently used of all the remedies is Bach Rescue Remedy, made up of Cherry Plum, Clematis, Impatiens, Rock Rose, and Star of Bethlehem. As the name suggests, it is the remedy for emergencies, for when you feel panic, shock, loss of control, and mental numbness. It is often the remedy that triggers the body's healing response during illness. Rescue Remedy can calm exam nerves and relieve the anxiety of flying or visiting the dentist. You can dab it on stings, bruises, and sprains, as well as taking it internally. Rescue Remedy cream is also available for external use.

RIGHT *Rock rose, one of the five ingredients of Rescue Remedy.*

early morning, when they are fresh and before the pattern of the day has become established; others choose the evening when the chatter of the world has ceased and everyone else is in bed. Remedies can be used:

- To treat the emotional outlook generated by disease
- To alter a temporary emotional response and situation
- To balance a particular recurring pattern in the personality
- As a preventive measure

An acute trauma may respond in a few days. A long-standing or chronic pattern might need supporting for three or four months. Try a new mixture for ten days and then reconsider patterns and moods before continuing.

Do not force yourself to take any remedy. It must feel right. Some people take their remedy regularly and then one day forget—a subconscious indication that they no longer need that particular remedy. Another may be needed but the original pattern has passed.

Flower remedies can be taken with other remedies, and will not interfere with orthodox treatment or any of the natural remedies mentioned in this book.

BELOW *Babies and children respond very well to flower essence remedies. The remedies can be administered internally or externally.*

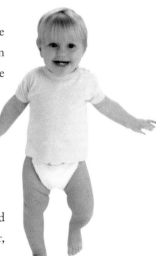

Babies, Children, and Special Needs

Flower remedies are especially suitable for children. Babies, very old people, and pets also respond very well. A few drops of remedy, diluted in a tumbler of water, can be put in children's drinks. The skin can be anointed or the remedy put on the pulse point of the wrist, neck, or temples. It is important to make sure that the remedies are appropriate for the child and gathered from accurate observations and not a projection of adult fears and feelings. If you feel that a child needs a remedy it may be worth taking Red Chestnut, Rescue Remedy, or Chicory your-self, to make sure that you are thinking, feeling, and acting appropriately.

New Flower Remedies

Since 1976, the Australian company Gurudas has been working on developing flower essences based on American plants, and there are now 150 remedies. They deal with the transformation of subtle energies to create a pain-free pattern, finding a balanced expression between polarities of life. Dr. Bach expressed his ideas in Christian terms. Gurudas integrates ideas from Eastern philosophies.

BELOW *shows a selection of the sources of classic Bach remedies.*

Australian Essences

Australian naturopath and herbalist Ian White has been working to develop essences from the unique Australian flora. He calls them Australian Bush remedies. There are over sixty to date.

White believes that essences have a very important role to play in our lives as catalysts, in helping people heal themselves, noting that:

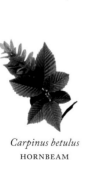

Centaurium erythrea
CENTAURY

Carpinus betulus
HORNBEAM

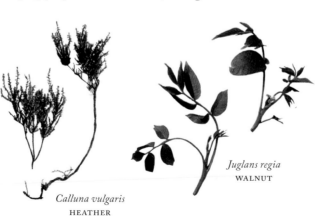

Calluna vulgaris
HEATHER

Juglans regia
WALNUT

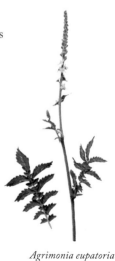

Agrimonia eupatoria
AGRIMONY

"The essences allow people to turn inwards and understand their own life plan, their own life purpose and direction. They also give people the courage and confidence to follow that plan. Illness, disease and emotional problems are only indicators that we have strayed off our individual path. The essences, as well as helping us return to that path, can assist us to work through and resolve our problems and imbalances. They can also help to give us an understanding of why these difficulties came about in the first place and what needs to be done to clear them, by unleashing the positive qualities inherent in us."

This is very similar to the roles that Dr. Bach ascribed to the actions of his remedies. The Australian remedies deal with subtle emotional states, but also with fears and situations that were unknown during Dr. Bach's time, for example, techno-fear or protection against radiation poisoning. There is an Australian version of the Rescue Remedy and its key lesson is "comfort."

Making Flower Essences

*R*emedies are prepared in two ways: the sun method and the boiling method. The methods are easy to follow. Cleanliness is essential and all utensils should be sterile. Wash your hands well with unscented soap and rinse several times with plenty of water. Sterilize utensils by boiling gently for twenty minutes in pure water, preferably rain water. Allow them to drain dry, and then wrap them in a clean cloth. Do not touch the inside of the bowl with your hands. Decide beforehand on the plants you will need, where to pick them, and where to place the bowl. Wait for a suitable sunny day. The best time of day is between 9 a.m. and midday, when the sun has dried the dew and the flowers are open but still fresh. Picked flowers should be put in water as soon as possible. Picking movements should be quick and sure so that the flowers are in contact with your hands for as short a period as possible. A large leaf, preferably of the plant being picked, should be used to cover

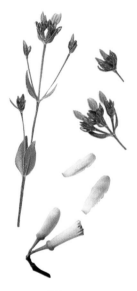

ABOVE *Whatever flowers you choose to make your own essence, touch them as little as possible to avoid damage.*

THE SUN METHOD

1 *If possible use water fresh from a local spring. If not available, use bottled spring water from a reputable source. Pour into a clean glass bowl.*

2 *Float the flowers on the water until the whole surface is covered. Use a twig or leaf to arrange them. Since the bowl is uncovered it is important that it is placed away from shadows and any possible contamination.*

3 *Leave the bowl out in the open where it will receive direct sunshine for three hours.*

4 *After three hours remove the flowers with a twig and pour 1.5fl. oz. (50ml.) of the water into the bottle with the brandy. Shake and label with the name of the stock flower essence and the date.*

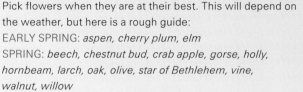

Pick flowers when they are at their best. This will depend on the weather, but here is a rough guide:

EARLY SPRING: *aspen, cherry plum, elm*
SPRING: *beech, chestnut bud, crab apple, gorse, holly, hornbeam, larch, oak, olive, star of Bethlehem, vine, walnut, willow*
LATE SPRING: *mustard, pine, red chestnut, water violet, white chestnut*
SUMMER: *agrimony, centaury, honeysuckle, mimulus, rock rose, sweet chestnut, wild rose*
LATE SUMMER: *chicory, clematis, heather, impatiens, scleranthus, vervain, wild oat*
AUTUMN: *cerato, gentian*

To make a 3fl.oz. (100ml.) bottle of stock flower essence, you need:

- 2pt. (1l.) bottle of spring water
- A shallow glass bowl
- A 3 fl. oz. (100ml.) dark-glass bottle containing 1.5 fl. oz (50ml.) brandy

This stock essence, made by the method shown on the right, will keep for many years.

the palm and protect the flowers from the heat of your hands and contamination with sweat. The remedy water should never be touched. Use twigs for stirring and separating.

For the boiling method, it would be ideal to try to boil the flowers in the open, as near as possible to their source. That way you do not compromise their freshness. You can do this using a camping stove if it is permissible to light a fire near your collection site. If not, get back home as quickly as possible after picking your flowers.

THE BOILING METHOD

Pick when the flowers are at their best (*see page 42*). Again, cleanliness is vital to avoid contamination. Sterilize utensils as described (*see page 41*).

1 Touch the plants as little as possible. Pick twigs or flowers until the saucepan is three-quarters full.

2 Put the lid on the saucepan. When over a source of heat cover the flowers and twigs with cold water and bring to a boil, and then simmer for half an hour, occasionally stirring with a twig.

3 After half an hour remove from the heat and stand outside to cool.

YOU NEED:

- 6pt. (3l.) saucepan with lid. Use an enamel, glass, or stainless steel pan; avoid copper, aluminum, and Teflon-coated pans

- A glass measuring pitcher

- 2pt. (1l.) cold water. Rain water is preferable but tap water will do

- A 3fl. oz. (100ml.) dark-glass bottle containing 1.5fl. oz. (50ml.) brandy

- Natural, unbleached filter paper

4 When cool remove the twigs and stand until any sediment has settled at the bottom. Then carefully filter the water into the measuring pitcher.

5 Put 1.5ft. oz. (50ml.) of the flower water into the bottle with the brandy.

6 Label with the name of the stock flower essence and the date. This will be used to make personal remedies.

The Future

More essences are likely to be discovered from various countries as more plants are studied, and as we learn from nature to seek solutions to the emotional fears that lead to disharmony and disease. There will be more and different fears as humans and nations face the ever-changing and uncertain future. Whatever the future holds, we have the stability of Dr. Edward Bach's twelve basic healers, the helpers, and the other remedies to help us grow and deal with negative responses to life.

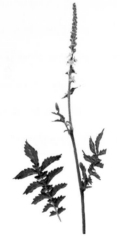

ABOVE *Agrimony flowers are readily available for picking and making flower essences at home.*

Aromatherapy

*T*he word aromatherapy comes from a combination of two words: "aroma," which means smell or fragrance, and "therapy," which means a treatment for the body or mind or social condition of a person to assist or facilitate a process where healing and change can take place. The science and art of aromatherapy is based on the various treatments by which essential oils can be used effectively and safely. Aromatherapy also plays an important role in the main branches of complementary medicine, where it acts as a link between orthodox medicine, homeopathy, osteopathy, and therapeutic counseling.

The History of Aromatherapy

The art of aromatherapy has been practiced for thousands of years. The first evidence of its use comes from China where, in 4500 B.C., a medical book was written by an emperor named Kiwant Ti on the aromatic and healing properties of plants. Between 4000 B.C. and 200 B.C., Egypt developed a reputation for its use of essential oils for medicine, pharmaceuticals, perfumery, and cosmetology, all of which was placed under the protection of the god Horus. The Egyptians believed in reincarnation and used essential oils such as cedarwood, incense, and myrrh to keep the body in good condition for embalming. They also used oils on a therapeutic basis in their everyday life. Tombs have revealed alabaster vases still full of aromatic preparations. Intricate carvings and detailed hieroglyphics can still be seen on many temple walls such as those on the island at Philae, at Edfu, and Deir el-Bahari, the temple dedicated to Hathor by Queen Hatshepsut. The ancient Egyptians described formulas and showed scenes where vessels were being used for perfumes and oils in ritual and dance.

BELOW *A Chinese garden; essential oils play an important part in traditional Chinese medicine, which embraces massage and herbalism as well as acupuncture.*

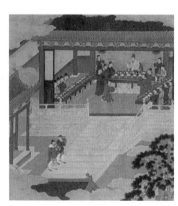

Egyptian priests were also doctors. They knew how to extract aromatic essences from plants, and they dedicated essences to their gods and to the astrological planets. Myrrh, for example, was dedicated to the Moon, incense to the Sun, and lavender and marjoram to Mercury. It was from their Egyptian captors that the Hebrews gained knowledge of the uses of aromatic and essential oils in medicine and in religious ritual.

In Greece, the revered surgeon and physician Hippocrates (460-377 B.C.) believed that, for medicine to be successful, the whole person had to be treated and not just the disease. He was known to have used saffron, thyme, cumin, peppermint, and marjoram in his work. Greek soldiers used to carry ointment made of myrrh into battle to put on their wounds. Later, many Greek doctors were employed by the Romans as military surgeons. Galen (A.D. 130-200), one of the most famous surgeons, treated many gladiators with his essential oils and remedies. He also invented the original "cold cream."

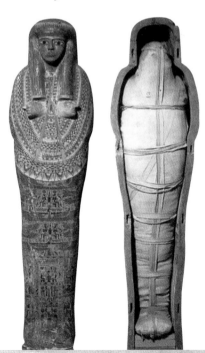

BELOW *The Egyptians understood the power of plant oils. Several kinds were used in the process that preserved the bodies of the ancient dynastic kings and queens before they were embalmed and mummified.*

Pedanius Dioscorides (A.D. 40-c.90), another great Greek physician who lived during the reign of Nero collected many medicinal plants and transcribed the results of his labors in his memorable work De Materia Medica. After the fall of Rome, his work was translated into Arabic and Persian and other languages. Texts spread from Constantinople to the famous medical library at Alexandria and on to the Arab world where aromatics and the art of distillation became widely practiced. One of the most famous medical authorities of these times was the Persian scholar, Avicenna (A.D. 979-1037), born Abu Ali al-Husayn Ibn ab Allah Ibn Sina, who is credited with the first distillation of essential oils.

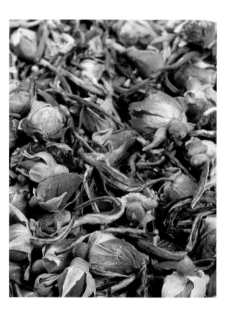

RIGHT Before the days of synthetic air-fresheners, flowers and roots played an essential role in the household to minimize smell and repel insects.

Medieval Medicine

Theophrastus Bombastus von Hohenheim, better known as Paracelsus (1494-1541), was a German physician and alchemist who pioneered the use of chemistry in medicine and studied the healing components of medicinal plants. He was an unconventional medical man and believed that everyone had an "inner doctor" and a life force; his contributions to the healing sciences, acclaimed in our century by the psychiatrist and psychologist C. G. Jung (1875-1961), were to provide the foundations of an empirical science of mental and physical health that continues to this day.

The use of essential oils continued to blossom around the European world; in Italy it was expanded under the patronage of the Medici family; in England Elizabeth I enjoyed aromatic oils; and in Germany and in France essences such as rosemary, lavender, camphor, mint, and sage were often used to fight off epidemics.

Aromatherapy in Modern Times

A French chemist named Rene Gatteffosé wrote his first thesis on "Aromatherapy" in 1928 and this was to become a cornerstone in the study and practice of the uses of essential oils. During the course of his work he discovered the healing properties of lavender for burns, when he treated himself for burns to the hand sustained in his laboratory by plunging his hand into water containing lavender essence.

In Paris from the 1920s to the 1940s, Dr. Jean Valnet conducted groundbreaking studies on aromatherapy and in 1964 published his authoritative book *The Practice of Aromatherapy*. At the same time, Madame Marguerite Maury, an Austrian who was working with her homeopath husband, became the first nonmedical person to study the powerful effect of aromatherapy on health. She wrote *Secrets of Life and Youth* in 1964.

Present-day aromatherapists, such as Madame Micheline Arcier and many other excellent teachers and practitioners, have continued to refine and develop the ancient art of using essential oils.

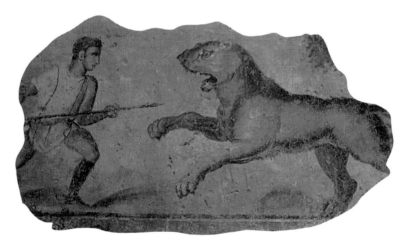

LEFT *A gladiator faces a ferocious lion; any gladiators who survived the arena had their wounds healed with herbal remedies and essential oils.*

Natural Healing Powers

The value of aromatherapy has been known since ancient times, but it is only in the last decade that it has become widely accepted as an important and useful part of healthcare. Aromatherapy offers us a way to get in touch with our bodies, by enjoying the effects of uplifting or calming aromas. It is a gentle healing art that is available to men, women, and children of every age, and of every state of health or physical fitness.

Imagine for a moment walking in a lush green meadow or a field full of beautiful purple lavender; imagine standing in a colorful rose garden, smelling the warm, heady sweet scent that fills the air. The positive feelings such imagined pleasures bring allow you to experience for a moment how beneficial and healing to the whole person—the body, mind, and spirit—an aromatherapy treatment can be. Aromatherapy encapsulates the wonderful smells and their healing properties in essential oils that have been extracted from the branches and twigs, leaves, petals, flower tops, roots, and resins of individual plants. These oils can be used as part of our everyday lives, and the power of their rich fragrances can work to enhance health and well-being.

Essential oils are an exciting and versatile way of treating ourselves on every level. They are a gift of nature, which we can enjoy and use in our day-to-day lives. Essential oils can penetrate our senses, through their sensual aromas. They are effective in many ways—through vapors that can be released into the atmosphere, through feeding the skin in the form of an aromatherapy massage, through the sensual effects of languishing and relaxing in an aromatic bath, and through their use as natural, pure perfumes in cosmetics or in cooking. Essential oils can be blended, combining the unique energy and life force of each oil to address a multitude of health problems. Care must always be taken when using essential oils at home: they are a powerful tool, and they must be used sparingly and in the correct circumstances and situations. If you have any doubts at all about the use of an oil, or its functions, consult a qualified practitioner for advice.

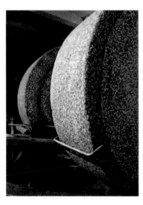

ABOVE
A traditional oil press for the extraction of virgin olive oil in industrial quantities.

What are Essential Oils?

Essential oils are the substances that give plants or parts of them—their petals, leaves, flower heads, seeds, stalks, bark, gums, or resins, for example—their aroma. Some plants yield different oils from their various parts; the bitter orange tree, for instance, yields neroli oil from its blossom, orange oil from its fruit peel,

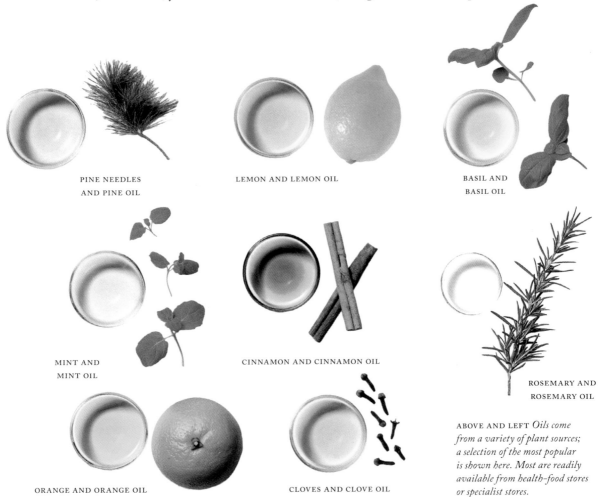

PINE NEEDLES
AND PINE OIL

LEMON AND LEMON OIL

BASIL AND
BASIL OIL

MINT AND
MINT OIL

CINNAMON AND CINNAMON OIL

ROSEMARY AND
ROSEMARY OIL

ORANGE AND ORANGE OIL

CLOVES AND CLOVE OIL

ABOVE AND LEFT *Oils come from a variety of plant sources; a selection of the most popular is shown here. Most are readily available from health-food stores or specialist stores.*

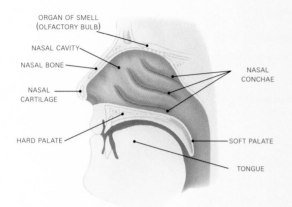

ORGAN OF SMELL
(OLFACTORY BULB)

NASAL CAVITY

NASAL BONE

NASAL
CARTILAGE

NASAL
CONCHAE

HARD PALATE

SOFT PALATE

TONGUE

SENSE AND SENSITIVITY

The nasal cavity showing where the organ of smell is located. A large area of the brain is allocated to the decoding of the sense data from nasal receptors; the scents and smells seem to work very directly on emotions and mood. A certain scent can evoke long-forgotten memories.

and petitgrain from its leaves and twigs. But other plants contain very little essential oil. These essences contain that living element, often referred to as the "soul" of the plant, which provides each plant with its own life force, its own energies and healing powers.

Essential oils vary in their natural qualities and constituencies. Most oils are not greasy and are thin in texture, with the exception of a few oils that become thicker in consistency over time. The color of the oil varies from clear, through pale to dark yellow, amber, pink, reddish brown, and pale to dark olive green to blue. Each essential oil, volatile by nature—which means that it will evaporate quickly when coming into contact with the atmosphere—must be contained in a dark-glass bottle in order to preserve it. Only a few drops of an essential oil are used at one time.

The effective molecular structure and powerful natural healing qualities of an essential oil enable it to penetrate the skin and enter the bloodstream within twenty to seventy minutes after treatment, so that the essential oil's life force can meet our own life force and exert its therapeutic effect upon different areas of our physical, psychological, and spiritual well-being.

Extracting Oils

There are five different methods of extracting and preparing essential oils today: distillation, enfleurage, maceration, expression, and solvent extraction.

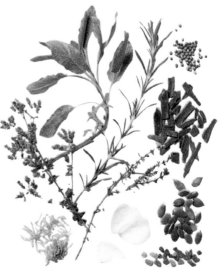

ABOVE *Petals, leaves, stalks, seeds, bark, resin, and roots are all used in the manufacture of essential oils.*

Distillation: The technique called distillation is the main way essential oils are extracted from plants. Steam is passed over the leaves or flowers that have been placed in a still. The steam or vapor then passes into a condenser where it produces a liquid that contains both oil and water. The oil is then easily separated because, depending upon the weight of the oil, it either rests on the surface of the water or sinks to the bottom.

Enfleurage: The method used to extract the most delicate essences from petals and flowers such as rose, jasmine, and neroli is called enfleurage. Each flower or petal must be collected at the time of the day when its aroma is at its most pungent, often at sunset or sunrise. The petals or flowers are spread out on a sheet of glass on which fat has been spread. The glass is mounted in a wooden frame, then twenty-four hours later, when the fat has absorbed the essential oil from the petals, the petals are blown off and the process is repeated. The fat, known as a pomade, is then washed in alcohol, which evaporates, leaving the essential oil.

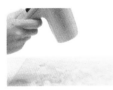

ABOVE *Enfleurage is a gentle method used to extract the oil from delicate petals and blossoms.*

Maceration: This process is applied to plants that do not yield their essential oils naturally after being harvested. The flowers are soaked in hot oil in order to break down the cells, so that the fragrance is released into the oil. This is then purified and the essential oils extracted into a pomade. The enfleurage method is then used to complete the process.

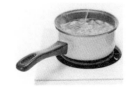

ABOVE *Maceration is a process used to prepare tough plants for oil extraction.*

Expression: This method is known as the sponge process, which was the way essential oil was extracted from the citrus family: orange, lemon, grapefruit, tangerine, and bergamot. Citrus oils used to be squeezed from the plant or fruit by hand on to a sponge. Machinery now carries out this work.

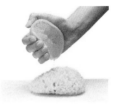

ABOVE *Expression is the traditional method for the extraction of citrus oils. The oil comes from the rind of the fruit.*

SAFEGUARDS AND CAUTION

The following notes are important for safe usage of essential oils.

SKIN: Before using an essential oil, do a skin test. Dot some oil on the wrist pulse point; if the skin becomes irritated or inflamed, wash off the oil with water and do not use.

PHOTOTOXICITY: Some oils can cause an adverse reaction in strong sunlight. This is called phototoxicity. Test a little on the inside of your wrist before using any oil outdoors.

TOXICITY: Check for toxicity, which can occur when oils are overused or are contraindicated for some conditions or people. For example, clary sage can be toxic when used for treating PMS, and peppermint or frankincense may overstimulate the nervous system.

ASTHMA: Special care must be taken to check each oil if you suffer from asthma. It is safer not to use inhalations because of the risk of suffering palpitations.

BLOOD PRESSURE: Caution is required if you suffer from low blood pressure; oils such as eucalyptus and lavender should be avoided. If blood pressure is high avoid oils such as cypress, peppermint, rosemary, hyssop, sage, clary sage, and thyme.

HOMEOPATHY: Always check with the homeopathic practitioner before using essential oils because they may nullify the effect of the remedies. Oils particularly important to avoid during homeopathic treatment are camphor, eucalyptus, black pepper, and peppermint.

PREGNANCY AND BABIES: The body is particularly sensitive in both pregnancy and infancy, and special care must always be taken before any oil is used.

PREGNANCY: Only "safe oils" should be used during pregnancy since it is not known what effect the natural essences have on the placenta that feeds the growing fetus. Even when using safe oils it is important to remember to mix at half the measured amount. One very relaxing and safe way of using essential oils during pregnancy is on a burner in the room rather than directly on the skin.

Solvent extraction: Used for resins and gums as well as some flowers, this involves placing the appropriate parts of the plant in a vessel and covering it with solvent. It is then electrically heated to produce an odiferous paste called a concrete, which is mixed with alcohol and chilled, then filtered. The alcohol is evaporated away, leaving a substance that is known as a resinoid.

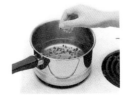

ABOVE *Gums and resins must be dissolved in chemical solvent before they yield their oils.*

Safe oils in pregnancy include black pepper, eucalyptus, chamomile (Roman), frankincense, geranium, ginger, lavender, mandarin, rose otto, tangerine, tea tree, and ylang-ylang.

Oils to be avoided in pregnancy include basil, cinnamon, citronella, clary sage, clove, cypress, hyssop, juniper, marjoram, myrrh, rosemary, sage and thyme.

BREAST-FEEDING: It is best to avoid all essential oils during breast-feeding. For the purpose of skin maintenance, however, a light carrier oil massaged over the breasts can be helpful in reducing stretch marks. If in doubt, always consult a practitioner.

BABIES AND CHILDREN: There are various ways essential oils can be beneficial in treating babies and children, particularly for sleep disorders, irritability, colic, colds, and coughs. Oils are best used on a burner in the room, in a bath, in massage, and in herbal teas, but it is very important to use only safe oils and check for toxicity.

For babies of 0-12 months use 1 drop of essential oil in 1 teaspoon of light carrier oil.

For children of 1-5 years use 2-3 drops of essential oil in 1 teaspoon of light carrier oil.

For children of 6-12 years use half the measured amount as for adults.

Safe oils for babies and young children include chamomile (Roman or German), lavender, mandarin, neroli, rose and tangerine.

THE ELDERLY: Aromatherapy is a wonderful way of relaxing and treating elderly people, but check carefully for toxicity and in general use half the measured amount. All oils that are safe for children are excellent for the elderly.

EPILEPSY: Avoid essential oils such as clary sage, sage, hyssop, and fennel since they work very powerfully on the nervous system.

Aromatherapy in Action

*T*here are a number of different ways to use essential oils in aromatherapy. These range from massage through baths and inhalations to sprays and compresses for specific healing needs.

Massage

A professional aromatherapist would favor a technique of therapeutic massage. This is also easy to do at home, with a friend or partner and on one's own. Specific areas of the body can gain particular benefit from massage—especially tired and aching muscles. Gentle massage over the abdomen will help relieve period pains. A gentle massage over the lower back will help relieve backache. And because of the aphrodisiac qualities and the sensual dimensions of a massage, lovers can gain extra pleasure from using essential oils within a caring relationship.

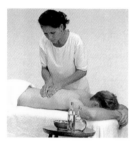

ABOVE *A luxurious and relaxing massage at the hands of a professional is one of the most pleasant ways to enjoy the power of essential oils.*

In aromatherapy massage, the oils are blended with a carrier oil, which will dilute the essential oils for the purposes of massage without actually dispersing their active ingredients.

It is a good idea to choose an oil that appeals to your own personal sense of smell, and you may wish to blend two oils together. For example, to make a 1.5fl. oz. (50ml.) bottle of oil, use:

• 1 teaspoon of jojoba or calendula oil

• 1 teaspoon of avocado or hazelnut

• Add a balancing oil, such as grapeseed or sweet almond oil

The secret of blending essential oils becomes easier with practice; it also enhances an individual's sense of smell. For example, an aromatherapy oil to relieve stress and tension can be made using 2 tablespoons of carrier oil in an egg cup or small bowl, combined with 2 drops clary sage, 3 drops lavender, and 3 drops rose.

Always remember to store aromatherapy oils in dark glass bottles to preserve them.

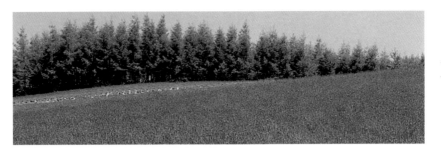

Baths

A simple, beneficial, and very enjoyable way of using essential oils is in a bath. The warmth of hand-hot water releases aromatic vapors that are a joy to the senses. For 1 teaspoon of bath oil, add 5-10 drops of essential oil to a carrier oil such as peach kernel, apricot, or sweet almond oil. This method helps to condition the skin and is safe if not more than a teaspoon of the blended oil is added to the bath. Only nonirritant essential oils, such as lavender, tangerine, and Roman chamomile can be added directly to a bath, but take care not to use more than 4-6 drops. You may wish to mix these first in a carrier oil before adding to the bath. There are oil dispersants available, which will ensure that the oil is spread throughout the bathwater, not just on the surface.

Hand bath

A bowl of warm water containing 3-4 drops of an essential oil can be a useful way of obtaining the therapeutic effects of aromatherapy.

Foot bath

Take an average size washing-up basin, fill it with hand-hot water and add 4-6 drops of essential oil. Soak the feet for ten minutes. This is good for swollen, tired, aching feet as well as for athlete's foot and fungal infections, and is an excellent means of using essential oils, particularly in the very young or old.

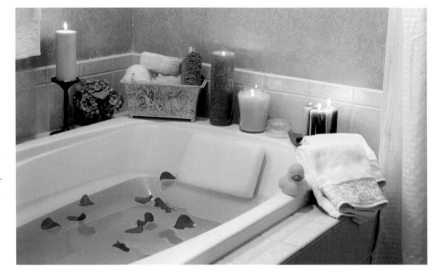

RIGHT *A deep, warm bath scented with aromatic oils is one of the best ways to enjoy aromatherapy at home. Avoid mixing essential oils with commercial bubble bath products.*

Sitz bath

A half-full bathtub or large bowl full of warm water using the same proportions as for a normal bath can be used for many conditions, including thrush, hemorrhoids, perineal stitches, or genital and urinary ailments. A douche can be made of 3-5 drops of essential oils such as tea tree or lavender in warm water.

Shower

After a shower, pour a little prepared essential oil and carrier oil onto a sponge then squeeze this over the body and massage it into the skin.

Sauna

Add 20-30 drops of eucalyptus, pine, or cypress essential oil to a large pan of water and pour this over the coals, then lie back and imagine being in a pine forest. Most aromatherapy oils can be used in this way.

CARRIER OILS

The following is a list of some fine oils:

SWEET ALMOND OIL (*light – for all skin types*)

AVOCADO OIL (*thick – for dry, aging skin*)

APRICOT KERNEL OIL (*light – good for all skin types*)

ARNICA OIL (*for injuries and bruises, but not on broken skin*)

CALENDULA OIL (*for feminine problems, PMS, menopause*)

COCONUT OIL (*solid – for dry skin*)

COMFREY OIL (*for rheumatism, aches and pains*)

CORN OIL (*medium – for dry skin*)

EVENING PRIMROSE OIL (*rich – for dry and aging skin*)

GRAPESEED OIL (*light – good base oil for all skin types*)

JOJOBA OIL (*medium – a balancing oil, for dry skin; best if diluted*)

OLIVE OIL (*thick – needs to be diluted*)

PEACH KERNEL OIL (*medium – for dry skin*)

SOYBEAN OIL (*light – good for all skin types*)

ST. JOHN'S WORT OIL (*antiseptic and pain relieving; good if diluted*)

SUNFLOWER OIL (*light – a good base oil, for all skin types*)

WHEATGERM OIL (*thick – good for stretch marks; best if diluted*)

Inhalations

For coughs, colds, chest infections, and skin cleansing, put 6-12 drops of essential oil in a bowl of boiling hot water, cover your head with a towel, and deeply inhale the vapors. Two or three drops of essential oil put on a handkerchief or a pillow while sleeping can also be very helpful to reduce coughing at night and to encourage sleep. This is good for children.

Caution must be used for people who are either asthmatic or epileptic.

Gargles

For the treatment of bad breath, mouth ulcers, sore throats, and other conditions, add 3-4 drops of essential oil, such as Roman chamomile or tea tree (which is bitter but effective) to a glass of warm boiled water and gargle or use it as a mouthwash.

Aromatherapy at Home

Aromatherapy and essential oils are not restricted to a healing role or just for personal use. The therapeutic powers of essential oils can also be enjoyed communally. There are many ways to scent the different rooms in your home, to establish certain moods or a special atmosphere: a calming scent in the evenings, a more bracing version at the start of the day, an elegant fragrance for a dinner party, something seasonal at Christmas, someone's favorite scent on their birthday. You can use the oils on their own or in combination. Many essential oil manufacturers give advice and recommend suitable blends.

There are various ways you can create a scented atmosphere. Some you can make yourself: a room spray, traditional bowls of pot pourri; others are easy to find commercially; fragrancers, scented candles, and ring burners. You can even wear some kinds of essential oils as perfumes, but take advice first since not all of them are suitable. And they have a role in the kitchen: lemon and orange oil, used very sparingly, are traditional ingredients in delicate desserts and cakes.

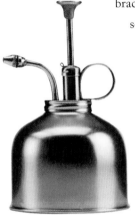

ABOVE *You can make your own environmentally friendly room spray using a pump-action plant spray.*

Fragrancers

A number of excellent fragrancers are commercially available. Some can be plugged into the electricity supply to warm a dish containing a mix of a teaspoon (5ml.) of carrier oil and 6-8 drops of essential oil such as frankincense, so this can evaporate slowly in a room. Others are made of pottery or porcelain, lit by a night light candle. As the dish warms up, water is added with 3-4 drops of essential oil to send beautiful aromatic vapors throughout a room. Another technique is simply to add a few drops of essential oil to a small bowl of boiling water and put it on top of a radiator. But in all cases, be sure to keep the fragrancer well out of the reach of children.

FIRST-AID

Essential oils, especially lavender, have a useful place in the family first-aid box.

COMPRESSES

A cold compress is good for treating bruises, sprains, headaches, and migraines. Soak a facecloth in a bowl of cold water with 5-6 drops of essential oil added, then wrap this around ice cubes from the freezer for a very soothing and effective balm. To make a hot compress for aches, pains, abscesses, or severe muscular tension, dip a facecloth into a bowl of hot water to which 5-6 drops of essential oil, such as lavender, have been added, then place this on the affected area.

INSECT BITES AND STINGS

Because of their natural plant properties, tea tree and lavender oil can be effective in relieving pain if they are used neat on insect bites, wasp stings, bruises, and wounds. Soak a Q-tip in the essential oil and dab on the affected area.

Room Sprays

Part fill a clean, empty plant spray with water then add 30-50 drops of, for example, lavender, lemon and citronella, geranium, or tea tree. This can be used to spray a fine mist into a room to act as a room fragrancer or insect repellent, depending upon your choice of essential oils. Citronella will deter cats from spraying.

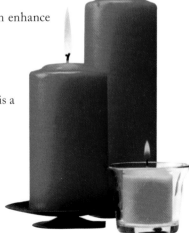

BELOW *Scented candles produce a gentle fragrance as they burn.*

Scented Candles

Adding 1-2 drops to the pool of wax of a burning candle can enhance the atmosphere.

Humidifiers

Adding 4-6 drops of essential oil to the water of a humidifier is a good way of experiencing the effects of aromatherapy oils.

Ring Burners

Small porcelain rings placed over a lit lightbulb dotted with a few drops of essential oil gently send a vaporous aroma around a room.

MAKING POT POURRI

Pot pourri is easy to make at home. You can design it to fit your color scheme and to create whatever mood you want, whether it be sensuous, exhilarating, calming, relaxing, or refreshing.

Whatever you choose, mix the measures so that the scents do not conflict. A mixture of rose petals, assertive herbs such as mint, and pungent spices such as cinnamon makes a pleasant room sweetener. A recommended proportion is 2½ cups each of your main ingredients to 4 tablespoons of secondary ingredients; add between ½ and 2 teaspoons of spice, depending on your taste. Always add orris root—about 2 tablespoons is generally enough in these proportions.

Add essential oil by the drop (around 10 drops should be sufficient), and choose oils that reflect your choice of flowers. Mix everything together, place it in a paper bag, seal the top, and leave in a dark place for 4-6 weeks to cure. When it is ready, display it in a suitably beautiful dish and refresh with your chosen essential oil when necessary.

LEFT *Pot pourri is a traditional and economical way to scent a room since its power can be periodically boosted by the addition of a few drops of oil.*

Pot Pourri

Make your own pot pourri or enliven the aroma of an existing one by adding 4-6 drops of essential oil such as rose, frankincense, geranium, or any other oil you enjoy.

Perfume

A few selected essential oils can be used neat as perfume. The pure essence of rose, neroli, lavender, ylang-ylang, jasmine, and sandalwood are good examples because they will not usually irritate the skin.

Cooking

In cooking, use only one or two drops for flavor since the essential oils are very strong. One drop of lemon or one drop of chamomile added to tea will be enough for several strong cups. Tangerine and lemon oils are good for using in cakes and desserts.

ABOVE *The pure essence of lavender can be used as perfume since it won't irritate the skin.*

From the Larder

The fact that many foods and culinary ingredients eaten and used in daily life have specific therapeutic applications, either in the prevention of disease or as a potential remedy, is not a recent discovery. Some foods have a long history of use as folk medicines throughout most parts of the world—corn, for example, was used by the Aztecs as a medicine for the heart; the medicinal uses of garlic, of which there are many, were mentioned in Chinese texts as long ago as around A.D. 500. Today, there is an ever-increasing knowledge about why a particular food may work for some conditions but not for others, knowledge that is the result of scientific analysis of the constituents of foods.

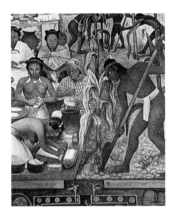

ABOVE *The cultivation of maize, or corn, was central to the lives of the Aztecs of Meso-America. Corn was used both as a food and a medicine.*

The therapeutic actions of natural foods and ingredients arise from the nutrients and other complex chemicals of which they are composed, and which have a direct effect on the body. Of the nutrients, the most widely known are the vitamins and minerals. These are the substances that we hear most about, particularly in connection with the debate about supplements—whether we get enough of all the nutrients by eating a balanced diet, or whether, for a variety of reasons, there are some nutrients we lack and should supplement by taking the appropriate tablet or pill to make up any deficiency.

Vitamins and Minerals

Of the many vitamins and minerals scientists have identified, there are five main vitamins (the group of B vitamins counting as one) and between six and eighteen minerals and trace elements that are universally recognized as essential nutrients that we should, ideally, receive from the food we eat. These nutrients, which play such a significant role in the maintenance of a healthy body, are described on *pages 274-277*, together with the appropriate recommended daily allowance (RDA) for an average healthy adult. A discussion of the most important vitamins and minerals—in this context, meaning those that are present in such significant amounts as to have an effect on health—provided by specific foods can be found under the individual food listings in Part Three.

Antioxidants

Many foods, including a large number of healing herbs, contain antioxidants, substances that provide protection against destructive molecules called free radicals. These molecules, when present in excessive numbers, can cause damage to the body's cells. They are manufactured in the body as a result of

HEALTHY EATING

Fruit supplies vitamin C, B complex, biotin, folic acid, potassium, calcium, magnesium, and other trace minerals, but is most important in the daily diet for vitamin C and potassium. Berries and citrus fruits contain high amounts of vitamin C.

GRAPEFRUIT   APPLE   BANANA

Vegetables are a good source of carotene, vitamin E and the B vitamins, folic acid, and the major minerals. Many also contribute significant amounts of vitamin C. Greenleaf and root vegetables should be included in the diet, and some should be eaten raw because cooking destroys some vitamins and leaches out minerals.

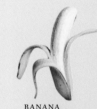

CABBAGE   CARROT   BROCCOLI

Protein is essential in the diet. It should make up 11 percent of a main meal. Fish supplies both protein and polyunsaturated oils; meat from poultry gives protein without fat; eggs contain the B vitamins and all the essential minerals.

EGGS   FISH   CHICKEN

metabolization or from environmental pollutants that enter the body during respiration. Three vitamins, A, C, and E (often referred to as the ACE vitamins), in conjunction with the mineral selenium, are antioxidants that prevent the formation of free radicals or act as scavengers that mop up these undesirable agents. Research seems to indicate that antioxidants, particularly vitamin E, can be of particular benefit in protecting health when supplements are taken.

There is also some evidence that foods rich in the vitamins A and C, when eaten regularly and in fairly abundant quantities, may protect against cancer of the gastrointestinal tract and respiratory system.

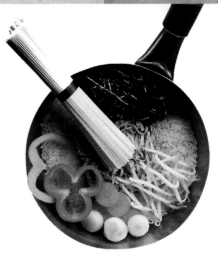

ABOVE *The traditional stir-fry cooking method used by the Chinese is an excellent way to preserve as many as possible of the vitamins and minerals in fresh ingredients.*

HEALTHY EATING

Beans, peas, and lentils supply carotene, vitamin E, the B complex, potassium, and trace minerals. They are low in sodium and contain substantial amounts of protein. They are also a good source of dietary fiber.

BLACK BEANS   NAVY BEANS   LENTILS

Cereal products supply bulk carbohydrate, the starchy element of the daily diet. They can be eaten in their natural forms, like oats, or eaten in bread (preferably wholewheat) or pasta. Carbohydrates should form at least 50 percent of your daily intake.

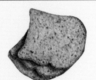

WHOLEWHEAT BREAD   OATS   PASTA

Milk is a good source of vitamins, rich in calcium and potassium and low in sodium. Products made from milk have the same qualities; those worried about the fat content should choose skim-milk products. Goat's or sheep's milk can be substituted for cow's if there is an allergy.

BUTTER   CHEESE   YOGURT

Natural Foods and Supplements

*T*here is really no question about how best to obtain the nutrients and other benefits foods can supply: fresh is almost always best (although in a few cases dried fruit may contain higher amounts of a nutrient than the fresh fruit). But how fresh is fresh, and how safe? Much of the so-called fresh fruit and vegetables we buy have been in storage for weeks, sometimes months. Whereas once most fruit and vegetables were available only in season, now most of them can be purchased year round—and this is not always because fresh produce has been air-freighted the day before from foreign producers. Storing foods, even at low temperatures, usually results in the loss of valuable nutrients. Then there is the matter of herbicides and pesticides that accumulate in fruit and vegetables from sprays that are applied during the growth of the plant, plus the addition of waxes and other substances that are used after harvesting to lengthen the shelf-life of food. Buying organically produced food, locally grown and available in season, is probably the best way to ensure that food really is fresh, and that it is free from herbicides and other food "enhancers."

When buying any fresh produce, choose those with leaves and roots that are crisp, not wilted; vegetables should not have any yellow or brown leaves or spots, and both fruit and vegetables should not have any sign of bruising.

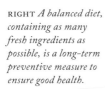

RIGHT *A balanced diet, containing as many fresh ingredients as possible, is a long-term preventive measure to ensure good health.*

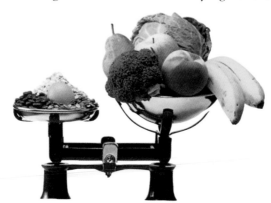

REACTIONS AND SIDE EFFECTS

As with all medicines, natural remedies must be treated with respect and taken with due regard to any potential adverse effects. This may seem to be overcautious: after all, on the surface of it, what could be safer and healthier than a freshly picked, homegrown strawberry or an organically grown cabbage? Unfortunately, however, natural does not necessarily mean safe. All foods may produce side effects or adverse reactions, particularly when taken in excess. Side effects may be desirable or undesirable, but are not usually life-threatening—for example, a side effect of eating beans is flatulence, which may be socially undesirable, but is not dangerous. Adverse reactions, however, produce undesirable effects that endanger health; eating strawberries, for example, can cause the classic symptoms of allergy in susceptible people, mainly skin rash, swelling of the face, eyes, and lips, hay-fever-like symptoms, and upset stomach.

Other foods may interact with prescribed drugs. Bananas and pickled cabbage, for example, may interfere with drugs of the MAOI (Monoamine-oxidase inhibitor) type, prescribed for ailments such as hypertension and depression, and can result in critical hypertension.

If you are taking prescribed drugs for an illness see your general practitioner before self-medicating with any natural medicine. Pregnant and lactating women, people with chronic gastrointestinal complaints, and the elderly should also seek the advice of a reputable, qualified practitioner, as should parents who are thinking of treating their children with natural medicines.

RIGHT *Strawberries can cause an allergic reaction and an irritating skin rash in susceptible people.*

Wherever possible, buy food that has been organically grown and eat within two or three days of purchase. Store in cool, dark conditions, preferably in the refrigerator or in a cold pantry. Eggs should always be refrigerated, never left at room temperature.

Wash fruit and vegetables very thoroughly. Although it is better to leave skins on fruit and vegetables—many of the nutrients are found just beneath the skin—washing may not remove the chemical residues of produce that has been sprayed, and it is probably best to peel them. This should not be necessary with organic produce. Just as fresh food is preferable to preserved food, so raw food is more beneficial than cooked food. If it is difficult to eat raw foods or, as in the case of cabbage, you would have to eat a large volume to obtain any therapeutic

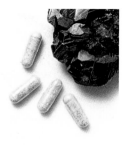

LEFT *Iron is essential in the diet as it is a constituent of hemoglobin, the oxygen carrying pigment in blood. Between 3 and 5g should be present in a healthy body. Good food sources include shellfish, wheat bran, liver, cocoa, soya, dried fruit, and cereal. Pregnant women and anemic people may need supplements, which should combine iron with vitamin C.*

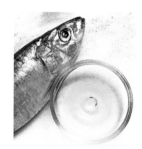

LEFT *Oily fish, such as herring, mackerel, eel, sardine, and tuna, is an excellent source of polyunsaturated fatty acids, which help to prevent blood clots and reduce blood fat levels. If you do not like eating fish, fish oil supplements are readily available in liquid or capsule form. Cod liver oil tablets are the most popular.*

benefits, drinking the juice is an equally good alternative, provided there is already sufficient fiber in the diet. An electric juicer is ideal for vegetables such as cabbage, carrots, and beets, the juices of which are not always readily available commercially. Make sure you consume bought fruit and vegetable juices soon after opening. Some nutrients, especially Vitamin C, deteriorate very quickly once exposed to the air, even if the container is closed tightly and stored in a refrigerator.

Vitamin C can be destroyed by heat, especially during cooking processes such as boiling. Fat-soluble nutrients may leach out into the water or oil they are cooked in, which is then discarded. Losing valuable nutrients in this way can be overcome by stewing fruit or vegetables, or using them to make soup; the nutrients that have leached out will still be present in the liquid.

Prepackaged Products

It is sometimes more convenient or efficient to use commercially prepared natural medicines rather than the food itself, where these are available. This is particularly the case where large quantities of a food would be needed to obtain therapeutic benefits, or where commercially prepared medicines cannot realistically be

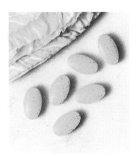

LEFT *Folic acid is a water soluble vitamin belonging to the B complex. It is very important in pregnancy since it combats anemia in the mother and builds up resistance to infection in the baby; women who take contraceptive pills should ensure they get enough folic acid. It occurs in greenleaf vegetables, soya flour, brewer's yeast, and is available as tablets.*

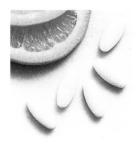

LEFT *Vitamin C is an anti-oxidant, promotes iron absorption, activates folic acid, and supports the body's immune system. The body cannot store it and so it has to be taken daily. Citrus fruit, blackcurrants, and green peppers are good sources of vitamin C but it is also available in soluble tablet or capsule form.*

prepared at home. There is a wide range of such medicines available in different forms, as any visit to a healthfood store or purveyor of natural remedies can testify. Ginger, for example, is usually available as tablets, capsules, extracts, tinctures, and concentrated drops, while celery can be purchased as concentrated drops, tablets, and tinctures.

When buying these products there are several things to bear in mind. Always buy products prepared by well-known manufacturers whose preparations have proved to be safe. Always read the instructions carefully and take as directed in the recommended dosage. If adverse reactions occur stop taking the product immediately and seek medical advice as soon as possible.

Be aware that tablets, capsules, and so on have—of necessity—ingredients other than the natural therapeutic substance, and these may not be listed on the packaging. For example, capsules may contain gelatines and tablets that will include binding agents that serve to hold all the ingredients together; they may also have a sugar coating to make them more palatable. While most of these are safe, any of them might be potentially harmful to those who are sensitive to certain substances.

BELOW *Garlic is a medicine chest in itself; if you do not like the taste, it is now available in pill form.*

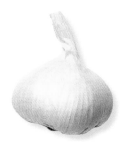

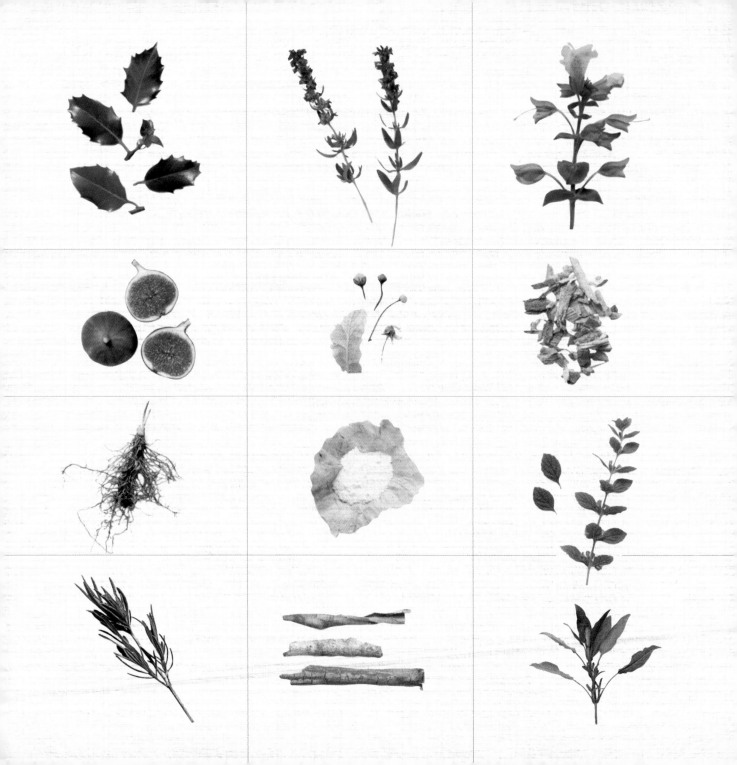

PART TWO

The Ailments

This part covers common family ailments, grouped together under the particular body system they affect: for instance, indigestion is discussed under The Digestive System. Each body system is introduced and described before the ailments are listed. Each ailment is accompanied by a panel indicating which natural therapies can be applied beneficially in the home, and how to use them safely. Tips on self-help are included in this panel. A special section at the end covers children's and babies' problems and the routine illnesses of childhood.

The Immune System

The immune system is the body's defense against attack. It repels unfriendly bacteria and viruses, and fights off infection. All infections and allergies are diseases involving the immune system, which is why it is always advisable to support the system during illness and to maintain its strength and vitality at other times.

Strengthening the Immune System

The immune system forms part of the lymphatic system, which runs parallel to the circulatory system. Its function is to fight off foreign substances such as viruses, bacteria, and allergens that invade the body. This is achieved by white blood cells (lymphocytes), which are produced in the bone marrow. Lymphocytes known as B-cells produce antibodies, which enable the body to protect itself against invading organisms when the immune system is healthy and functioning properly. A weakened immune system makes us susceptible to ailments such as colds and other infectious diseases and can produce the feeling of generally being run down.

 HERBALISM

• Echinacea root stimulates the immune system and strengthens a weakened one. Take as a tincture, decoction, or tablets.

 AROMATHERAPY

• Siberian ginseng enhances resistance to disease.

• Ginger oil burned in a room is a preventive that encourages immunity to colds, flu, bronchitis, catarrh, blocked sinuses, and headaches. Ginger oil in the bath is very helpful. Juniper oil strengthens the immune system.

 FROM THE LARDER

• Supplements of the ACE vitamins, plus selenium, play an important role in strengthening the immune system. Vitamin B6 may also help promote a healthy immune system.

SELF-HELP

• Regular exercise and a nutritious diet are essential for maintaining the general health of the body, including the immune system.

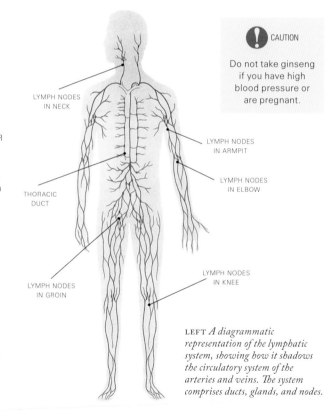

LYMPH NODES IN NECK

LYMPH NODES IN ARMPIT

LYMPH NODES IN ELBOW

THORACIC DUCT

LYMPH NODES IN KNEE

LYMPH NODES IN GROIN

! CAUTION

Do not take ginseng if you have high blood pressure or are pregnant.

LEFT *A diagrammatic representation of the lymphatic system, showing how it shadows the circulatory system of the arteries and veins. The system comprises ducts, glands, and nodes.*

HIV and AIDS

Human immunodeficiency virus (HIV) can cause a breakdown in the immune system, resulting in acquired immunodeficiency syndrome (AIDS). Both HIV-positive people and AIDS sufferers need the care of specialist medical practitioners. However, some aspects of these diseases can also be managed by natural therapies (*See also Strengthening the Immune System page 70*).

SYMPTOMS *People who are HIV positive do not usually have symptoms. The symptoms of AIDS are many and varied; they include chronic diarrhea, infections, enlargement of the glands, fever, and weight loss. Dementia may occur in the later stages.*

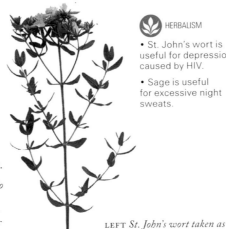

 HERBALISM

• St. John's wort is useful for depression caused by HIV.

• Sage is useful for excessive night sweats.

LEFT *St. John's wort taken as tea or tincture can help lift a depressed mood.*

 AROMATHERAPY

• Juniper oil strengthens the immune system and may be useful for HIV sufferers.

• Orange essential oil reinforces the immune system.

• Tea tree oil is useful for both HIV and AIDS patients.

 CAUTION

St. John's wort should not be taken in cases of severe depression. High doses of concentrated tablets may cause skin rash when the skin is exposed to sunlight.

Allergies

Allergies are reactions to allergens, susbstances such as pollen and cat hair that trigger physical symptoms in people who have been sensitized to them.

SYMPTOMS *These vary according to the type of allergy. For example, air-borne allergens usually cause runny eyes and noses, sneezing, and chest congestion: food allergies may cause upset stomachs, diarrhea, swollen lips, and skin rashes.*

 CAUTION

• Avoid agrimony if you are suffering from chronic constipation.

• Astragalis should not be used by severely debilitated patients unless supervised by a herbalist.

 HERBALISM

• Arigomony tea or tincture is beneficial for those suffering from multiple allergies, but must be taken over a long period.

• Milk thistle seed is helpful for food allergies.

• Alternatively, try astragalis root tincture or decoction.

• Add gensing powder to herbal drinks to help reduce the frequency of attacks.

 HOMEOPATHY

• Apis mel. is used to treat allergic reactions following a bee or wasp sting, particularly when breathing becomes difficult.

 AROMATHERAPY

• The essential oil of patchouli is anti-inflammatory and may ease the symptoms.

RIGHT *Oyster can cause a violent allergic reaction in some people.*

 FROM THE LARDER

• Vitamin B6 may help reduce sensitivity in the case of food allergy, but because it can cause adverse reactions in large doses, you should seek advice of a nutritionist or naturophatic practitioner.

 SELF-HELP

• Common sense dictates that avoiding the allergen will minimize or eliminate problems.

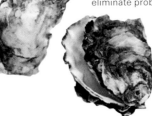

Infectious Mononucleosis or Glandular Fever

Infectious mononucleosis is an acute ailment. It is caused by a virus that usually affects young people.

SYMPTOMS *Listlessness, fatigue—sometimes complete exhaustion—headache, and chills. These are followed by fever, sore throat, and swollen lymph glands.*

 HERBALISM
• Astragalus root tincture or decoction may be beneficial.

 FROM THE LARDER
• Vitamin C supplements will help to strengthen the immune system.

• Hot lemon and honey drinks may relieve sore throat and lower the temperature.

 SELF-HELP
• Keep warm and get plenty of bed rest.

• Hot-water bottles will help with chills.

Shingles

Shingles is a form of herpes, *Herpes zoster*, the same virus that causes chickenpox. Shingles occurs most frequently in older people who did not have chickenpox as children.

SYMPTOMS *A red rash on the chest, accompanied by fever. There is usually severe pain in the nerves lying beneath the skin rash. It can occur prior to the rash.*

 HERBALISM
• Take echinacea root decoction or tincture three times a day.

 FLOWER ESSENCES
• Rescue Remedy may prove helpful when symptoms are at their worst. It can also be applied as a cream.

 AROMATHERAPY
• Eucalyptus can be beneficial in the treatment of herpes.

• Dip a Q-tip into tea tree oil and gently dab on to the affected area.

• Lavender can be used in much the same way.

 FROM THE LARDER
• A plantain compress will soothe the rash.

• Drink plenty of fresh, pure fruit and vegetable juices.

• Soothe the affected area with the juice of leeks.

 SELF-HELP
• Frequent cool showers may help relieve the pain.

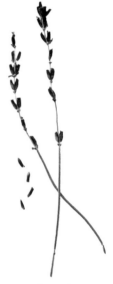

ABOVE *Lavender oil applied directly to the affected skin can help to soothe the itch and pain of shingles.*

Tonsillitis

Tonsils are lymphatic tissue that have a role in protecting the body against infection. When they become infected—usually by a streptococcus bacterium—they cause pain and discomfort.

SYMPTOMS *Sore throat, enlarged glands, pain on swallowing, a raised temperature, and swollen, inflamed tonsils, often speckled with white patches. There may be referred pain, causing earache, vomiting, and general malaise. Children may complain of stomachache rather than a sore throat.*

 HERBALISM
• Gargle and clean the mouth out with a mouthwash of echinacea root decoction or tincture.

• Marigold flower used as a mouthwash and gargle can also help relieve the pain and swelling.

 HOMEOPATHY
• Take Apis mel. when the throat is bright red, dry, and swollen.

• Belladonna is particularly good for children who suddenly become ill.

 FROM THE LARDER
• Strengthen the immune system by taking vitamin supplements (ACE vitamins plus selenium).

• Garlic capsules may also help to relieve some of the symptoms.

 SELF-HELP
• A cold compress (made with a length of cloth long enough to go around the neck once only) wrapped around the neck at night will often reduce the swelling.

The Circulatory System

The circulatory system keeps blood flowing around the body, delivering nutrients and oxygen wherever needed. The system comprises the heart and a network of arteries, veins, and smaller vessels. Obstructions to the smooth flow of blood, damage to the heart and blood vessels, and deficiency in the blood itself are the main diseases.

Anemia

There are more than half a dozen types of anemia. One of the most common is iron-deficiency anemia; deficiencies in the bone marrow or stomach are among the other causes. Where the condition is serious, as in pernicious anemia, seek medical help. Pernicious anemia is usually treated with injections of vitamin B12.

SYMPTOMS *Breathlessness, a pale appearance, and lethargy, sometimes associated with palpitations. In severe cases there may be dizziness, fainting, jaundice, constipation, and thirst. The symptoms of pernicious anemia include nosebleeds and "pins and needles" in the hands and feet.*

 HERBALISM

• Chinese angelica root may be helpful. Take as a tea, tincture, or decoction.

 HOMEOPATHY

• Ferrum phos. is useful for anemia caused by profuse bleeding during menstruation.

• If the patient is cold and exhausted, Natrum mur. may be beneficial.

 AROMATHERAPY

• Lavender is helpful where the condition is associated with palpitations and dizziness.

• Massage with the essential oil of Roman chamomile.

 FROM THE LARDER

• Eat iron-rich foods such as oats, egg yolks, pumpkin seeds, and watercress. Eat foods rich in vitamin C, such as eggs, broccoli, citrus fruit, and pineapple, to help the body absorb iron and iron supplements.

• Nettle soup or tea is also helpful.

 SELF-HELP

• Rest, plenty of fresh air, and a wholefood diet help to improve general health.

 CAUTION

Angelica should not be taken in pregnancy without professional advice. It may cause a skin rash when handled in sunlight.

RIGHT *Eating iron-rich foods like oats are essential for a strong circulatory system.*

Hypertension

Hypertension, or high blood pressure, occurs when pressure exerted on the walls of the arteries by the passage of blood is raised above the normal level over an extended period.

SYMPTOMS *Hypertension does not always produce symptoms, at least in the initial stages. Often it is diagnosed during a routine blood pressure check. When symptoms do occur they may include dizziness, swollen ankles, and shortness of breath. Severe symptoms include blackouts and minor strokes. Left untreated, hypertension may result in a debilitating stroke or heart attack.*

 HERBALISM

• If swollen ankles are symptomatic, take dandelion leaf tea. Drink frequently, taking enough to produce a good flow of urine.

• Garlic, eaten daily or taken as pills, provides additional benefits.

• Gingko leaves will help to protect against stroke.

 AROMATHERAPY

• A massage with lavender oil helps control dizziness and is a good general remedy.

• Use petitgrain if the ankles are swollen.

• Massaging with marjoram, or putting a few drops of marjoram oil in the bath, may also be beneficial.

 FROM THE LARDER

• Bananas, celery juice, nettle, and cinnamon tea may help reduce high blood pressure.

• Both olive leaves and garlic are sometimes prescribed.

• Increasing potassium and fiber in the diet and eating a vegetarian diet have all had beneficial results.

• Decrease salt intake.

• The minerals in hard water may prevent the occurrence of high blood pressure.

 SELF-HELP

• Daily exercise, such as walking and gentle aerobics, sustained for twenty to thirty minutes, has been proved to help lower raised blood pressure.

Chilblains

Chilblains are common on the feet but may also occur on the fingers, ears, and nose.

SYMPTOMS *Irritation and pain. The affected area becomes red and swollen.*

 CAUTION

• Ginger and geranium oils should be used in half measures by pregnant women and children.
• Do not use ginger in the bath because it may irritate sensitive mucous membranes.
• Avoid yarrow in pregnancy.

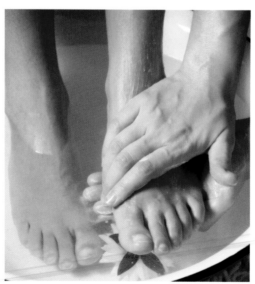

LEFT *Add a few drops of ginger oil to a warm footbath to soothe chilblains.*

 HERBALISM

• Yarrow is good for the circulation and warms cold hands and feet.

 AROMATHERAPY

• Put a few drops of geranium oil in the bathwater.

• Ginger footbaths will soothe and soften the dry skin.

 FROM THE LARDER

• Niacin (vitamin B3) has proved to be beneficial. This can be taken in the form of yeast tablets.

• To relieve the irritation, make a paste of honey, flour, and egg white. Smooth over the affected area and cover with a clean bandage.

• An application of mustard oil may also be beneficial.

• Rub a cut, raw onion over the chilblains to soothe and relieve itching.

Atherosclerosis and Arteriosclerosis

Atherosclerosis is caused by the deposit of atheroma, a greasy substance consisting mainly of cholesterol, along the walls of an artery. This may eventually cause the artery to thicken and harden and become narrower, so the passage of blood is restricted, a condition known as arteriosclerosis. Blood may also become attached to the artery walls, creating a blood clot (thrombosis). Both conditions require the attention of a qualified medical practitioner, but natural therapies can give additional support.

SYMPTOMS *Atherosclerosis is a disease that can have fatal consequences if left untreated. There are few ill effects to indicate its development. Raised blood pressure and poor circulation to the part of the body concerned can be early symptoms. Atherosclerosis is a factor in heart disease and thrombosis, stroke, and angina.*

 HERBALISM

• Bladderwrack, used regularly, often prevents further damage when the arteries have begun to harden.

 AROMATHERAPY

• Marjoram oil massaged into the skin assists in the treatment of hardening of the arteries.

 FROM THE LARDER

• Alcohol in small quantities may help to prevent diseases of the arteries, while apples, globe artichokes, oats, and yogurt can contribute to lowering levels of cholesterol in the blood.

• The antioxidant vitamins (ACE) and selenium are recommended as a preventive.

• Garlic, eaten daily or taken in capsule form, can be helpful for both atherosclerosis and arteriosclerosis.

 SELF-HELP

• Eating foods low in cholesterol may help prevent atherosclerosis.

Varicose Veins

Varicose veins occur in the superficial veins in the legs, the veins that lie between muscle and skin. Veins that are varicose allow blood to flow back down the leg, which is not possible when the veins are healthy. This causes blood to collect and the wall of the vein to stretch.

SYMPTOMS *Swollen, raised veins, blue in color, most commonly in the legs.*

 HERBALISM

• Gingko leaf tea, tincture, or tablets will help.

• For painful veins, apply a compress of marigold flowers.

 HOMEOPATHY

• Take Calcium fluor. to prevent and treat varicose veins in pregnancy.

 AROMATHERAPY

• Massage the legs with basil oil.

• For ulcerated veins, massage with frankincense essential oil.

 FROM THE LARDER

• Vitamin E, bell peppers, and lemons may be helpful in treating varicose veins.

• An old remedy for ulcerated varicose veins is to make a poultice with equal parts honey and cod liver oil. Bandage in place overnight.

 SELF-HELP

• To prevent varicose veins, try to avoid standing still.

• When sitting, raise your feet off the floor and rest them on a stool or chair.

• Raise your feet when in bed.

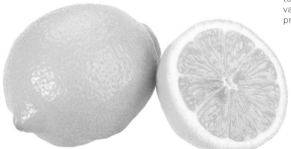

LEFT *Lemons may be helpful in treating varicose veins.*

The Respiratory System

*T*he respiratory system supplies the blood with oxygen. Air is breathed into the lungs via the windpipe, passing down ever smaller tubes until it reaches the alveoli, where oxygen is taken in and carbon dioxide given out. Infection or obstruction causes illness. Mucus is created by the body to rid itself of infection, so should not be suppressed.

Common Cold

The common cold involves infection and inflammation of the mucous membranes lining the nose and throat. It is caused by a virus.

SYMPTOMS *A tickle in the throat, shivering, aching joints, a sore throat—any or all of these can mark the beginning of a cold. Fits of sneezing, headache, congestion of the nasal passages, watery eyes, and a runny nose soon follow.*

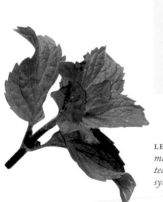

CAUTION

Peppermint leaf should not be used during pregnancy.

LEFT *Peppermint makes a warming tea to relieve cold symptoms.*

 HERBALISM

• A mouthwash and gargle of marigold flowers will soothe a sore throat.

• A tea made from peppermint leaves, elderflower, and yarrow acts on mucous membranes, relieving a blocked nose and other cold symptoms.

 HOMEOPATHY

• Use Aconite for feverishness alternating with chills during the night.

• Sabadilla is useful for fits of sneezing.

 AROMATHERAPY

• Essential oil of bay, burned in the room or inhaled from a bowl of steaming water, will ease cold symptoms.

 FROM THE LARDER

• Taking frequent doses of vitamin C may help to relieve symptoms. One-gram tablets, dissolved in water, or large doses of vitamin C powder, are particularly beneficial. This remedy is sometimes recommended for the prevention of colds.

• Drink plenty of fluids (avoid milk and other dairy products, which will encourage the buildup of catarrh). Hot drinks of honey and lemon, honey and vinegar, or onion juice and honey can be soothing.

 SELF-HELP

• Bed rest and warmth will help relieve some of the symptoms.

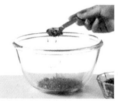

1 *Put three teaspoons of eucalyptus leaves in a heatproof bowl. Other herbs can also be used; pine is useful.*

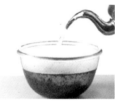

2 *Pour 4¼pt. (2l.) of boiling water directly onto the herbs. Leave to soak for a minute or two.*

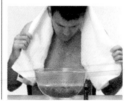

3 *Place your head over the bowl and cover it and the bowl with a towel. Inhale through the nose for about ten minutes.*

Coughs

Coughing can be symptomatic of a mild illness such as a cold or just a natural, involuntary response to clear the air passages of foreign material. Persistent coughs with other symptoms such as fever, however, can be indicative of a serious respiratory illness and should be referred to a qualified medical practitioner.

 HERBALISM

• Angelica leaf and root are expectorants and antiseptics. Use as a tea or tincture.

• Codonopsis root tincture, decoction, or powder is useful for chronic coughs.

• Licorice is good for nonproductive coughs.

• Take comfrey tea and syrup for dry coughs that will not go away.

 HOMEOPATHY

• For coughs characterized by whooping take Drosera.

• If the cough is loose and rattling, producing little or no phlegm, take Antimonium tart.

• Ferrum phos. is beneficial for tickly, hard, dry coughs.

 AROMATHERAPY

• Inhaling jasmine or pine, or burning the essential oil in a room, may ease a cough.

 FROM THE LARDER

• Carrot juice mixed with honey and a little warm water is a traditional Russian remedy for coughs. Take by the spoonful throughout the day.

 SELF-HELP

• Raise the end of your bed to help ease the coughing at night.

• A room vaporizer or humidifier will keep the air moist, which will help to soothe airways and make breathing easier.

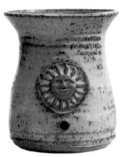

RIGHT *The warm scent of pine oil in a burner will help ease a constricted throat and soothe a tight cough.*

 CAUTION

• Do not give comfrey syrup to children.
• Pregnant women should avoid angelica.
• Licorice, used for extended periods, acts as a laxative. Anyone with high blood pressure should avoid licorice since it will exacerbate the condition.
• If coughing is accompanied by chest pains and other symptoms, consult a qualified medical practitioner.

Chronic Catarrh

Catarrh is a common but uncomfortable complaint caused by irritation or inflammation of the mucous membranes lining the nose and throat.

SYMPTOMS *A runny nose, followed by dryness when the nose becomes blocked.*

RIGHT *Catarrh is produced in all parts of the mouth, nose, throat, and windpipe. This view of the throat and nose from the back shows how all the parts are intimately connected.*

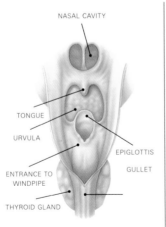

NASAL CAVITY
TONGUE
URVULA
ENTRANCE TO WINDPIPE
THYROID GLAND
EPIGLOTTIS
GULLET

 HOMEOPATHY

• Kali bich. is recommended when the nose is blocked and mucus is thick, yellow-green. It also helps in postnasal catarrh.

• Pulsatilla is suitable for catarrh that becomes worse in a stuffy room. It is particularly suitable for children who are prone to glue ear.

 AROMATHERAPY

• Inhaling or burning jasmine essential oil can be beneficial.

• Niaouli massaged around the chest and lung areas may reduce congestion caused by catarrh.

 FROM THE LARDER

• Garlic capsules may help relieve the symptoms.

• Cayenne capsules or drops will act as a decongestant.

 SELF-HELP

• Regularly blowing the nose will help to clear some of the mucus.

• Fresh air and exercise may bring temporary relief.

CAUTION

Chronic catarrh, which lasts beyond six weeks, should be treated by a qualified therapist or general practitioner.

Hay fever

Hay fever is an extremely common allergy that in severe cases can drastically disrupt daily life.

SYMPTOMS *Irritation, sneezing, and a watery discharge from the nose and eyes are mild symptoms. More serious ones include sore throat, blocked nose and sinuses, a feeling of stuffiness and heaviness in the head, itchy and streaming eyes.*

 CAUTION

During pregnancy avoid patchouli except when used in a vaporizer. Not suitable for infants and babies.

 HERBALISM

• Elderflower tea or tincture is particularly good for a runny nose.

• Alternatively, make a tea of peppermint leaf and yarrow.

• Take steps to improve your immune system, which can reduce the severity of symptoms.

 HOMEOPATHY

• Use Euphrasia when the eyes are hot and irritated by burning tears.

 AROMATHERAPY

• Patchouli oil is anti-inflammatory and therefore useful for hay-fever symptoms of blocked nose and sinuses.

 FROM THE LARDER

• Drink cider vinegar and honey to relieve congestion in the nose and sinuses.

• Honey contains traces of pollen. Eating a local honey in the early spring, before the hay fever season begins, may help to desensitize you to pollens in your area.

SELF-HELP

• There is some evidence that an increased intake of vitamin C may reduce symptoms because of its effect on the immune system.

BELOW *The brilliant chrome yellow of a rape field in full bloom may signal high summer, but can be anathema to hay-fever sufferers.*

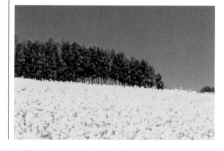

Asthma

Asthma is an increasingly common disease, especially among children. Some authorities blame the rising incidence and intensity of air pollution as the reason for the increase, but allergies still account for a large number of cases.

SYMPTOMS *Heavy, labored breathing, especially on breathing out, which may become very severe and disabling.*

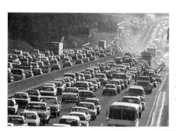

LEFT *Pollution from car exhaust fumes is one of the factors leading to the increase of asthma among children.*

 HERBALISM

• For chronic cases, codonopsis root can be helpful.

• Gingko leaves help to reduce the dependency on prescription drugs. However, do not stop taking or alter the dosage without consulting your medical practitioner.

 HOMEOPATHY

• Mag. phos. is recommended for asthma brought on by nervousness.

• Use Ipecac to relieve symptoms brought on by anger or irritability.

 AROMATHERAPY

• The essential oil of cajeput is excellent when inhaled. Eucalyptus, marjoram, and melissa are also useful.

 FROM THE LARDER

• Apricots strengthen the mucous membranes and may be of some

help in preventing asthma attacks.

• A drink made from vinegar and honey is an old remedy for asthma. It may help to clear congestion of the lungs.

• Aniseed tea may also bring some relief from symptoms.

 SELF-HELP

• Asthma is often exacerbated by stress, and steps to reduce stress will discourage attacks.

• Make sure your house is free of dust, pollen, and pet hairs, which may lead to an attack.

 CAUTION

• Cajeput is a stimulant and should not be used before bedtime. It is unsuitable for babies.

• Aniseed should not be used during pregnancy or by anyone with a digestive problem.

Influenza

The virus that causes influenza is remarkable in that it is able to change its appearance in an effort to hoodwink the immune system. So it presents in a different strain every twelve months or so, although on rare occasions it will emerge in a form similar to one it took previously. The latter occurrence means that some people will have an immunity to the virus. Every thirty to forty years, changes to the strain produce an entirely new virus, causing a worldwide epidemic.

SYMPTOMS *Fever, aching joints and muscles, shivering, headache, sore eyes, and a runny nose. These are sometimes combined with diarrhea and/or vomiting. Severe forms of influenza can be fatal, particularly for the elderly and the very young.*

 HERBALISM

• Elderflower tea or tincture should help to relieve symptoms, particularly if the elderflower is combined with equal parts of peppermint and yarrow. Drink a cup every two hours.

• Echinacea encourages resistance to illness.

 HOMEOPATHY

• For feverishness alternating with chills at night, take Aconite.

 • Gelsemium is helpful when the whole body aches, chills run up and down the spine, and burning heat alternates with shivering.

 AROMATHERAPY

• To ease aching limbs, add juniper oil to the bathwater.

• A massage with juniper is both comforting and soothing.

RIGHT *A soothing massage can help ease the aches and pains that accompany influenza.*

 FROM THE LARDER

• Taking large doses of vitamin C may help to relieve symptoms.

• Lemon acts as a tonic to the immune system and helps to reduce fever.

• Onion stimulates and warms the body.

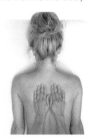

 SELF-HELP

• Get plenty of bed rest, warmth, and fluids, including energizing, sugary drinks.airways and make breathing easier.

 CAUTION

• Avoid peppermint during pregnancy.

• Serious cases should be referred to a qualified medical practitioner.

Pneumonia

Pneumonia most often occurs as a result of bacterial infection. Other causes include viral or fungal infection, or, more rarely, the inhalation of a foreign object.

SYMPTOMS *Symptoms depend on the type of pneumonia. In those caused by a bacterium, coughing is the common symptom; other symptoms may include feverishness, the production of sputum, and chest pain. In pneumonia caused by agents other than bacteria, symptoms include cough, fever, and breathlessness (in the newborn), with very little or no sputum.*

RIGHT *A steam inhalation of hot water with pine, bay, or eucalyptus oil in it can help support conventional treatment for pneumonia.*

 HERBALISM

• Echinacea root stimulates the immune system to fight infections.

• Garlic and thyme syrup may be helpful.

 AROMATHERAPY

• Bay, when inhaled, acts as a pulmonary antiseptic.

• Inhaling eucalyptus may also be beneficial.

• Pine is a powerful antiseptic for the lungs. Use as an inhalation in a bowl of steaming water. It can be burned in a vaporizer and placed in a baby's or child's room.

 FROM THE LARDER

• Vitamin C can help to strengthen the immune system.

• An onion compress or mustard plaster placed on the chest may help to reduce inflammation.

SELF-HELP

• After receiving conventional medical attention there are many remedies that will help make you more comfortable, encourage healing, and prevent further attacks. Bed rest is essential. Drink plenty of fresh juices and cool water to flush the system.

CAUTION

This is a serious disease that requires treatment by a qualified medical practitioner.

Ears, Nose, and Throat

*P*robably the most recurrent ailments we deal with in the home concern infections in the ears, nose, and throat, where the inside of the body is exposed to external influences and pollution. This is usually treated as one "system" because each area is closely connected to the other: a cold can lead to an ear infection, blocked ears to a sore throat. Ailments include earache, laryngitis, tonsillitis, and sinusitis.

Earache and Infections

Infection of the ears, or otitis, takes several forms. Otitis media is an infection of the middle ear usually caused by a viral or bacterial infection in the nose and throat. It is commonly known as glue ear and often affects infants and young children. Left untreated, it may cause mastoiditis. Otitis externa is inflammation of the outer ear, caused by a fungus or a bacterium. Earache may be caused by inflammation of the lymph nodes in the neck or by an illness such as mumps. There may be an ear infection in the inner, middle, or outer parts of the ear. Occasionally a boil can crop up in the outer ear, which can be very painful. Ear infections can cause a great deal of pain, and the pressure may burst the eardrum, causing a discharge. There may be fever and a sore throat.

SYMPTOMS *In otitis externa, the outer ear is red and itchy. There may be a watery discharge. In acute conditions of otitis media there is a buildup of pus, which may cause excruciating pain and fever. There is usually some hearing loss. If the condition is not treated early, the eardrum may perforate. Chronic conditions of otitis media cause persistent earache, sometimes accompanied by fever and a slight discharge of pus.*

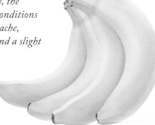

RIGHT *Bananas are rich in vitamin C and vitamin B6, both of which help promote a healthy immune system.*

 HERBALISM

• Garlic has antibiotic properties. A few drops of garlic oil in the ear canal should ease the pain of earache.

• Mullein flower infused oil used as eardrops will relieve itching in otitis externa.

• A mouthwash of marigold flowers used as a gargle may be helpful for chronic ear infection.

 HOMEOPATHY

• Belladonna is beneficial in cases of otitis media, particularly when there is sudden onset of throbbing, stabbing pain.

• Merc. sol. can be taken for earache that is accompanied by a thick, yellow discharge.

• Aconite may help if the earache comes on suddenly.

 AROMATHERAPY

• For mild cases of earache soak a piece of absorbent cotton in cajeput essential oil and place it carefully in the outer ear.

• Carefully dab neat lavender oil into the ear canal to soothe and encourage healing in both external and middle ear infections.

 FLOWER ESSENCES

• Rescue Remedy cream can be rubbed in around the ear canal, or Rescue Remedy can be taken internally to relieve pain and discomfort.

 FROM THE LARDER

• Foods rich in vitamin C and vitamin B6 (pyridoxine)—citrus fruit, bananas, wholewheat bread, brewers' yeast—help promote a healthy immune system, which will fight infection.

• A small bag of warm salt placed against the ear should ease the pain of earache.

 SELF-HELP

• A warm compress on the affected side will ease pain and help to bring out the infection.

Wax in the Ear

Ear wax protects the inner ear from infection. It consists of oils secreted by small glands in the skin of the outermost part of the ear canal, pieces of skin, and dust particles. In ordinary circumstances wax constantly moves into the outer ear and is washed away. When it accumulates in the ear canal it can cause problems.

SYMPTOMS *Irritation, temporary deafness, and a buzzing or ringing sound in the ear (see Tinnitus, right). It rarely causes pain.*

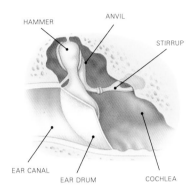

HAMMER ANVIL STIRRUP EAR CANAL EAR DRUM COCHLEA

ABOVE *A cross-section of the complicated arrangements of the middle ear. A buildup of wax in the ear canal can disturb balance, affect hearing, and seal in infection.*

 SELF-HELP

• Prevent the buildup of wax by keeping the outer ear clean. Never try to remove wax from the ear canal yourself; this should be done by a medical practitioner. DO NOT DO THIS YOURSELF.

• Hopi ear candle therapy is a safe and natural way to remove obstinate ear wax, but must be carried out by a trained practitioner.

• A specially made candle is placed in the ear and lit. Old wax softens and is drawn out and healing herbal vapors penetrate the ear.

Tinnitus

Tinnitus is symptomatic of an ear disorder. It may be a result of wax that has become impacted in the ear canal, or a fungal or bacterial infection in the external ear. Middle ear infections and inner ear disorders, such as damage to the cochlea, may also cause tinnitus. If tinnitus is accompanied by giddiness so severe that the sufferer vomits or falls down, consult a medical practitioner; this may be caused by Ménière's disease, a periodic affliction of the inner ear.

 HERBALISM

• Lycium fruit decoction or tincture is useful for weakness associated with tinnitus.

• Gingko leaf tea, tincture, or tablets may help in cases of tinnitus.

 HOMEOPATHY

• Ignatia is recommended for ringing in the ears that is relieved by listening to music.

• Calc. sulf. in the 6c dosage, may help; a homeopath may recommend Chininum sulf. or Kali iod., both in the 6c potency.

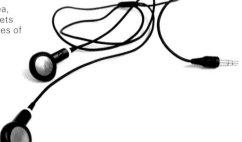

LEFT *Personal stereos played at high level can increase the risk of tinnitus.*

Cold Sores

Cold sores are a viral infection caused by the microorganism Herpes simplex, usually following a cold, flu, sore throat, or chest infection.

SYMPTOMS *Tiny, inflamed blisters fill with a yellowish-white fluid. They are itchy, tender, and often painful. During the healing process the blisters dry up and a crust forms on the top. This should not be removed: it will fall off when the blisters have healed.*

 HERBALISM

• Use echinacea root with damiana leaf as a tincture or decoction.

• Use St. John's wort tincture with a few drops of essential oil of myrrh as a lotion.

 HOMEOPATHY

• Take Natrum mur. or Rhus tox. for blisters that itch and burn.

 AROMATHERAPY

• The essential oil of bergamot will help to heal the sores.

• Dab lavender oil neat on the sores to encourage healing and attack the virus.

 FROM THE LARDER

• Vitamin C and bioflavinoids, available as supplements and found in green bell peppers, blackcurrants, and citrus fruit, will aid in the healing. Both vitamin C and vitamin B6 (pyridoxine) help promote a healthy immune system.

• A few drops of undiluted lemon juice, applied several times a day, may help in the healing process.

SELF-HELP

• A peculiar old remedy for "cold blisters" advises the sufferer to "rub a slug on it."

• Cold sores are a sign that you are run down: consider more rest and a better diet.

RIGHT *Undiluted lemon juice dabbed onto a cold sore will sting but help to heal.*

Mouth Ulcers

Ulcers in the mouth are caused by a viral infection. If left untreated, they may cause problems in other parts of the body. Children may get mouth ulcers as a result of the same virus that causes cold sores in susceptible adults.

SYMPTOMS *Yellowish or white patches that are surrounded by red sore areas. This may be accompanied by halitosis.*

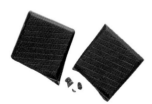

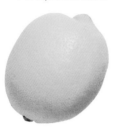

 HERBALISM

• Make a mouthwash with echinacea root. Use frequently to gargle and to rinse out the mouth.

 HOMEOPATHY

• Merc. sol. may be helpful for mouth ulcers.

 AROMATHERAPY

• Use myrrh or orange essential oils as a mouthwash.

 FROM THE LARDER

• Rinsing the mouth with cabbage juice.

 SELF-HELP

• Avoid chocolate, oranges, tomatoes, pineapple, and other acid foods until the condition improves.

LEFT *Chocolate and citrus fruit should be avoided if there are ulcers in the mouth.*

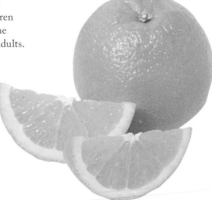

Halitosis

Bad breath has a number of causes, including smoking, tooth decay, and indigestion. Crash dieting can also cause halitosis. Ketones, produced by the body during the breakdown of fats and carried in the bloodstream, have a sickly, sweet odor that is noticeable on the breath.

 HERBALISM
• Use aniseed tea as a mouthwash.

 AROMATHERAPY
• Myrrh, prepared as a mouthwash, will sweeten the breath.

 FROM THE LARDER
• Gargling with a solution of baking soda and water should eliminate bad odors. Repeat as necessary.

 SELF-HELP
• Identifying the cause of halitosis and eliminating the problem is the best solution.

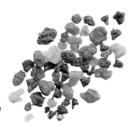

RIGHT *Tincture of myrrh diluted to form a mouthwash helps to sweeten sour breath.*

Oral Thrush

Oral thrush is caused by the same agent as vaginal thrush—the fungal yeast Candida, particularly *Candida albicans*.

SYMPTOMS *Small white patches on the gums, tongue, inside the lips and cheeks. There may be soreness when eating or drinking.*

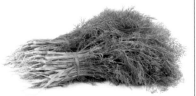

ABOVE *The antifungal properties of fennel make it ideal for an oral thrush attack.*

 HERBALISM
• Use raspberry leaf tea as a mouthwash.

 FROM THE LARDER
• Live sheep's or goat's yogurt has proved to be successful in treating thrush. Eat it or apply it to the area.

• Garlic can be chewed for local effect.

• Try cinnamon to boost the immune system.

• Fennel has antifungal properties and can be drunk or chewed raw during an attack.

 SELF-HELP
• Where possible, eliminate dairy products from cows, yeast products, and wheat from the diet until the symptoms have disappeared.

Gum Disease

There are two types of chronic gum disease: gingivitis and pyorrhea. Left untreated they can lead to the premature decay and eventual loss of teeth.

SYMPTOMS *Symptoms of gingivitis are bleeding gums caused by a mild inflammation. The gums will become swollen and pus will form if the condition is not treated. With trench mouth, a form of gingivitis, grayish sores appear and there may be a temperature. In pyorrhea, crevices form in the gum in which bacteria flourish and plaque accumulates.*

 HERBALISM
• To soothe sore gums, use a mouthwash made with tincture of aloe vera.

• Try a sage mouthwash.

 AROMATHERAPY
• Rinse the mouth out with a mouthwash of myrrh or orange. Myrrh is particularly good for pyorrhea.

 FROM THE LARDER
• Vitamin C supplements are beneficial; they promote healthy gums.

• A gargle of vinegar (1 tablespoon) in a glass of water may help to treat the condition.

 SELF-HELP
• Cleaning the teeth properly and having regular dental checkups will help prevent recurrences.

ABOVE *A regular and thorough dental hygiene routine will prevent gum disease from ever taking hold.*

Laryngitis

Both common and acute laryngitis may be caused by overuse of the voice, violent shouting, irritation from cigarette smoke, dust, or other pollutants, and infection.

SYMPTOMS *In acute laryngitis, the larynx may be tender and painful and the sufferer may have difficulty speaking. Sometimes the ability to speak is lost completely.*
Acute laryngitis usually clears up in a day or two. In chronic conditions there is hoarseness, the feeling of "a frog in the throat" and tenderness that continues unabated for some time. This condition requires medical attention.

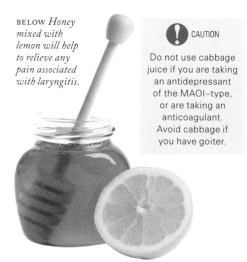

BELOW *Honey mixed with lemon will help to relieve any pain associated with laryngitis.*

 CAUTION

Do not use cabbage juice if you are taking an antidepressant of the MAOI–type, or are taking an anticoagulant. Avoid cabbage if you have goiter.

 HERBALISM

• Try a sage gargle.

 HOMEOPATHY

• Kali bich. will help when the voice is hoarse and there is a dry cough

 AROMATHERAPY

• Frankincense burned in a room or myrrh used in a vaporizer will soothe the throat

• Cabbage juice may alleviate hoarseness.

 FROM THE LARDER

• Honey mixed with lemon will help to relieve any pain, and if there is a bacterial infection present, honey will work as an antibiotic.

 SELF-HELP

• Resting the voice is one of the best cures.

• An old remedy advises chewing rowanberry and pimpernel.

Sinusitis

Sinusitis can be a chronic or acute condition. It is the inflammation of the mucous membranes that line the sinuses of the nose.

SYMPTOMS *Blocked nose, cough, some pain, and nasal discharge are symptoms of chronic sinusitis. In acute cases the pain is more severe, and the sufferer may experience this as a headache or as pain in the cheekbones. There is little or no discharge. The senses of smell and taste may be affected. If the eyes are affected the patient may experience double vision.*

RIGHT *A cross section of the nose and throat. The sinuses are a continuation of the nasal cavity.*

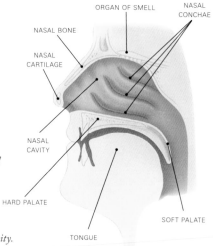

ORGAN OF SMELL

NASAL CONCHAE

NASAL BONE

NASAL CARTILAGE

NASAL CAVITY

HARD PALATE

TONGUE

SOFT PALATE

 HERBALISM

• Drink elderflower tea or tincture. Elderflower can also be taken as a syrup or as tablets.

• Yarrow tea is beneficial.

• Steam inhalations of pine or eucalyptus can help. (*see page 76*).

 HOMEOPATHY

• Kali bich. is recommended when there is a localized hot, burning pain.

 AROMATHERAPY

• Use the essential oil of bay, either inhaled or vaporized.

 FROM THE LARDER

• Garlic can be beneficial in relieving the symptoms.

• Increase your intake of vitamin C, B complex, iron, and zinc.

 SELF-HELP

• Humidify bedrooms and living rooms.

Eyes

*T*he eyes are particularly vulnerable to strain, inflammation, allergic reaction, and physical damage (*see also The Respiratory System on pages 76-79*). Always consult your general practitioner if problems persist for more than twenty-four hours, or if there is a foreign body in the eye that cannot be removed with an eye bath or by rapid blinking.

Conjunctivitis

Conjunctivitis, or pink eye, occurs quite frequently in children. These cases are generally mild. A more severe form of the disease can result in loss of sight.

SYMPTOMS *Painful, inflamed eyes and watery discharge or pus. There may be an intolerance to strong light and the eyelids may become swollen.*

 HERBALISM

• German chamomile makes an effective eyewash.

• A compress soaked in cornflower, chamomile, or marigold infusions will soothe.

• Diluted witch hazel can be used on sore, red (closed) eyes.

 HOMEOPATHY

• Use Argentum nit. (silver nitrate) for eyes pink with pus and with a bland discharge.

• Euphrasia is useful for red, inflamed eyes.

 FROM THE LARDER

• Take vitamin C and vitamin B complex supplements to boost the immune system.

• To relieve itching, lie down and place cucumber slices over the eyes.

 SELF-HELP

• Rinse the eyes frequently with cooled, boiled water.

• Rub a little olive oil into your lashes before you go to bed to prevent them from sticking together.

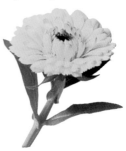

BELOW *Marigold infusion on a compress can soothe inflamed eyes.*

Eyestrain

Eyestrain is usually caused by close work in poor lighting conditions and by poor eyesight.

SYMPTOMS *Headache behind the eye or at the front of the head. The eyes may feel tired and a little sore.*

 HERBALISM

• Make a marigold flower compress for sore eyes.

• Chamomile tea can be used as a compress to cool sore eyes.

• Dampened rosehip teabags may be used to relieve symptoms.

 HOMEOPATHY

• Euphrasia will soothe tired eyes, refresh and brighten them.

• Use Ruta grav. when the eyes are hot, sore, and itching and when the condition is aggravated by reading, sewing, or working in dim light.

 FROM THE LARDER

• Cold tea bags placed over the eyes may also help alleviate eyestrain.

• Slices of cucumber placed on each eyelid will cool and refresh the eyes.

SELF-HELP

• Palming—closing your eyes and cupping them in your palms, with the heels of the hand resting on the lower orbital bone—can soothe tired eyes.

• Rest your eyes frequently when working.

The Digestive System

*T*he digestive system begins at the mouth and ends at the anus; it is a huge, complex organization whose job is to break down food into its constituent nutrients and distribute them. It is intimately linked with the endocrine and nervous systems, which is why anxiety so often results in digestive distress.

Heartburn and Indigestion

Heartburn, like hiccups, can be a nuisance but is not serious. The cause is not really known but may result from acid rising from the stomach into the gullet. It is quite common in overweight people and pregnant women. Indigestion has many causes, among them eating too quickly, stress, and anxiety.

SYMPTOMS *Heartburn is felt as a burning pain in the center of the chest. Indigestion may be felt in the same area as a dull ache or stabbing pain. It may also be felt as stomachache.*

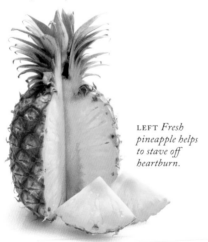

LEFT *Fresh pineapple helps to stave off heartburn.*

 HERBALISM

• Take agrimony or horsetail tea or tincture for indigestion.

• Take a combination of meadowsweet (to lower acid production), comfrey (to heal acid "burn"), marshmallow (to soothe), and chamomile (to reduce stress and inflammation).

 HOMEOPATHY

• Arsenicum alb. is used to treat heartburn that creeps up into the chest and throat.

• Carbo veg. is useful when indigestion is accompanied by flatulence.

• For cramping pains in a hard, bloated abdomen after eating beans, onion, cabbage, and other "windy" foods, take Lycopodium.

• Kali mur helps indigestion caused by eating fatty foods.

 AROMATHERAPY

• Clove oil massaged over the stomach is useful for dyspepsia.

• Mandarin essential oil aids digestion.

 FROM THE LARDER

• A glass of milk may relieve the pain of heartburn.

• Indigestion may be relieved by drinking soda water and prevented by drinking sparkling mineral water with the meal.

• Eat fresh pineapple following a meal to prevent an attack of heartburn—canned pineapple does not have the same effect. This is particularly useful during pregnancy.

 SELF-HELP

• Weight loss will probably effect a cure in heartburn if obesity is the underlying problem.

• Indigestion brought on by stress or anxiety may respond to relaxation exercises.

• Relaxing while eating may prevent indigestion; avoid eating while moving around.

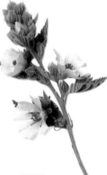

ABOVE *Marshmallow tea can soothe indigestion.*

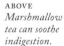 CAUTION

• If indigestion causing pain in the chest area lasts for a number of hours, you should seek medical advice, particularly if pain is also felt in the arms, neck, or jaw, with vomiting, sweating, or shortness of breath.

• Avoid agrimony if you are suffering from chronic constipation.

• Avoid comfrey in pregnancy.

Nausea and Vomiting

Nausea and vomiting have many causes, including overindulgence in food and drink, food poisoning, pregnancy, and travel sickness. They may also be symptoms of a more serious underlying illness. If these symptoms continue for more than twenty-four hours, see a qualified medical practitioner.

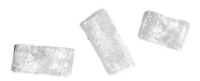

ABOVE: *Chewing crystallized ginger can help quell feelings of nausea.*

 HERBALISM

• German chamomile or peppermint tea or tincture will ease nausea.

• Hang fresh angelica leaves in the car or ship's cabin when traveling.

 HOMEOPATHY

• Cocculus is useful for travel sickness.

• For vomiting and nausea attributable to the early months of pregnancy, try Sepia, or Kali mur. if white phlegm is vomited.

 AROMATHERAPY

• Orange oil helps to prevent travel sickness.

 FROM THE LARDER

• Chewing a piece of raw or crystallized ginger or drinking ginger tea may help.

• Drinking barley water or clove tea may help relieve both nausea and vomiting.

 SELF-HELP

• Swallowing cracked or crushed ice may help relieve morning sickness.

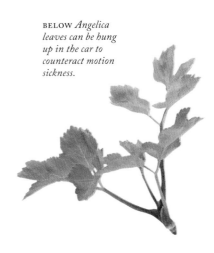

BELOW *Angelica leaves can be hung up in the car to counteract motion sickness.*

Irritable Bowel Syndrome

Irritable bowel syndrome occurs when digested food and waste material pass through the bowel too quickly. Anxiety, stress, and food intolerance may be a contributing factor in the onset of this ailment.

SYMPTOMS *Diarrhea or constipation, severe abdominal pain, bloating, and stomach rumblings. There may be long periods without any symptoms before they recur. Emotionally, sufferers may appear to be depressed.*

 CAUTION

Do not take peppermint in pregnancy. Nervous and overexcitable people may find that it is too stimulating.

 HERBALISM

• Slippery elm drinks or tablets are soothing and helpful for most bowel irritations.

• Fennel seed tea or tincture and teas made from mint and peppermint may be helpful.

• Try a tea made from yellow dock root, chamomile, and marshmallow.

 FROM THE LARDER

• Drinking at least eight glasses of water a day and increasing fiber intake in the form of wholegrains and cereals may help.

• Avoid foods with gluten—for example wheat and rye—if a gluten allergy is suspected.

SELF-HELP

• If anxiety and stress are a causative factor, exercise, in the form of a sport, or relaxation may be helpful.

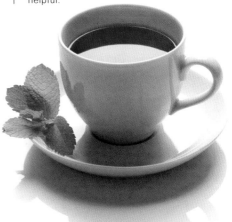

RIGHT *Teas made from mint or peppermint might be helpful to people who suffer from irritable bowel syndrome.*

Constipation

Constipation may be caused by an inadequate diet or a change in lifestyle, such as going on vacation, as well as ill health.

SYMPTOMS *Infrequent passing of stools. It is usually associated with some degree of discomfort.*

 HERBALISM

• For constipation in pregnancy, try a decoction of dandelion root. Add 2oz. (50g.) peeled licorice root to 2pt. (1l.) cold water. Bring to a boil, then simmer for ten minutes. Drink three wineglassfuls a day until the condition improves.

 HOMEOPATHY

• Calcarea carb. may help to resolve the problem.

 AROMATHERAPY

• Try a massage with geranium oil.

• Massage over the abdominal area.

 FROM THE LARDER

• Gradually increase bran intake, beginning with a heaped teaspoon each day for three days. Increase water intake by drinking an extra 10fl. oz. (300ml.) for each additional teaspoon of bran you eat.

• Eating one or two apples a day will help prevent constipation in the future.

 SELF-HELP

• Fresh air and exercise may be helpful.

Crohn's disease

Crohn's disease—also known as ileitis—and ulcerative colitis affect the bowel. Medical practitioners refer to both conditions as inflammatory bowel disease.

SYMPTOMS *Swelling in any part of the bowel as a result of ulceration or inflammation is characteristic of Crohn's disease. The ileum, the final part of the small intestine, may be particularly affected. Sometimes the passage of feces is obstructed. In ulcerative colitis only the large intestine is inflamed and there may be copious diarrhea. These conditions require the attention of a qualified medical practitioner.*

 HERBALISM

• Try meadowsweet, chamomile, and licorice as a tea or mixture of tincture.

• Slippery elm as tablets or a drink is soothing.

 AROMATHERAPY

• Lemongrass, massaged over the abdomen, is helpful when there is gastric infection.

 FROM THE LARDER

• Eat foods that are high in fiber, such as wholegrain cereals, pulses, fruit, and vegetables.

• Take natural yogurt, sweetened with a little honey, several times a day.

 SELF-HELP

• Keep a record of foods that appear to aggravate the condition and avoid them in future.

 CAUTION

Avoid licorice in pregnancy or if you have high blood pressure.

Peptic ulcers

Peptic ulcers occur in the stomach (gastric ulcers) and duodenum (duodenal ulcers) and less commonly in the esophagus. They are caused by the action of stomach acid on the lining or mucous membranes of these structures. Heavy drinking, smoking, stress, and aspirin may all contribute to the formation of an ulcer.

SYMPTOMS *Pain (dyspepsia) that occurs in bouts over a period of one to two weeks.*

 HERBALISM

• Astragalus root tincture or decoction helps relieve stomach ulcers.

• Alternatively, drink tea made from comfrey, chamomile, and meadowsweet.

 AROMATHERAPY

• For gastric ulcers, massage the abdomen with Roman chamomile.

 FROM THE LARDER

• Short-term relief may be gained from drinking five glasses of cabbage juice every day.

• Banana powder may help to heal

ulcers and prevent peptic ulcers caused by aspirin.

• For advice on diet it is best to consult a nutritionist or natural healthcare practitioner.

 SELF-HELP

• Bed rest has been shown to be beneficial in the treatment of peptic ulcers.

 CAUTION

Comfrey should not be taken in pregnancy. Do not give to children.

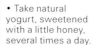

Diarrhea

Loose, watery stools may be symptomatic of an underlying condition. It may also be caused by eating an excess of high-fiber foods or infection by bacteria in food, among other things.

 CAUTION

Diarrhea that lasts for more than forty-eight hours should be reported to your physician. Children and the elderly are particularly at risk of dehydration; ensure adequate intake of liquids.

 HERBALISM

• Agrimony tea or tincture may ease the condition.

• In cases of chronic diarrhea, take codonopsis root as a decoction, tincture, or powder.

 HOMEOPATHY

• Phosphoric acid is useful for painless, watery diarrhea that is not debilitating, although the patient may feel weak afterwards.

• Take Calcarea carb. when the diarrhea is caused by infection and Graphites for a fluid diarrhea with undigested food particles.

 AROMATHERAPY

• Geranium oil massaged over the stomach area may be beneficial.

• Use neroli for diarrhea related to stress.

 FROM THE LARDER

• Grated apple mixed with live yogurt may be helpful.

• Potassium supplements may be indicated in cases of chronic diarrhea.

• An old remedy for diarrhea advises eating white bread with cinnamon and drinking black tea—with no other food—until the condition improves.

 SELF-HELP

• Restrict foods to soups, such as barley soup, and soft foods, such as pureed or mashed fruit and vegetables, until the condition clears.

Hemorrhoids

Hemorrhoids, or piles, are varicose veins that occur in the anus. They can be particularly troublesome and, if severe, may need medical attention. They may be caused by straining when passing stools.

SYMPTOMS *Painful, protruding veins around the anus. Bleeding and itching.*

 HERBALISM

• Try devil's claw as a tincture or decoction.

• Elder leaf ointment helps relieve painful piles.

 HOMEOPATHY

• Use Nux vom. for throbbing piles.

 AROMATHERAPY

• Neroli essential oil may bring relief.

 FROM THE LARDER

• A wholefood, high-fiber diet may prevent a recurrence of this condition.

• Witch hazel can be applied neat to the hemorrhoids to reduce swelling and itching.

• Apply garlic directly to the affected area and ensure that you have plenty of garlic and onions in your diet, which increase the elasticity of the veins.

 SELF-HELP

• Keep the area clean, washing gently after each bowel movement.

• Sitting on a cushion with the legs raised may bring some temporary relief. Some people find that a hot-water bottle, wrapped in a towel and placed over the bottom, also helps relieve pain when applied before a bowel movement.

Gallstones

Gallstones are made of bile pigments, calcium salts, and cholesterol. They usually go unnoticed while they remain in the gallbladder, but if they begin to pass into the intestine through a bile duct, they may get trapped, causing irritation and inflammation of the gallbladder, bile ducts, or pancreas.

SYMPTOMS *Vomiting, severe pain in the abdomen, chest area, or right shoulder. There may be a rise in body temperature.*

 HERBALISM

• Take a decoction of milk thistle seeds.

 HOMEOPATHY

• Natrum phos. should be taken when there is sour vomit.

 AROMATHERAPY

• Try a massage with peppermint oil.

 FROM THE LARDER

• A fairly drastic (but reportedly effective) remedy for passing gallstones painlessly is as follows. Take a dose of Epsom salts. One hour later, drink a wineglassful of olive oil. Follow this with a small glass of lemon juice. Continue taking the Epsom salts, olive oil, and lemon juice every five minutes until 10fl. oz. (300ml.) of oil and the juice of six lemons have been taken.

 SELF-HELP

• A wholefood diet with a high-fiber, low-sugar content may aid in the prevention of gallstones.

 CAUTION

Persistent or recurring symptoms should be reported to your physician.

The Nervous System

The body has three nervous systems, all interlinked: the central, the peripheral, and the autonomous nervous systems. Anxiety, stress, depression, and headaches respond well to natural treatments, but physical or degenerative problems of the nervous system or severe depression must be treated by a medical practitioner.

Anxiety

Abnormal forms of anxiety—those that go beyond the normal worries and cares experienced by everyone—can be debilitating. Severe states of anxiety usually benefit from counseling or therapy.

SYMPTOMS *Increased heart rate, raised blood pressure, and rapid breathing are common symptoms of abnormal anxiety states. In some cases the sufferer may have panic attacks and a strong feeling that they are losing control. There may also be a sense of detachment from the surroundings and loss of appetite.*

 CAUTION

Severe cases of anxiety should be treated by a qualified medical practitioner or therapist.

 HERBALISM

• Hawthorn berries and valerian or linden flowers will help relieve palpitations associated with anxiety attacks.

 HOMEOPATHY

• Arsenicum alb. helps those who feel out of control. You may have phobias or be obsessive and may break out in a cold sweat when anxiety is at its worse.

• Kali mur. may be beneficial where anxiety is linked with depression, irritability, and a nervous dread.

 FLOWER ESSENCES

• Take Aspen for vague anxieties that apparently have no cause.

• Cherry Plum is helpful for fear.

• Rock Rose helps overcome panic attacks.

• Rescue Remedy is excellent for relieving anxiety and promoting a feeling of calm.

 AROMATHERAPY

• Essential oils with a calming effect include Roman chamomile, lavender, neroli, or marjoram. Use in the bath, or during massage.

• Petitgrain is useful for those with panic attacks.

• Cedarwood, burned in a room or used in a vaporizer, balances anxiety and nervous tension.

 FROM THE LARDER

• In mild cases, oats, which contain thiamine and pantothenic acid, are a gentle tonic for the nerves.

• Supplements of vitamin B complex and zinc may also be beneficial.

 SELF-HELP

• Learn and practice deep breathing and relaxation techniques. Meditation may also be helpful.

Stress

Some level of stress appears to be inevitable in modern life. When it becomes excessive and prolonged it can be dangerous to mental and physical health.

SYMPTOMS *Stress may manifest itself in physical ailments, and the underlying cause may not always be immediately apparent. Headaches and skin complaints such as eczema are just two common ailments that can result from unmanageable levels of stress. Mental and emotional effects include mental fatigue, confusion, lack of concentration, and poor memory.*

 HERBALISM
- Chinese ginseng helps the body to cope with stress. For cases in which stress is prolonged, take Siberian ginseng.
- Motherwort and vervain aids anxiety associated with stress.

 AROMATHERAPY
- Frankincense is excellent for achieving calm and relaxation; it also aids meditation, as it slows and deepens breathing.

 FROM THE LARDER
- Foods rich in zinc—blackstrap molasses, egg yolk, sesame seeds—and zinc supplements may help to alleviate stress.

SELF-HELP
- Learn and practice deep breathing and relaxation techniques. Meditation may also be helpful.

CAUTION

Ginseng should not be taken during pregnancy. Do not give to children unless advised to do so by a qualified herbalist. Avoid if you have high blood pressure.

Insomnia

Short spells of sleeplessness affect most people, often as a result of temporary depression or anxiety. Chronic insomnia requires the advice of a qualified practitioner who will look for the underlying cause.

SYMPTOMS *Inability to fall asleep on first going to bed, or waking during the night and being unable to get back to sleep.*

CAUTION

Coffea is an antidote to many homeopathic remedies.

 HERBALISM
- As a general remedy, try German chamomile tea or tincture before retiring.
- Skullcap, hops, and vervain are soothing; take as a tea at bedtime.
- A tea or tincture of. wild oats is helpful for restless sleep and sleeplessness.

 HOMEOPATHY
- Use Coffea when you cannot unwind and sleep because your mind is too active.

- Kali phos. helps insomnia that results from excitement or mental stimulation.

 AROMATHERAPY
- A massage with mandarin oil, or a few drops in bathwater, will help sleeplessness in children.
- Adults suffering from insomnia should try marjoram as a massage or bath oil.
- Lavender oil is soothing—try a few drops on the bedclothes or in a bath just before retiring.

 FROM THE LARDER
- Supplements of niacin (vitamin B3) can have a sedative effect, but take only as directed.
- A hot, milky drink taken before bed may help promote sound sleep.
- An old remedy for sleeplessness is to wash the head in a decoction of dill seed prior to retiring and to smell the decoction frequently.

 SELF-HELP
- Learning and practicing deep breathing and relaxation techniques can be very helpful in inducing sleep.
- Eat your final meal of the day several hours before going to bed.
- Avoid stimulants such as tea and coffee in the evening and limit alcohol consumption.

Meningitis

Meningococcal meningitis, caused by a bacterium, is the most severe form of this disease. It is highly infectious and can be fatal. It requires immediate medical attention. Viral meningitis is generally milder but also needs treating by qualified medical professionals.

SYMPTOMS *Severe headache and feverishness are symptoms of viral meningitis. Meningococcal meningitis begins with coldlike symptoms, such as snuffles, and a high temperature (102°F/39°C). The patient then becomes drowsy, confused, and has severe headaches. There may be a stiff neck and an inability to tolerate bright lights. A red rash may appear on the buttocks, legs, and trunk.*

 HERBALISM

• Echinacea root is very useful for a weak immune system and for fatigue following a viral infection.

 FROM THE LARDER

• Supplements of the ACE vitamins, plus selenium, play an important role in strengthening the immune system. Vitamin B6 may also help promote a healthy immune system. Foods rich in these vitamins and in selenium, such as offal, fish, shellfish, dairy produce, fruit, vegetables, and cereals, should be eaten regularly to maintain a healthy immune response.

Depression

Depression has a number of causes and exhibits itself in many different ways.

SYMPTOMS *Like the causes, the symptoms vary in kind and in intensity, from feeling in low spirits for a few days to feelings of intense despair that continue for a prolonged period. Sleeplessness is common, as is apathy, fatigue, lack of confidence, and manifestations of physical illness.*

 HERBALISM

• Damiana leaf is a stimulant for the nervous system. Take as a tea or tincture.

• Marigold flowers are helpful in depression that occurs during the menopause.

• Skullcap can be helpful for postexam depression.

• Take vervain tea or tincture for chronic nervous depression.

 HOMEOPATHY

• Actaea racemosa helps with feelings of overwhelming gloominess, for example when it feels as if a black cloud has settled over the head.

 FLOWER ESSENCES

• Take Gorse for feelings of helplessness.

• Mustard is useful in cases of deep depression, melancholy, and sadness.

 AROMATHERAPY

• Bergamot oil is uplifting and jasmine increases self-confidence, the lack of which may be at least partly responsible for the depressed state.

• Melissa has healing powers and may be helpful.

 FROM THE LARDER

• In mild cases, oats, which contain thiamine and pantothenic acid, are a gentle tonic for the nerves; they are available in capsule form.

• Supplements of vitamin B complex and zinc may also be beneficial.

• Food containing the amino acids phenylalanine, tryptophan, and tyrosine, such as turkey, can supply help to ease symptoms.

 SELF-HELP

• Take care of yourself. Gentle exercise and relaxing baths should promote a feeling of well-being. You may find it helpful to seek counseling, which allows you to talk about your feelings.

CAUTION

• Bergamot should not be used during pregnancy. In sunlight and hot climates it may produce a rash when applied to the skin.

• Clinical depression should be treated by a qualified medical practitioner or therapist.

Headache

Headache can result from minor ailments or tension, from factors such as lack of sleep, hay fever and other allergies, or loud, sustained noise. It can also be a symptom of a more serious disease.

SYMPTOMS *Stiffness and pain in the neck and back of the head, around the eyes and forehead. Migraine headaches usually begin with an "aura"—a visual disturbance such as flashing lights or zigzagging lines in the left or right eye—followed by severe pain. In the most serious attacks there may be vomiting, numbness down one arm, and an inability to communicate successfully.*

 HERBALISM

• A tincture made from the fresh leaves of feverfew eases migraine. Used with valerian it is useful for migraine and other severe headaches caused by anxiety.

• Chamomile is the best remedy for milder headaches.

• For persistent headache, combine feverfew with skullcap and valerian.

 HOMEOPATHY

• Coffea is beneficial when headaches are caused by exhaustion from insomnia or from overstimulation.

• Phosphoric acid is used for crushing headache in the temples, with pressure on the top of the head.

 AROMATHERAPY

• Inhale basil oil for migraine.

• Melissa in the bath or as a massage oil is uplifting and calming, both for migraine and other headaches.

 FROM THE LARDER

• A mustard footbath is a traditional remedy for headache.

 SELF-HELP

• Avoiding foods such as chocolate, red wine, and cheese may help prevent migraine attacks where migraine is caused by food allergies. Other foods implicated in migraine include oranges, rhubarb, coffee, and spinach.

• Cold compresses on the forehead and back of the neck may bring some relief; this can be done for migraines as well as ordinary headache.

• A light headache caused by congestion may be alleviated by taking a brisk walk in the fresh air.

 CAUTION

• Coffea may reverse or eliminate the effects of other homeopathic remedies; coffee will have the same effect, so it is advisable not to drink it while taking homeopathic remedies.

• Feverfew leaves, when eaten fresh, should be wrapped in bread to eliminate the possibility of mouth ulcers. Feverfew should not be taken during pregnancy and by people who are taking drugs such as warfarin to thin the blood.

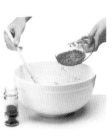

LEFT *Headaches can cause neck pain.*

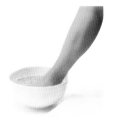

1 *Lightly crush 4oz. (100g.) black mustard seeds in a bowl big enough to fit your feet. You can use ordinary mustard powder if you do not have seeds.*

2 *Pour on enough boiled, hot water to half fill the bowl, leaving sufficient room for your feet. Soak for as long as feels comfortable.*

Neuralgia

The localized pain that occurs in neuralgia is caused by irritation of a nerve and its subsequent malfunction. This is a condition that results from one of several diseases, including neuritis and shingles (*see also Immune System*), emotional upsets, or minor complaints such as a tooth abscess, or sitting in a cold draft.

SYMPTOMS *In facial neuralgia severe pain causes the facial muscles to go into spasm. Neuralgia caused by shingles may occur several days before the red rash appears.*

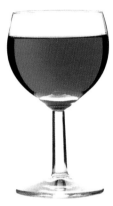

ABOVE: *Elderberry wine, a herbal remedy for neuralgia.*

 HERBALISM
- St. John's wort rubbed into the painful area often helps.
- Elderberry wine is a traditional herbal remedy for neuralgia.

 HOMEOPATHY
- Take Chamomilla to relieve intolerable neuralgic pain.
- Mag. phos. relieves shooting pains.
- Cajeput oil in the bath relieves pain.

 AROMATHERAPY
- For neuralgia caused by anxiety and stress, try Roman chamomile.

 FROM THE LARDER
- Eating eggs was an old remedy for eliminating the pain from neuralgia.

 SELF-HELP
- A cold compress can help ease the pain.

 CAUTION

Cajeput oil placed directly and undiluted on to the skin can be an irritant: use sparingly. Do not use before going to bed unless it is mixed with a sedative oil, since cajeput is a powerful stimulant.

ME (Myalgic Encephalomyelitis)

ME, once called "yuppie flu," has been classified by the World Health Organization as a disease of the nervous system. It can be seriously debilitating and may last for years. The cause is still unknown, but it appears that illnesses such as chickenpox, tonsillitis, and infectious mononucleosis may trigger the disease. Some authorities believe that a viral infection or a failure of the immune system may be partly responsible, since food allergies are often part of the syndrome.

SYMPTOMS *Depression, physical exhaustion, memory lapses, Candida, chronic muscle fatigue, and pain are among the many reported symptoms.*

 HERBALISM
- Use sage for nervous exhaustion, postviral fatigue, and general debility.
- A decoction of rehmannia root is useful for weakness and lack of energy.
- Take a wild oat tea or tincture when there is anxiety.
- Vervain is a useful general tonic.

 HOMEOPATHY
- Carbo veg. is beneficial when there has been a poor recovery from an infectious disease, and may be helpful in cases of ME.

 FLOWER ESSENCES
- Rescue Remedy may be beneficial when symptoms are at their worst.
- Take Gorse for feelings of helplessness.

- Mustard is useful in cases of deep depression, melancholy, and sadness.

 AROMATHERAPY
- Juniper oil strengthens the immune system: lavender strengthens the nervous system.
- Palmarosa and rose may assist ME sufferers.

 SELF-HELP
- Foods that may be implicated in the occurrence of ME include dairy products, wheat, rice, and chicken.

 CAUTION

Avoid sage in pregnancy and when breast-feeding. Do not use if you are epileptic.

Skin and Hair

*T*he skin is the largest organ of the body and is our protection against the outside world. It is remarkably strong, resilient, and self-healing. Hair is the result of the development of the specialized skin cells that also form our nails. Many of the minor ailments of skin and hair can be safely treated at home using natural remedies.

Eczema

Eczema is a discomforting skin condition that is often associated with allergies but may also be caused by stress.

SYMPTOMS *Itchy, weepy rash, rough, red patches on the skin. The affected area may become infected.*

  HERBALISM

• Applications of aloe vera gel or cream on the affected area may be helpful.

• Chickweed ointment may stimulate healing and can be used to soften the skin.

• German chamomile used as lotion or cream is also beneficial.

 HOMEOPATHY

• Graphites is useful when the skin is hard, rough, and cracked with a honeylike discharge. Recommended for infantile eczema.

• When blisters are filled with a white fluid, take Kali mur.

• Natrum mur. will promote healing in cases of raw, inflamed eczema; Kali sulf. is indicated for weeping eczema.

• Use Calendula cream to soothe.

 FLOWER ESSENCES

• Rescue Remedy cream can be applied to all skin irritations to soothe and promote healing.

 AROMATHERAPY

• A massage or bath using Roman chamomile may soothe the skin.

• Melissa will benefit eczema that is stress-related.

 FROM THE LARDER

• Cucumber juice and cabbage poultices may be beneficial.

• An oatmeal bath can help to soothe the skin. Put one or two handfuls of oatmeal in a cheesecloth bag and place under the hot water faucet when running the bath.

• Both sesame oil and apricot kernel oil are useful for moisturizing and soothing the skin. A few drops of vinegar in the bath may also help soothe irritated skin.

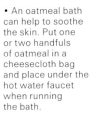 SELF-HELP

• Except in severe cases it is not recommended that you use hydrocortisone cream, which has numerous side effects.

• Wear cotton clothing and use soap powders without stain digesters.

• See a doctor or therapist about allergy tests.

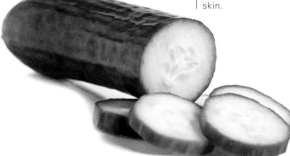

LEFT: *Cucumber juice might be beneficial to those who suffer from eczema.*

Dermatitis

Dermatitis is a general term for any skin rash. It has many causes, including contact dermatitis in which a rash results when the skin comes into contact with an irritating substance. Dermatitis may also be an allergic reaction. In atopic dermatitis the skin rash is an allergic response that occurs when the affecting substance comes into contact with a part of the body other than the skin; for example, eating strawberries produces hives (urticaria) in some sensitive people.

SYMPTOMS *Red, itchy skin, sometimes rough patches. Atopic dermatitis causes patchy, mild inflammation.*

RIGHT *Strawberries may cause allergic dermatitis.*

 HERBALISM

• Marigold flower cream or lotion will relieve itchiness.

 HOMEOPATHY

• Sulfur is useful for severe itching when the skin is hot and bleeds easily when scratching to relieve the itch,

• Calendula cream will soothe itching and soften skin.

 FLOWER ESSENCES

• Rescue Remedy cream can be applied to all skin irritations to soothe and promote healing.

 AROMATHERAPY

• Local massage with neroli soothes sore, sensitive skin and helps it to heal.

• Apply lavender oil and chamomile, in a suitable carrier oil, directly to the affected area to relieve discomfort and promote healing.

 FROM THE LARDER

• Nettle tea, taken three times a day, may be beneficial in cases of contact dermatitis.

• Both sesame oil and apricot kernel oil are useful for moisturizing and soothing the skin. A few drops of vinegar in the bath may also help soothe irritated skin.

• Make a paste of baking soda and apply to the affected area.

 SELF-HELP

• Avoid perfumed soaps and soap powders with stain digesters. Wear cotton clothing whenever possible and try to avoid known allergens.

! CAUTION

Sulfur should be used cautiously for skin complaints. It may initially aggravate the condition. For severe cases, consult a homeopathic practitioner.

Ringworm

Ringworm is a common skin disease caused by infection with a fungus. It often occurs on the scalp.

SYMPTOMS *A raised and red circle on the skin that usually dries in the center as the active infection spreads outward. It is usually very itchy. There may be temporary loss of small clumps of hair when ringworm occurs on the scalp.*

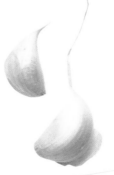

LEFT *Fresh garlic juice rubbed directly on the site may help it to heal.*

 HERBALISM

• Apply aloe vera gel or cream to the affected area.

 FROM THE LARDER

• Fresh garlic juice may help the healing process.

• Covering the infected area with a thick layer of honey is messy but may help the healing process. Repeat as many times as necessary during the day and before retiring for the night. Leave uncovered.

SELF-HELP

• Eliminate sugars and yeast from the diet until the infection has been treated successfully.

• Tincture of iodine is a traditional remedy.

Athlete's Foot

Athlete's foot is caused by a fungus that thrives in warm, moist conditions. It is easily transmitted in public places such as swimming pools and gyms.

SYMPTOMS *Patches of dry flaky skin and itching. The skin may crack and bleed, allowing bacteria to enter.*

RIGHT *To relieve athlete's foot, bathe your feet in warm water with an added essential oil like eucalyptus, myrrh, or patchouli.*

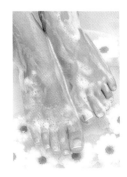

 HERBALISM

• Apply tincture of myrrh twice a day. It should be diluted if the skin is broken.

 HOMEOPATHY

• Sulfur may help reduce itchiness and redness.

 AROMATHERAPY

• Bath the feet in warm water to which you have added eucalyptus, myrrh, or patchouli essential oils.

 FROM THE LARDER

• To keep the skin dry, powder between the toes with arrowroot.

• A footbath of apple cider vinegar (about 2 tablespoons in a bowl of warm water) will often soothe areas where the skin is broken.

 SELF-HELP

• Wear cotton or woolen socks.

• Dry the area between the toes thoroughly after bathing, swimming, and showering.

Dandruff and Dry Scalp

Dandruff occurs when excessive amounts of skin scales are sloughed off the scalp, accumulating on the scalp and, sometimes, on other hair–covered parts of the body. It is a particular problem in adolescence when the sebaceous glands in the skin may be overactive. Dry scalp is merely dry skin that flakes off easily.

SYMPTOMS *Scaling of the skin of the scalp, sometimes accompanied by itching.*

 HERBALISM

• Massage the scalp daily with rosemary tea.

• Rinse your hair with a few drops of thyme tincture, or rinse with an infusion of marigold or nettle.

• Burdock and nettle can be taken internally as a tonic for the scalp.

 HOMEOPATHY

• Rub the scalp with Calendula cream.

• Suitable remedies include Arsenicum, Graphites, and Kali mur., or Sepia.

 AROMATHERAPY

• Massaging the essential oil of bay into the hair can be beneficial. It also assists growth.

 FROM THE LARDER

• Rinsing the hair with nettle tea may help to remove dandruff.

RIGHT *Avoid harsh shampoos if you have a sensitive scalp, since they may cause flaking. Rinse the hair thoroughly after shampooing, using a marigold or nettle infusion in the final rinse.*

 SELF-HELP

• Taking cod liver oil or halibut liver oil improves lackluster hair and dry scalp.

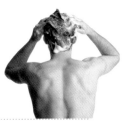

Warts

Warts are harmless growths that are caused by a virus. They are contagious and are particularly likely to occur on the hands—especially in childhood—the neck, and the genitals. A plantar wart, or verruca, is a similar growth on the foot.

RIGHT *Dandelion sap is a folk remedy for warts.*

 HERBALISM

• Dabbing the white sap from dandelion flower stalks on to the wart may help if done on a regular basis.

• Rub elderberry juice on warts to break them down.

 HOMEOPATHY

• Sepia is useful for dealing with brown, itchy warts.

 AROMATHERAPY

• Massage the wart with basil essential oil. Tea tree oil is useful for plantar warts.

FROM THE LARDER

• An old remedy is to rub the wart with pure, undiluted lemon juice first thing in the morning.

• Dampen the wart and sprinkle a little salt over it, then cover with a small band-aid.

• Fresh pineapple contains an enzyme that can break down warts—apply several times a day until they have gone.

• The juice from the white cabbage can be used in the same way.

SELF-HELP

• A country remedy is to rub the wart with fig leaves and bury the leaves in the garden. The belief is that the wart will disappear as the leaves rot.

Psoriasis

Psoriasis is a fairly common, noncontagious disease affecting the outer layer of skin. Usually the scalp, back, and arms are most affected. Fortunately this condition rarely affects the face. Each case of psoriasis is different and requires different remedies. Some of the more common ones are given below.

SYMPTOMS *Red, thickened blotches with a scaly surface. It may be painful and it is always distressing because it is so disfiguring. In rare cases the condition spreads very rapidly and becomes dangerous.*

 HERBALISM

• Use licorice internally and as an ointment for psoriasis that is inflamed.

• Yarrow used twice weekly in the bath has proved to be beneficial in some cases.

• Burdock root is the most useful drink, but you need to persist for many months.

 AROMATHERAPY

• Bergamot essential oil, cajeput, and Roman chamomile can all be used to some benefit as a massage oil. They also bring about some comfort when used in a vaporizer.

 FROM THE LARDER

• Nettle tea and products based on nettles may be helpful.

• Take at least one tablespoonful of olive oil a day and at least one raw vegetable salad.

 SELF-HELP

• Sunbathing and dry skin brushing can help improve the condition.

> **! CAUTION**
>
> • Avoid licorice if you have high blood pressure or in pregnancy.
>
> • Do not take burdock root during the first six months of pregnancy without expert advice.
>
> • Do not apply bergamot oil when-exposing the skin to sunlight.

Impetigo

Impetigo is a highly contagious bacterial infection requiring immediate medical treatment with antibiotic creams, injections, or tablets. To avoid contaminating others, affected individuals should keep their own towels, hair brushes, combs, and so on away from those used by other family members. These should be cleaned frequently until the infection clears. Impetigo is very common in children, particularly around the nose area.

SYMPTOMS *Clusters of small abscesses on the surface of the skin. Discomfort in the lymph glands of the neck.*

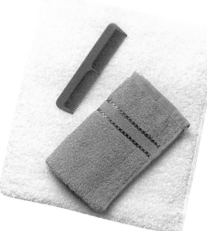

LEFT *Impetigo is highly contagious; keep towels, facecloths, and combs separate from those of the rest of the family.*

 HERBALISM

• Apply marigold cream or lotion to the affected area.

• Aloe vera gel or cream may also promote healing. Wash hands thoroughly after touching the skin.

 FROM THE LARDER

• Additional vitamin C, available in fresh citrus fruits and kiwi fruit, will help strengthen the immune system.

• A course of multivitamins and minerals will supplement nutrients that are depleted by antibiotics.

Urticaria

Urticaria, nettle rash, and hives are all names for the skin complaint caused by a reaction to an allergen or an irritating substance. Urticaria is a type of dermatitis. Nettles are a common cause (hence one of its popular names, nettle rash). The hairs, or stings, of nettles cause the release of histamine when they are touched, and it is the histamine that gives rise to the problem.

SYMPTOMS *Red, itchy, or painful blotches on the skin.*

 HERBALISM

• Apply German chamomile as a lotion or cream.

 AROMATHERAPY

• Massage using chamomile or melissa may prove beneficial.

RIGHT *Fresh fruit and vegetables help to cleanse the system.*

 FROM THE LARDER

• Eat at least four servings of fresh, raw fruit and vegetables every day.

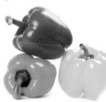

 SELF-HELP

• The stinging rash caused by nettles can be soothed by rubbing the area with a crushed dock leaf, usually found growing nearby.

• Anyone sensitive to the salicylates in aspirin may get an allergic reaction—urticaria—to foods containing these substances. These include tomatoes, citrus fruits, berries, potatoes, cucumbers, and bell peppers. The food coloring tartrazine (E102) contains a large amount of salicylates. Eliminating these foods from the diet may prevent urticara.

Boils, Spots, Abscesses

Boils, spots, and abscesses are all localized infections of a hair follicle or wound. They are caused by bacteria. Large abscesses on the skin, and tooth abscesses, should be treated by a qualified medical practitioner as soon as possible.

SYMPTOMS *Boils and abscesses are extremely painful, producing raised red areas on the skin or gums.*

 HERBALISM

• Echinacea purifies the blood; take with marigold or burdock root to treat boils and spots. Drink as a tea.

• Make a poultice of marigold flowers, marshmallow, and chamomile. Apply frequently to aid in the healing of boils.

• Marigold tea or tincture is also helpful.

• Use echinacea root as a gargle and mouthwash for tooth abscesses.

 HOMEOPATHY

• Treat boils and abscesses that give rise to pricking pain and are red and swollen with Hepar sulf.

• Use Calc. sulf. for discharging abscesses that have come to a head.

• Kali sulf. is useful for irritating spots with a yellow, weepy discharge.

• Silica is useful when boils come in crops, heal slowly, and leave a scar.

 AROMATHERAPY

• For tooth abscesses, apply a little clove oil to a piece of pure absorbent cotton and dab gently on to the affected area.

 FROM THE LARDER

• A cabbage poultice will help in the treatment of both boils and minor abscesses. Bandage in place.

• Cucumber juice may be beneficial in healing spots.

• Use warm bread poultices for boils.

• An old remedy advises using the skin of an egg to heal boils. Remove the shell carefully so that the skin remains on the egg. Gently lift off the skin, wet it, and apply to the boil.

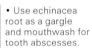 SELF-HELP

• Treating boils with magnesium sulfate paste (which can be bought over the counter at drugstores) is very effective.

• Doctors quite rightly caution against squeezing or lancing a boil, since this can spread the infection.

MAKING A CABBAGE POULTICE

1 *Pull fresh large leaves from a white cabbage.*

2 *Wash well, dry lightly and bruise slightly with a rolling pin.*

3 *Lay them on the boil or abscess and keep in place with a bandage. Replace after twenty minutes.*

Acne

Acne can be a distressing condition, particularly during adolescence when it usually occurs in its most aggressive form.

SYMPTOMS *Whiteheads, blackheads, and red spots, most frequently on the face, upper back and chest, and back of the neck. Scars may remain once the condition has cleared.*

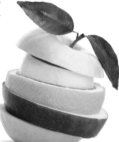

RIGHT *Fresh fruit in the daily diet helps keep acne at bay.*

 HERBALISM
• Applications of aloe vera gel or cream can be helpful.

 HOMEOPATHY
• Calc. sulf. is useful when spots are red, hot, and tender with oozing yellow heads.

 FLOWER ESSENCES
• Crab Apple is a useful flower remedy for skin conditions.

 AROMATHERAPY
• Massage with bergamot, cajeput, or grapefruit essential oils is a general remedy for acne.

• Juniper oil helps with open pores and blackheads.

• Use mandarin in a vaporizer for acne and oily skin.

 FROM THE LARDER
• Eat plenty of fresh fruit and vegetables. Supplements of vitamins E, zinc, and selenium have proved to be beneficial in some cases.

• Vitamin B6 may be helpful where acne worsens during or prior to menstruation.

 SELF-HELP
• Cleanse the skin gently but thoroughly in the morning and before going to bed.

• Wash your hair frequently

and keep combs, brushes, and all grooming equipment scrupulously clean.

• Exercise regularly and get as much fresh air as possible.

⚠ CAUTION
• Do not take zinc supplements if you have been prescribed tetracyclines. Those with kidney complaints should seek their general practitioner's advice before using zinc.

• Avoid bergamot during pregnancy and do not use on the skin when going out in the sun.

• Aloe vera and echinacea root should not be taken internally during pregnancy.

Baldness and Hair Loss

Baldness is generally an inherited characteristic, male-pattern baldness especially so. Sudden hair loss, as occurs in alopecia, is largely determined by emotional factors. Abnormal amounts of hair may also be lost after pregnancy—a temporary situation—and hair may become thinner following the menopause. Long-term vitamin and mineral deficiencies may lead to hair loss, as will certain drugs and radiotherapy used in the treatment of some cancers.

SYMPTOMS *In alopecia the hair is usually lost in one area, producing a bald patch on one side of the head.*

 HERBALISM
• Rosemary with horsetail and skullcap can be beneficial for hair loss caused by anxiety and stress.

• Make an infusion of nettles and rub into the scalp twice a day, as a remedy for baldness.

LEFT *Male-pattern baldness is an inherited trait.*

• Make a hair rinse with yarrow and use after shampooing to control sudden hair loss.

 HOMEOPATHY
• Use Arnica for hair loss after injury.

• Use Phosphoric acid for hair loss following an emotional upset.

• Baryta carb. for hair loss due to age.

• Lycopodium for hair loss after childbirth.

 AROMATHERAPY
• For hair loss as a result of alopecia, massage cedarwood into the scalp.

 FROM THE LARDER
• Supplements of vitamins C and A are prescribed where hair loss is caused by chronic deficiencies of these nutrients.

• Hair loss as a result of zinc and

iron deficiencies also responds to supplements of these minerals.

• Old remedies for restoring hair loss include rubbing brandy and salt into the scalp, or rubbing the bald area with the juice of an onion until the skin becomes red.

 SELF-HELP
• Rubbing a teaspoon of castor oil into the scalp before shampooing may stimulate hair growth.

Excessive Perspiration

Perspiration is vital for regulating the body's temperature. It is produced by sweat glands—eccrine glands and apocrine glands—in the skin. The sweat glands are controlled by the nervous system and hormones. Excessive perspiration can therefore be caused by emotions such as fear and excitement, and by an hormonal imbalance. Other causes include an unhealthy diet.

SYMPTOMS *The unpleasant smell of body odor is often associated with excessive perspiration from the apocrine glands, which are situated in the armpits, groin, and areola of the breast. These glands become active in adolescence, a time when excessive perspiration can be particularly troublesome and embarrassing.*

 HERBALISM

• Sage tea taken regularly often reduces excess perspiration.

• For smelly feet, take a daily footbath to which you have added 1oz. (25g.) of horsetail plus a spoonful of sea salt. Bathe the feet for ten to fifteen minutes, rinse in cool water and dry.

 AROMATHERAPY

• Soak the feet in a footbath using essential oil of pine, a natural deodorant.

• Lemongrass in the bathwater cleanses and deodorizes the whole body.

 FROM THE LARDER

• Perspiration can produce body odor when it is allowed to remain on the skin. For persistent body odor, wash the underarms, breasts, and genital areas twice a day with warm water, to which you have added a capful of apple cider vinegar.

 SELF-HELP

• Clean cotton clothing or clothing in other natural fabrics next to the skin allows air to circulate more freely; it also absorbs moisture.

Cellulite

Cellulite is fat stored just underneath the skin. It has a dimpled appearance, which is caused by a network of collagen fibrils that attach the skin to muscles. This network is a bit like a trellis; the fat fills up the gaps in the trellis causing the skin to look puckered. Women are particularly likely to have this type of fat on their thighs and buttocks. It may become more noticeable with age as the skin loses its elasticity.

RIGHT *Cellulite is a term used for a type of fat, which is best burned off by following a sensible diet and choosing a regular exercise that you enjoy doing.*

 HERBALISM

• Bladderwrack capsules, tablets, or powder may aid weight reduction.

• Where the metabolic rate has slowed down as a result of aging, kelp tablets may help in weight control through their action on the thyroid gland.

 AROMATHERAPY

• A massage with essential oil of grapefruit is cleansing and balancing.

• Mandarin is an excellent diuretic.

 FROM THE LARDER

• Grapefruit aids in the digestion of fatty foods.

 SELF-HELP

• Diet and exercise may help. Eat a healthy diet based on grains, pulses, fresh fruit and vegetables. Restrict the daily fat intake to 30 percent. Avoid foods high in fat, and exercise regularly—at least thirty minutes sustained exercise a day.

• Current evidence suggests that losing weight and maintaining your correct weight results from exercising and from changing your eating habits, rather than following a punishing low-calorie regime.

The Musculoskeletal System

*B*ones and muscles linked together by joints, tendons, and ligaments form the mechanical structure of the body. There are 206 bones in the adult human body, supported and moved by more than 650 muscles. Most ailments are the result of wear and tear, injury, or aging and may be helped or relieved using natural remedies.

Sciatica

Sciatica is usually caused by a slipped disk, which puts pressure on the sciatic nerve at the bottom of the spinal column.

SYMPTOMS *Pain in the lower back initially, followed by severe, sharp pain in the legs.*

 CAUTION

See your physician if you have prolonged sciatica.

 HERBALISM
• Elderberry wine is a traditional remedy for sciatica.

 HOMEOPATHY
• Lavender oil is antispasmodic and antiinflammatory; use it in the bath or in local massage.

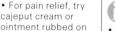 HERBALISM
• For pain relief, try cajeput cream or ointment rubbed on the affected area.

 FROM THE LARDER
• Taking a warm bath to which nettles have been added may help relieve the pain.

SELF-HELP
• Sciatica and other forms of back pain may be eased by lying on the floor for fifteen minutes. Prop the head up on a small pile of paperback books and keep the knees bent. Repeat daily.

Backache

Backache can result from injury to the spine, or occur as a symptom of a number of ailments and diseases, including arthritis, kidney infection, sciatica, and menstrual problems.

SYMPTOMS *Pain in any area of the back, often accompanied by referred pain in the legs or, sometimes, the arms, and neck.*

 HERBALISM
• Massage cramp bark cream into the back. Alternatively, take cramp bark decoction, tincture, or capsules.

 HOMEOPATHY
• Take Calc. fluor. for backache that is worse when starting to move but eases with continued movement.

• Ruta grav. will help relieve pain at the nape of the neck and in the lumbar region.
• Use St. John's wort oil for a massage.

 AROMATHERAPY
• Relaxing in a warm bath to which lavender oil has been added can be very soothing.

 FROM THE LARDER
• It may be helpful to chew a small quantity of horseradish leaves daily to ease pain.

SELF-HELP
• Ice packs will help to relieve backache. You can use a package of frozen peas or ice cubes in a plastic bag if nothing else is handy. Wrap the frozen item in a clean cotton towel and leave in place for about three minutes. Repeat every thirty minutes.
• For chronic backache, try placing a warm, moist cloth over the area and leaving in place until it begins to cool. Repeat as necessary.

Bunions

Bunions are caused by wearing ill-fitting shoes over a prolonged period. This puts pressure on the big-toe joint where it meets the foot.

SYMPTOMS *Pain and enlarged joints.*

 AROMATHERAPY

• For inflamed bunions, add a drop of melissa or chamomile essential oil to the massage oil and rub in gently.

• Lavender or marjoram oil will relieve pain.

 SELF-HELP

• Ensure that shoes fit properly and are designed to suit the foot, not the fashion.

• High-heeled shoes and shoes with narrow toes are especially bad for the feet.

• Go barefoot as often as is practical, walking on a variety of surfaces to exercise the small bones in the feet.

• Practice picking up small objects, such as marbles, with the toes.

RIGHT *Go barefoot as often as possible to exercise the small bones in the feet.*

Cramp

Muscular cramp may be caused by low salt levels in the body—as a result of excessive sweating, for example—or by blood vessels temporarily narrowing and cutting off the blood supply to the muscles. Night cramp is a common occurrence, the reason for which is unknown.

SYMPTOMS *A painful spasm in which the muscle spontaneously contracts and sustains the contraction for a short period of time.*

 HERBALISM

• A decoction of cramp bark taken four to five times a day should bring relief. Cramp bark can also be taken as a tincture or in capsule form. The ointment made from it is useful for massaging into the affected area.

 HOMEOPATHY

• Take Mag. phos. (6c) every five minutes when cramp occurs. It is especially useful for writer's cramp and cramp that occurs after excessive exercise.

• For menstrual cramp, take Mag. phos. every half hour.

 AROMATHERAPY

• Lavender is antispasmodic and can be usefully employed for cramp as a massage oil.

 FROM THE LARDER

• To treat cramp brought on by low salt levels, take salt tablets as soon as possible. If symptoms persist, consult a qualified medical practitioner. Salt tablets are recommended when living in hot climates for any length of time.

 SELF-HELP

• Stretching the affected muscle will usually relieve night cramp.

• The condition may be prevented by taking lemon juice before going to bed, or by dissolving a pinch of salt on the tongue.

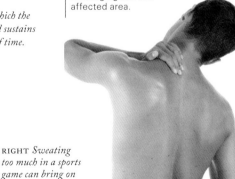

RIGHT *Sweating too much in a sports game can bring on a muscular cramp.*

Osteoporosis

Osteoporosis—often called "brittle bone disease"—is caused by bones becoming less dense and therefore more vulnerable to fracture. Women after menopause may become prone to osteoporosis.

SYMPTOMS *In many cases there are no symptoms, but some people suffer pain in the back or neck.*

RIGHT *Vitamin and mineral intake should be kept up in cases of osteoporosis; magnesium is thought to be especially helpful.*

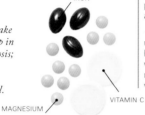

IRON

VITAMIN C

MAGNESIUM

 HERBALISM

• Drink a wineglassful of comfrey leaf and bay leaf tea three times a day.

• Many herbs contain estrogen-like substances, such as hops or sage, which can protect the bones against loss.

• If you are in pain, use analgesic herbs such as white willow, meadowsweet, or wild yam.

 HOMEOPATHY

• Ruta grav. will help relieve pain at the nape of the neck and in the lumbar region.

 FROM THE LARDER

• Recent evidence suggests that an increased intake of magnesium may help prevent the worst effects of osteoporosis. Magnesium sources include soybeans, nuts, and brewers' yeast.

• Calcium can also be very helpful.

Recommended doses are between 1,000 and 1,500mg. a day. To meet this, supplements would be necessary in addition to eating calcium-rich foods such as milk, cheese, and yogurt. (Those watching their weight should note that skim milk and low-fat cheese and yogurts have the same amount of calcium as full-fat products.)

• Vitamin D—obtained from cod liver oil, mackerel, eggs, and milk—helps the body absorb calcium.

• Foods containing boron, which reduces the body's excretion of calcium and magnesium, and increases the production of estrogen, should be taken. Such foods include beer, wine, cider, and edible plants.

• Fluoride may be useful for preventing and treating the condition because it stimulates new bone formation.

Arthritis

There are four common forms: osteoarthritis, or wear and tear on the joints, mainly occurs as part of the aging process; rheumatoid arthritis mostly affects women of all ages and is often crippling; ankylosing spondylitis occurs mostly in young men and can result in a "frozen" spine. A form of arthritis can follow injury.

SYMPTOMS *Painful joints, restriction of movement in the joints, disability, and some degree of deformity.*

 HERBALISM

• Bladderwrack capsules, tablets, or powder used regularly may prevent the progress of the disease.

• For aching joints, try a liniment made with tincture of comfrey and a few drops of black pepper essential oil.

• Dandelion root and horsetail tea or tincture is recommended for degenerative arthritis.

• For inflamed joints in the hand, take a decoction or tincture of devil's claw.

• Siberian ginseng is beneficial for rheumatoid arthritis.

 HOMEOPATHY

• Bryonia is useful for arthritis where stitching pains occur in swollen, pale or red joints.

 AROMATHERAPY

• Use juniper oil in the bath or as a massage. It is stimulating and anti-rheumatic.

• Massage petitgrain into the limbs for osteoarthritis.

 FROM THE LARDER

• There is some evidence to show that the antioxidants —ACE vitamins, plus selenium—may have beneficial effects on arthritis.

• Magnesium is required to form the synovial fluid, which surrounds the joints, and an adequate intake will promote health.

• Eating nettles or drinking nettle tea is an old remedy for arthritis. The "stings" in stinging nettles contain histamines, which are anti-inflammatory.

• Vinegar and honey is another old remedy.

 SELF-HELP

• Copper may help relieve the symptoms of rheumatoid arthritis, and many sufferers use copper bracelets.

Rheumatism

Rheumatism is a general term used to describe aches and pains experienced in the muscles, bones, and nerves of the body. Often the cause may be unattributed, but some muscular rheumatism is caused by inflammation of the tissue that surrounds the muscles and tendons.

SYMPTOMS *General aches and pains, occasionally accompanied by stiffness, headache, and, rarely, fever.*

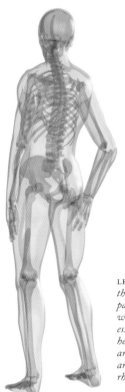

LEFT *Massaging the affected painful joints with a suitable essential oil can help ease the pain and stiffness of arthritis and rheumatism.*

 HERBALISM

• Useful herbs, which may be taken internally or applied as a compress to the affected part of the body, include bogbean, feverfew, meadowsweet and white willow.

• A poultice of slippery elm on the offending area may help.

• An infusion of celery seed may help reduce the level of acid in the blood, which can contribute to rheumatism.

 AROMATHERAPY

• There are many oils that can reduce swelling and inflammation and encourage the healing process. Try massage with pine, lemon or juniper, in a suitable carrier oil.

• Massage with oil of black pepper or eucalyptus can stimulate the circulation and relieve stiffness.

• Lavender oil is antiinflammatory.

 FLOWER ESSENCES

• Rub a little Rescue Remedy into the affected area.

 FROM THE LARDER

• Chew a tiny quantity of horseradish leaves, which is said to prevent attacks.

• Many cases of rheumatism respond to a dietary change, and it is suggested that the following foods are eaten as often as possible to reduce muscular and joint inflammation: cabbage, celery, turnip, lemon, dandelion, and oily fish.

• Drink plenty of water, which will flush the system and act as a detoxificant.

 SELF-HELP

• Eliminate members of the "Nightshade" family of plants from your diet, which can cause joint problems. These include potatoes, peppers, eggplants, and paprika.

• Evening primrose oil is a rich source of gamma linoleic acid, which is necessary for the production of prostaglandins, and may have an anti-inflammatory effect on the body's system.

• Copper deficiencies may be at the root of the problem, and wearing a copper bracelet may help—the copper is absorbed into the skin when it comes into contact with your perspiration.

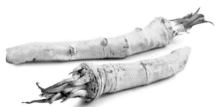

LEFT *Chewing a small quantity of horseradish leaves is said to relieve rheumatism attacks.*

The Endocrine System

*T*he endocrine system consists of various ductless glands, which secrete hormones, or chemical messages. Over-or-underproduction of the hormones, mistimed secretion, or damage to a gland causes diseases that need qualified medical attention, although home remedies can support orthodox medical treatment.

Obesity

Obesity has a clinical definition. It is measured by the body mass index (BMI), which is an individual's weight (in pounds) divided by their height squared (in feet). Obesity can lead to heart and kidney problems, osteoporosis, diseased gallbladder, diabetes mellitus, hypertension, and stroke.

 HERBALISM

• Take bladderwrack capsules, tablets, or powder.

 AROMATHERAPY

• A massage with essential oil of juniper is often helpful.

• Mandarin is an excellent diuretic.

 SELF-HELP

• Take regular exercise—at least thirty minutes sustained activity, five to six times a week.

• Reduce daily fat intake to 30 percent or less and eat fresh fruit and vegetables and wholefoods that are high in starchy carbohydrates.

• Drinking eight glasses of water a day will help to cleanse the digestive system.

• Current evidence suggests that losing weight and maintaining your correct weight results from exercising and from changing your eating habits, not from dieting.

THE BODY MASS INDEX

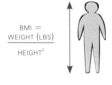

$$BMI = \frac{WEIGHT\ (LBS)}{HEIGHT^2}$$

IDEAL
BMI 20-25

OVER WEIGHT
BMI 25-30

OBESE
BMI 30+

UNDERWEIGHT
BMI 20 OR LESS

The Body Mass Index (BMI) is reached by dividing your weight in pounds by your height in meters squared. So, if you weigh 80kg. and are 2m. tall, your BMI is 80 divided by 2x2—80 divided by 4—which is 20. The graphic shows how the index works. If you have a BMI of 27 or more, you double the risk of high blood pressure, heart disease, and gallstones, and are 14 times more likely to contract diabetes. If it is over 30, you have 4 times the risk of heart disease, high blood pressure, and gallstones, and are 30-50 times more likely to contract diabetes. You are also 4 times more likely to get degenerative arthritis.

Diabetes

The two types of diabetes—Type I, insulin-dependent diabetes; and Type II, noninsulin-dependent—are serious, life-threatening conditions that need orthodox medical treatment. However, natural therapies can help the patient achieve a healthy lifestyle.

SYMPTOMS *Thirst, the need to urinate frequently, a sweet smell to the urine, and weight loss. The appearance of boils may also be symptomatic.*

 AROMATHERAPY
• Eucalyptus has grounding, harmonizing, and cleansing qualities. It is useful as a massage oil in cases of diabetes.

• Massage with juniper oil is detoxifying. It can help in challenging conditions.

 FROM THE LARDER
• Dietary restrictions (avoiding sugar and large amounts of alcohol) should not prevent diabetics from following a wholefood diet based on fresh fruit and vegetables, grains, and pulses.

• Foods containing chromium, such as egg yolks, molasses, brewer's yeast, hard cheese, liver, fruit juice, and wholewheat bread may help to control blood sugar levels. the affected area.

 SELF-HELP
• Regular physical exercise in conjunction with a healthy diet will help to strengthen the whole system.

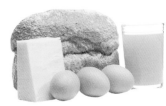
ABOVE *Foods containing chromium can help control their blood sugar levels.*

The Reproductive System: Male

*T*he male reproductive system consists of the two testes and the penis. It is responsible for the manufacture and delivery of sperm and the production of testosterone, the hormone responsible for male characteristics. Sexual organs are outside the body since sperm production needs a lower temperature than that inside the body.

Infertility

Infertility in males may result from a low sperm count or the failure to produce sperm. Other reasons for this condition are the inability of sperm to swim and an inability to deposit them in the vagina near the cervix (as in premature ejaculation).

ABOVE *A decoction made from the Chinese lycium fruit can help with premature ejaculation.*

 HERBALISM
• For infertility with premature ejaculation, use a decoction or tincture of white willow bark or lycium fruit.

 AROMATHERAPY
• Rose is a euphoric oil that can help those who are making a new beginning.

Massage with rose oil is recommended for infertility caused by premature ejaculation.

 FROM THE LARDER
• Vitamin E therapy may be beneficial in improving the mobility of sperm and their ability to fertilize the ovum.

• Zinc supplements are sometimes recommended for improved production of healthy sperm.

• Pumpkin seeds are an excellent source of zinc. They are available from healthfood stores and Chinese herbalists.

Prostate Problems

The role of the prostate is to secrete some of the seminal fluid in which sperm, produced by the testes, are suspended. Problems may arise if there is inflammation in the urinary system, enlargement of the glands, physical injury, or undue continuous pressure on the area.

SYMPTOMS *These include a frequent urge to urinate, obstruction of urine flow, and the presence of blood in the urine.*

 HERBALISM

• As a general remedy, drink damiana leaf tea twice a day.

• When the prostate gland is swollen, take a decoction of horsetail with equal parts of crushed saw palmetto berries. Saw palmetto on its own will help an enlarged prostate.

 AROMATHERAPY

• Pine massaged over the abdomen can be helpful.

• Jasmine is a relaxant and has a strong masculine scent. It is useful for a number of problems associated with the reproductive system, including those affecting the prostate. Massage with the oil is recommended.

 FROM THE LARDER

• Dandelion leaves— they can be eaten in a salad—are a traditional remedy for prostate problems.

Impotence

Most cases of impotence are psychological in origin, but a small minority are the result of a physical condition, for example the adverse effects of prescribed drugs.

 HERBALISM

• A Damiana leaf tea or tincture is recommended for impotence caused by underlying anxiety. Take ½ teacup or 1 teaspoon twice a day.

• Wild oats with saw palmetto may also help. Alternatively, take a decoction or tincture of lycium fruit.

 AROMATHERAPY

• Jasmine is a relaxant and has a strong masculine scent. It is useful for a number of problems associated with the reproductive system. Massage with the oil is recommended.

• Vetivert and clary sage are natural aphrodisiacs that help in the treatment of impotence.

 FROM THE LARDER

• Oatmeal has been a traditional remedy for impotence and sterility for many years.

• Cinnamon is warming and strengthening and may be beneficial.

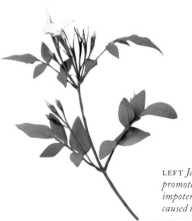

LEFT *Jasmine oil promotes relaxation; impotence is often caused by anxiety.*

The Reproductive System: Female

The female reproductive system consists of the womb (uterus), Fallopian tubes, two ovaries, the cervix, and the vagina. Eggs are present in the ovaries at birth; the ovaries also produce the hormones estrogen and progesterone, which regulate the menstrual cycle. Natural remedies can be helpful for menstrual and menopausal complaints.

Vaginal Thrush

Vaginal thrush is caused by the same agent as oral thrush—the fungal yeast Candida, particularly Candida albicans. Some antibiotics may create a favorable environment in which thrush can thrive.

SYMPTOMS *Itching, soreness, sometimes a burning sensation. There is usually a thick, creamy discharge.*

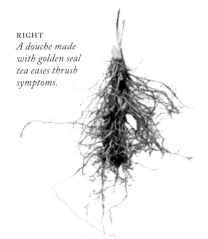

RIGHT
A douche made with golden seal tea eases thrush symptoms.

 HERBALISM

• Put a cup of German chamomile vinegar in the bath or dilute it with six parts warm water to make a tea; use this as a vaginal douche.

• Golden seal can be applied externally or infused and used as a douche to ease symptoms.

• Take steps to boost the immune system (*see page 70*).

 HOMEOPATHY

• Pulsatilla may be useful when the discharge is watery but cloudy, and smarting and soreness are worse around the time of the periods.

• Sepia is good for yellow, smarting discharge, a distended abdomen, and a stinging in the uterus.

• Carbo veg. is for yellowish, burning discharge.

 AROMATHERAPY

• Myrrh has antifungal properties. Use as a douche.

 FROM THE LARDER

• Eat plenty of garlic, parsley, onions, and live yogurt, and drink as much water as you can.

• Take multivitamin and mineral supplements to improve general health, particularly if you are taking or have been taking a course of antibiotics.

• Applications of live yogurt can be soothing and may help in the treatment.

• Garlic can be used as a poultice and applied locally.

 SELF-HELP

• Wear cotton underwear and avoid pantyhose and tight trousers, to allow the free flow of air around the area.

• Thrush is usually treated by following an anti-Candida diet, which means cutting out sugars and yeasts, and reducing alcohol, caffeine, citrus fruits, dairy produce, eggs, fat, hops, malt, mushrooms, and peanuts.

• Do not wash with irritating soaps or perfumes.

 CAUTION

Use myrrh at half strength if you are pregnant.

Breast Problems

Discomfort, pain, or lumps in the breast not associated with menstrual problems should be referred to a qualified medical practitioner. If an illness is diagnosed and treatment has begun, natural therapies may help the patient strengthen the system and return to health.

SYMPTOMS *Sore or tender breasts, mastitis, discharge from the nipple, inverted or puckered nipples, and lumps in the breast tissue—all should be reported to your general practitioner as soon as possible. In a large majority of cases, lumps in the breast are harmless and do not require medical treatment.*

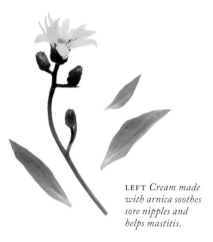

LEFT *Cream made with arnica soothes sore nipples and helps mastitis.*

 HERBALISM

• For lumpy, painful breasts, drink marigold flower tea or use marigold as a compress.

 HOMEOPATHY

• Arnica is helpful for treating mastitis and sore nipples that result from breast-feeding.

• Use Chamomilla for unbearably painful, inflamed nipples.

 AROMATHERAPY

• To minimize stretch marks on the breast as a result of pregnancy or weight loss, massage the breasts with the essential oils mandarin and neroli, or with palmarosa oil.

 FROM THE LARDER

• Eating sprouted barley may help to relieve swollen and painful breasts.

PMS (Premenstrual Syndrome)

Premenstrual syndrome can often be treated very productively by the therapies outlined below.

SYMPTOMS *The dominant symptoms of PMS may be anxiety, characterized by sweating, palpitations, dizziness, headache, cramp, sleeplessness, and fatigue. In other instances PMS may manifest itself in depression, with apathy, tearful outbreaks, aggression, and confusion. Some sufferers of PMS–H (hyperhydration PMS) complain of breast tenderness, sudden gain in weight, and bloating.*

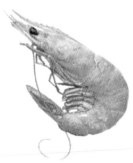

LEFT *Pasta and shellfish are good sources of magnesium; a deficiency of this trace element may contribute to PMS.*

 HERBALISM

• Agnus castus decoction or tincture is beneficial, especially if irritability, breast tenderness, mood swings, and water retention are severe.

• Fennel seed and sage tea help alleviate breast tenderness.

• For painful breasts caused by PMS, take fennel, sage, and marshmallow.

 FLOWER ESSENCES

• Scleranthus helps to balance cyclical symptoms.

 AROMATHERAPY

• Massaging the essential oil of marjoram, jasmine, or rose over the abdomen may help.

 FROM THE LARDER

• Vitamin B6 (pyridoxine), found in dairy products such as yogurt and eggs and cheese, is often helpful in eliminating symptoms in cases of PMS-H and those where anxiety is the dominant feature. For severe cases, supplements are probably the best choice to ensure the dose has therapeutic value.

• Where a craving for sweet foods is symptomatic, magnesium supplements may help. Good sources of magnesium are pasta, shellfish, wholewheat bread, peas, and other green vegetables, dried brewers' yeast, and nuts.

• Vitamin E may be beneficial where breast tenderness is a problem. Rich sources include wheatgerm, eggs, wholewheat bread, and green, leafy vegetables.

• Many women feel PMS is much improved by taking evening primrose oil.

 SELF-HELP

• Restricting amounts of alcohol and dairy products, keeping salt intake low, and avoiding caffeine may help eliminate some of the symptoms.

 CAUTION

• Avoid sage if you are breast-feeding or if you suffer from epilepsy.

• Agnus castus sometimes causes headaches. It should not be taken by anyone undergoing hormone treatment such as HRT (Hormone Replacement Therapy), or anyone taking oral contraceptives.

Menstrual Problems

Heavy, painful, and irregular periods, and a failure to menstruate regularly, should be referred to a qualified general practitioner, since they may be symptomatic of an underlying disease. Once this has been ruled out, complementary therapies may help in alleviating the problem.

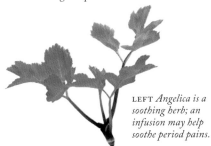

LEFT *Angelica is a soothing herb; an infusion may help soothe period pains.*

 HERBALISM

• Chinese angelica tea or tincture can help relieve painful periods.

• Lady's mantle with marigold flowers, taken on a regular basis, can also help with pain. Use Lady's mantle as a tea or tincture for heavy bleeding. Lady's mantle can be used with equal parts of shepherd's purse or yarrow for the same symptoms.

 HOMEOPATHY

• Chamomilla is recommended for heavy periods with dark clots and unbearable pain in the pelvic area, especially when associated with anger and irritability.

• Use Actaea racemosa for irregular, painful, and heavy periods.

• Graphites is beneficial for late periods that are scanty and associated with constipation and nausea.

 AROMATHERAPY

• Rose oil or cypress oil, massaged over the abdomen, helps with heavy periods.

• Try lavender to regulate scanty periods.

• Melissa will also act as a regulator.

• A massage with marjoram is beneficial for pain.

 FROM THE LARDER

• Frequent drinks of cinnamon tea may be beneficial for heavy periods.

• Evening primrose oil tablets, taken daily, will help to prevent menstrual pain and premenstrual symptoms.

 SELF-HELP

• A warm compress, placed across the abdomen, will help to relieve period discomfort.

• Avoid alcohol and caffeine the week before your period is due, to prevent uncomfortable symptoms.

Infertility

Infertility in women may occur as a result of disease, such as salpingitis, which blocks the Fallopian tubes, a failure to ovulate, or a problem with the cervix. Sometimes the cause is unknown, and in many cases it is linked to stress levels. Once any underlying problem has been found, treatment with drugs or surgery may be necessary.

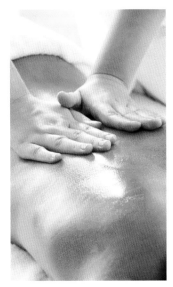

RIGHT *Relaxation and massage with aromatherapy oils help ease anxiety, a contributory factor in many cases of infertility.*

 HERBALISM

• Lady's mantle may be useful when there is no obvious cause.

• Marigold flowers are recommended for infertility caused by blocked Fallopian tubes or ovarian cysts.

 HOMEOPATHY

• Conium, Sabina, and Sepia may all help, depending on the cause.

 AROMATHERAPY

• Orange encourages a positive outlook and is useful for those undergoing treatment for infertility when they are becoming frustrated and doubtful about the results.

• An abdominal massage using rose essential oil may be beneficial.

 FROM THE LARDER

• Extra vitamin E may help to regulate the production of cervical mucus, so it is advised that you eat foods that are good sources— for example, wheatgerm and avocado.

 SELF-HELP

• Relaxation and deep breathing techniques can help to alleviate stress and anxiety. Frankincense can be helpful here as it deepens breathing.

• A good diet is essential to ensure healthy eggs and a welcoming home for a growing embryo. Cut out alcohol, tobacco, drugs, and caffeine, and eat plenty of wholefoods, rich in vitamins and minerals.

Menopause

Menopause usually occurs in the late forties and early fifties. Some women pass through it with few, if any, noticeable symptoms, other than a gradual decrease in the frequency and volume of menstruation, or irregular periods prior to total cessation. Other women seem to suffer from all of the classic ailments associated with the change of life.

SYMPTOMS *Hot flashes, headaches, sudden mood swings, inability to concentrate, "pins and needles" in the face, arms, and legs, and irritability—any or all of these may affect menopausal women.*

CAUTION

- Agnus castus sometimes causes headaches. It should not be taken by anyone undergoing hormone treatment such as HRT, or anyone taking oral contraceptives.
- Sage should not be taken when breast-feeding or during pregnancy.

 HERBALISM

- Agnus castus is particularly helpful for mood swings and depression. Combine with sage to help reduce hot flushes.

 HOMEOPATHY

- Use Lachesis for hot flushes and palpitations.

- Sepia is beneficial for hot flushes and dry vagina and vulva.

 FLOWER ESSENCES

- Walnut helps with times of change in your life.

AROMATHERAPY

- Roman chamomile will help control profuse sweating and hot flushes and act as a diuretic in fluid retention.

- Rose is an excellent oil for female complaints, including menopausal symptoms. Massage over the abdomen for greatest benefit.

 FROM THE LARDER

- Vitamin E supplements have had some beneficial results in trials. Many therapists also recommend calcium supplements to minimize the risk of osteoporosis.

- Oatmeal has an effect on the reproductive system and may be beneficial in alleviating some of the symptoms.

- Nettles are an excellent restorative during the menopause. Add them to soups and casseroles, or use them like spinach to make a sauce for pasta.

The Urinary System

The urinary system consists of the kidneys, ureters, bladder, and urethra. Urine is made in the kidneys as a carrier for soluble waste products and poisons, and then flows to the bladder, where it is stored. When full, the bladder empties via the urethra. The female urethra is shorter and more susceptible to infections than the male urethra.

Cystitis

Cystitis is inflammation of the bladder. It occurs most often in women, causing much discomfort. It may result from infection or bruising, particularly during sex, or as a result of taking the contraceptive pill. Recurrent cystitis or cystitis that does not respond to treatment should be referred to your general practitioner. If untreated, the infection may spread to the kidneys.

SYMPTOMS *A constant urge to pass water, pain on urinating, blood in the urine. This may progress to abdominal pains and dull backache.*

 CAUTION

Avoid agrimony if you suffer from chronic constipation.

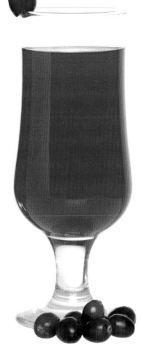

 HERBALISM
• Take agrimony with horsetail as a tea or tincture.

 HOMEOPATHY
• Cantharis will relieve the frequent urge to urinate.

 AROMATHERAPY
• Cedarwood is antiseptic and can be added to bathwater to clear infection and soothe symptoms.

• Niaouli can be used as a douche.

 FROM THE LARDER
• Cranberry juice, preferably unsweetened, is the first choice of many women who suffer from cystitis. Drink as much as you like.

• Hot nettle tea, barley water, and corn silk also seem to have a beneficial effect on cystitis.

 SELF-HELP
• Avoid wearing pantyhose, tight trousers, or jeans, and wear cotton underwear.

• Restrict alcohol intake until the symptoms have cleared up.

BELOW *Cystitis affects more women than men. Cotton underwear can help prevent discomfort.*

Kidney Infection and Stones

Kidney infections can have very serious, even fatal, consequences if left untreated. If there is any likelihood that the kidneys may be malfunctioning seek immediate medical attention. Kidney stones are caused by the abnormal deposit of calcium, phosphates, or oxalates in the kidney or, rarely, the crystallization of uric acid, sometimes as a by-product of gout.

SYMPTOMS *Pain in the loin or abdomen; blood in the urine or urine that is otherwise discolored; pain on passing urine; frequent urination; swollen ankles; thirst; dehydration—numbness or lack of feeling in the tips of the fingers is symptomatic of dehydration.*

RIGHT *Fresh asparagus in the diet is a delicious way to cleanse the kidneys.*

 HERBALISM

• Meadowsweet is a diuretic with a mild antiseptic action. It helps eliminate toxic wastes and uric acid.

• A syrup made from empty rose hip capsules helps in the treatment of kidney disorders.

 HOMEOPATHY

• Lycopodium is helpful for backache caused by kidney complaints.

 FROM THE LARDER

• Minor kidney infections may be improved by increasing consumption of fresh asparagus, grapefruit, and lemon juice.

• Drinking barley soup may help relieve inflammation of the kidneys.

• A cocktail of beet, carrot, and cucumber juices, used in conjunction with orthodox treatment, may be beneficial to those suffering from kidney stones.

• Corn silk, infused in hot water, may also be helpful for kidney stones.

• Magnesium supplements may help in the prevention and treatment of kidney stones, and vitamin B6 (pyridoxine) may also be a preventive.

 SELF-HELP

• An old remedy for dissolving kidney stones recommends taking a spoonful of glycerine on an empty stomach first thing in the morning.

Incontinence

Incontinence has a number of causes, some of which result from other disorders in the nervous system, such as multiple sclerosis, stroke, and injury to the spinal column. Disease or injury to the bowel and/or bladder may also result in incontinence.

SYMPTOMS *An inability to prevent urination or defecation.*

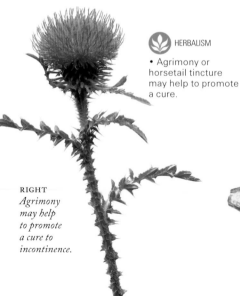

RIGHT *Agrimony may help to promote a cure to incontinence.*

HERBALISM

• Agrimony or horsetail tincture may help to promote a cure.

HOMEOPATHY

• Sepia is particularly good for stress incontinence.

• Phosphoric acid is beneficial for bedwetting, particularly when large amounts of urine are produced.

FROM THE LARDER

• Corn and its products may help in the treatment of childhood bedwetting.

• An infusion of cardamom seed is a useful tonic for incontinence.

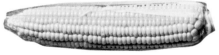

ABOVE *Corn in the diet can help prevent bedwetting in children.*

Children's Problems

This section covers most of the minor complaints that babies, infants, and children are likely to suffer. Most are uncomfortable rather than serious, but always check with your medical practitioner if symptoms persist for more than twenty-four hours or are sudden and violent. Common childhood illnesses are covered on pages 125-129.

Diaper Rash

Diaper rash occurs around the genitals and anus, and may extend up the abdomen or down the legs in more severe cases. It is caused by contact with urine or feces, which cause the skin to produce less protective oil and therefore provide a less effective barrier to further irritation. Friction may also exacerbate the condition.

 CAUTION

Any diaper rash that does not heal within a week or so should be seen by a physician.

 HERBALISM

• Marigold (calendula) ointment can be rubbed onto the diaper area to soothe and to reduce inflammation.

• Wash the diaper area with infusions of marigold, rosemary, or elderflower.

• Powdered golden seal can be applied to a clean diaper area before putting on the diaper.

• Give your baby lots of soothing drinks, such as diluted chamomile tea, to reduce the acidity of the urine.

 HOMEOPATHY

• Internally, you can try Rhus tox. for an itchy, blistered rash.

• Sulfur may be appropriate if the skin is dry and scaled.

 FLOWER ESSENCES

• Rescue Remedy cream may be gently massaged into the affected area to reduce inflammation and ease any pain or itching. A few drops of Rescue Remedy on pulse points will calm a baby who is distressed.

 AROMATHERAPY

• A few drops of lavender or rose oil in a peach kernel carrier oil can be gently rubbed into the diaper area.

 FROM THE LARDER

• Wash the bottom with a little diluted cider vinegar and allow it to dry before putting on the diaper.

• Spread live yogurt on the diaper area to soothe and to prevent thrush.

• Egg white can be painted on the sore bottom to encourage healing. Allow to dry before putting on a diaper.

 SELF-HELP

• Avoid using soap or other detergents on the diaper area. Rinse carefully with clean water at each diaper change.

• Frequent diaper changes are suggested, and using a disposable diaper liner may help to reduce irritation.

• Allow your baby to go for as long as possible with a bare bottom, to allow it to dry and heal.

• Give your baby plenty to drink.

Cradle Cap

Cradle cap appears on the scalp of babies as a thick, yellowish crust, sometimes in patches, and sometimes covering the entire surface of the scalp. Cradle cap is caused by overproductive sebum glands, and most babies who suffer from cradle cap have slightly oily skin. It can last for up to three years in some children, but as the hair grows in it becomes less noticeable. Many babies outgrow the condition in the first few months of life.

 HERBALISM

• Rinse the scalp after washing with an infusion of marigold, which acts as an anti-inflammatory and will reduce any itching.

• Burdock may also be used to rinse the scalp after washing.

 HOMEOPATHY

• Massage the scalp with Calendula ointment.

• Lycopodium, taken internally, is useful if the skin is dry but uninfected.

 FLOWER ESSENCES

• Rock Rose is useful if the itching causes distress.

• Rescue Remedy cream may be massaged into the scalp to reduce symptoms.

• Impatiens relieves irritation.

 AROMATHERAPY

• Massage a few drops of lavender or lemon oil, mixed in a light carrier oil, into the scalp before bedtime. Rinse gently each morning.

 FROM THE LARDER

• Olive oil can be massaged into the scalp each evening, and then gently shampooed away in the morning.

 SELF-HELP

• Cradle cap is not caused by inadequate hygiene, and overwashing will make the condition much worse. Gently brush away loosened crusts with a soft brush.

> **! CAUTION**
>
> Try not to loosen crusts that have not pulled away on their own—bleeding and infection may result.

Teething Problems

Most babies get their first teeth at about six months of age, and there may be problems with teeth coming through until the age of two or three. Most babies experience some discomfort, which can range from simply being clingy and fractious, to dribbling, loosened stools, and problems sleeping.

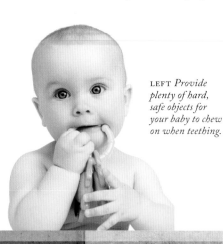

LEFT *Provide plenty of hard, safe objects for your baby to chew on when teething.*

 HERBALISM

• Syrup made from the marshmallow root will soothe inflamed gums, and a few teaspoons can be added to your baby's normal meals.

• Offer infusions of chamomile or fennel to calm, and to soothe.

 HOMEOPATHY

• Chamomilla is the standard remedy for teething and can be take up to six times daily.

• Calcarea phos. may also be useful. Rub a little Rescue Remedy directly into the gums, or apply to pulse points if your baby is crying inconsolably. A few drops at nighttime will help your baby to sleep.

• Rock Rose is also useful.

 FLOWER ESSENCES

• Put a few drops of lavender oil on the bedclothes to help your baby sleep.

 AROMATHERAPY

• Essential oils of chamomile and lavender can be added to the bathwater to calm a distressed baby.

• Rub the gums with a little chamomile oil mixed with a teaspoon of honey.

• Clove oil also acts as a local anesthetic and a minute amount can be diluted and rubbed into the gums.

 FROM THE LARDER

• Rub a little honey into the gums (make sure it is pasteurized) for relief.

• Give your baby a cold licorice root to gnaw on.

• Cold, raw carrots are useful teethers, but watch your baby carefully to make sure he or she doesn't bite off a piece and choke.

 SELF-HELP

• Offer your baby a cool teething ring to gnaw on, and rub his or her gums with a clean finger.

• If your baby has trouble sleeping, gentle rocking may help him or her get back to sleep.

> **! CAUTION**
>
> Fever and vomiting are not symptoms of teething. See your physician if your baby seems unwell.

Colic

Colic is a condition affecting almost a quarter of all infants, usually beginning at about two or three weeks, and often continuing until the baby is eight to twelve weeks old. It is characterized by inconsolable crying—usually at the same time each evening—wind, severe pain in the abdomen, which causes the legs to be drawn up against the body, and bloating. The cause is unknown, but may be caused by contractions of the colon, an allergy to something in the formula (if bottle-fed), or the mother's diet (if breast-fed), or simply excessive air gulped in through repeated bouts of crying.

 CAUTION

If colic is accompanied by vomiting or diarrhea, see your physician.

 HERBALISM

• Because colic is exacerbated by tension, relaxing herbs are often suggested—used in the bath, or infused, cooled slightly, and taken by bottle. Chamomile, lemon balm, and limeflowers are most effective.

• If you think your own stress or nervousness is causing your baby to become tense, drink a cup of passion flower or chamomile tea just before feeding.

• A warm bath with infusion of dill, fennel, marshmallow, or lemon balm will soothe a colicky baby.

• If you are breast-feeding, drinking fennel seed tea will promote milk flow and wind the baby automatically.

 HOMEOPATHY

• Chamomilla is useful for babies who seem better when they are held.

• Pulsatilla is used for babies who are better in the fresh air, and when they are rocked.

• Cuprum met. is used when the tummy rumbles and the child curls his fingers and toes in discomfort.

 FLOWER ESSENCES

• Rock Rose is excellent for distress and fright.

• Rescue Remedy can be used to calm and help to reduce any spasm.

 AROMATHERAPY

• A gentle massage of the abdominal area with one or a blend of chamomile, dill, lavender, or rose oil will help to ease symptoms and calm a distressed baby.

• If your baby is wakened by discomfort, place a cloth moistened with a few drops of lavender oil by the bed.

• Try a few drops of lavender or chamomile oil in a warm bath, just before evening feeds.

 FROM THE LARDER

• If you are breast-feeding, chew cinnamon sticks, which can be passed through the breast milk to aid digestion.

• Caraway water can be diluted and given to even a very young baby in a sterilized bottle. Offer a few sips just before a feed.

 SELF-HELP

• Most babies respond to being rocked and gently massaged.

• Colic can be very distressing for parents, and this can often be passed on to the baby. Try to stay calm. If you are breast-feeding, avoid dairy produce for a few days to see if this helps. Other foods to avoid are very spicy foods, citrus foods, gassy foods (beans, onions, cabbage, etc.), and sugar.

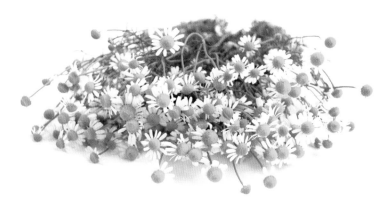

RIGHT *Relaxing herbs, like chamomile, are recommended for a colicky baby's bath.*

Vomiting and Diarrhea

There are many causes of vomiting and diarrhea in children including infections (such as gastroenteritis), eating rich or fatty foods (or, indeed, overeating), emotional upsets, food poisoning, and many others. These conditions are not usually serious unless they recur or carry on for more than about forty-eight hours.

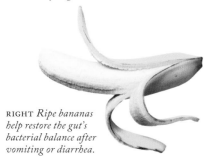

RIGHT *Ripe bananas help restore the gut's bacterial balance after vomiting or diarrhea.*

 CAUTION

Babies and children can very easily become dehydrated by vomiting or diarrhea and it is important that you seek medical treatment urgently. See your physician if there is blood in the vomit or feces.

 HERBALISM

• Depending on the cause, there are many herbs that can be used to treat these conditions.

• Use meadowsweet, with chamomile, if there is distress or inflammation.

• Chamomile, peppermint, and thyme can be drunk as infusions, or added to a bath when there is infection at the root of the illness.

• Chamomile and vervain can be taken internally to soothe a child whose illness is exacerbated or caused by emotional upset, or who is distressed by the vomiting.

 HOMEOPATHY

• China is useful for diarrhea with wind, particularly when the child is very irritable.

• Colocynth can help if the diarrhea is accompanied by episodic pain and is copious, thin, and yellow.

• Arsenicum is useful when there is burning and the child is restless, anxious, and cold.

• Use Veratrum alb. when there is vomiting and diarrhea with cold sweats.

• Pulsatilla can be taken after a rich, fatty meal, when there is no thirst.

 FLOWER ESSENCES

• Rescue Remedy will relieve the distress caused by vomiting and diarrhea.

• Olive is useful for recuperation.

• Holly or Beech may help if the vomiting is linked to emotional problems.

 AROMATHERAPY

• Massage the tummy and chest with a few drops of lavender or chamomile in a light carrier oil.

• Use essential oil of thyme or tea tree in a vaporizer for their antiseptic properties.

• A few drops of lavender in the bath or by the bedside will calm.

 FROM THE LARDER

• Following an attack of vomiting or diarrhea, offer lots of live yogurt and very ripe bananas to restore the bacterial balance of the gut.

• Garlic is excellent to fight infection, boost immunities, and cleanse the blood. It is also a natural antibiotic, so it is excellent in cases of bacterial infection.

• Drink fresh lemon juice, warmed and mixed with a little honey, to cleanse the gut.

• Drink blackcurrant juice, which will act as a gut astringent.

• Raw apple that has gone brown is useful for settling an upset stomach. Offer in small quantities.

• Milk and honey are excellent for treating food poisoning.

• Mustard is a natural emetic and can be taken internally, mixed with a few teaspoons of warm water.

 SELF-HELP

• Offer lots of fresh, cool water to drink, but make sure that your child drinks only small sips at a time. If your child is having trouble keeping even small sips down, freeze some chamomile or fennel tea in ice cube trays and give them to him or her to suck. These should only be given to children over the age of six.

• Avoid eating dairy products and solid food until the symptoms have passed.

• Fresh fruit juice, herb teas, and a mixture of salt and glucose mixed with a glass of water will prevent dehydration.

• If you are breast-feeding your baby, carry on, for breast milk provides all necessary nutrients, as well as your own antibodies. Breast-fed babies are less likely to develop gastroenteritis.

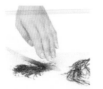

1 *Chop up fennel leaves to make an infusion (see page 20). Chamomile can be used if preferred.*

2 *Pour boiling water onto the herbs and leave for fifteen minutes. Transfer the infusion to a pitcher when it is cool.*

3 *Pour into an ice cube tray; freeze. Offer the cubes for your child to suck.*

Sleeplessness

All babies and children need different amounts of sleep, and most of them experience some difficulty sleeping at some point. Common causes of sleep problems in babies are diaper rash, teething, colic, illness, being too hot or cold, or simply being wakeful. Older children may be worried about something at school, or a stressful event in the family home. Illness usually disrupts sleep patterns in some way. Some children experience night terrors, which may cause them to waken suddenly, screaming and often wringing their hands.

 CAUTION

If you suspect that sleep problems are associated with illness, consult your medical practitioner.

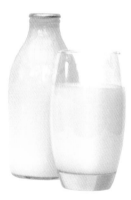

ABOVE *A soothing warm milky drink last thing at night can promote restful sleep. Do not offer milky drinks to children suffering from a cold, since dairy products stimulate mucus production.*

 HERBALISM

• A crying baby may be soothed with an infusion of chamomile, offered an hour or so before bedtime, or when he or she wakens.

• A strong infusion of chamomile, lavender, or limeflower can be added to a warm bath to soothe and calm a baby or child.

• Add about 10 drops of tincture of catmint to a little honey and give to a distressed child as required.

 HOMEOPATHY

• Night terrors are often treated with Calcarea carb. and Antimonium tart.

• Constant crying may be treated with Colocynth or Bryonia.

 FLOWER ESSENCES

• A distressed child or baby can be given Rescue Remedy, which will calm him.

• Offer Rock Rose for treating night terrors.

• A few drops of Mimulus will soothe a distressed or fearful baby or child.

• Walnut is helpful if insomnia comes at times of change, such as moving the baby to his own room.

 AROMATHERAPY

• A few drops of chamomile, geranium, rose, or lavender can be added to the bathwater.

• Lavender oil, on a handkerchief tied near the crib or bed, will help your baby or child sleep.

• Lavender or chamomile can be used in a vaporizer in your child's room.

• A gentle massage before bedtime, with a little lavender or chamomile blended with a light carrier oil, may ease any tension or distress.

 FROM THE LARDER

• A little milk before bedtime may help your baby to sleep.

• Older children may suck a zinc lozenge before bedtime to help them sleep.

• A little brewer's yeast mixed with honey and warm milk is a soothing bedtime drink for children from four upward.

 SELF-HELP

• Avoid a big meal before bedtime.

• For young babies, try to stick to a regular routine—for example, bedtime following a warm bath and story. Babies and children can become "programmed" to routines, which gives them a sense of security.

• Make an older child's bed a special place—let him choose the bedclothes and furnish it with his favorite comfort toys. Try to avoid sending your child to his room as a punishment because he will learn to associate it with unhappiness.

• Avoid computer games or television too close to bedtime.

• Allergies or food intolerance may be at the root of sleep problems, and your physician will be able to help with this.

BELOW *Restful sleep is essential for healthy growth and development.*

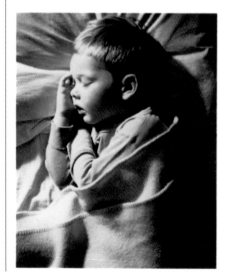

Colds

Small children are more susceptible than adults to the viruses causing colds and flu because their immune systems are immature and antibodies have not yet been developed against viruses. At school age children often have a new crop of illnesses as they come into contact with viruses carried by other children. Symptoms of a cold include a running nose, headache, and sometimes a cough. There may be a mild fever and a feeling of general malaise.

> **! CAUTION**
>
> Use only one drop of aromatherapy oil in a baby's bath, and take care not to allow the bathwater to come into contact with the eyes.

ABOVE: *Mercury is the source of the homeopathic remedy Merc. sol. which can be prescribed if your child's cold is accompanied by earache and swollen glands in the neck.*

 HERBALISM

• Elderflowers, drunk as an infusion, will reduce catarrh and help to decongest.

• Peppermint is another decongestant and will also work to reduce a fever.

• Rosemary and thyme will help to clear congestion and work as antiseptics, which may help to prevent a secondary infection of the tonsils or bronchi (bronchitis).

• Chamomile will soothe an irritable child and help it to sleep. Chamomile also has antiseptic action, which will help to rid the body of infection, and it works to reduce fever and feverish symptoms.

• Try a strong infusion of chamomile or yarrow in the bath.

• Mullein or comfrey can be drunk, or used as a compress around the neck to soothe a sore throat.

• Herbs to strengthen the immune system (*see page 70*) can be taken throughout a cold, and afterward to stimulate healing and prevent subsequent infection.

 HOMEOPATHY

• Pulsatilla is useful if your child is clingy and irritable, and when there is thick yellow discharge.

• Bryonia helps an irritable child who is thirsty and want to be left alone.

• Merc. sol. is for a child with an earache and swollen lymph nodes in the neck.

 FLOWER ESSENCES

• Rescue Remedy will soothe any distress—rub the cream into the chest area to calm.

 AROMATHERAPY

• Try a few drops of lavender or tea tree oil in a warm bath to encourage healing and help to open up the airways. Use only one drop for babies.

• Use chamomile, cloves, lavender, pine, lemon, and thyme together or separately in a room vaporizer to help ease symptoms and promote healing.

• Place your child's head over a steaming bowl of water with a few drops of essential oil of cinnamon.

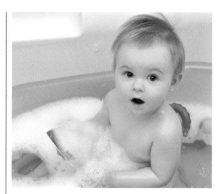

ABOVE: *A warm bath with one drop of lavender or tea tree oil added to it can help unblock a stuffy nose and cheer up a baby made miserable with a cold.*

Place a towel over the head to make a tent, and let the child sit there for four or five minutes to ease congestion.

• Massage a few drops of pine or eucalyptus in a light carrier oil into the chest area.

 FROM THE LARDER

• Blackcurrant tea is excellent for catarrh and infections.

• Eat plenty of fresh garlic and onions, to reduce catarrh and cleanse the blood. Garlic is also antibiotic and boosts the immune system.

• Hot lemon and honey will help to clear catarrh, prevent a secondary infection (such as tonsillitis or bronchitis), and soothe discomfort.

 SELF-HELP

• Encourage your child to drink plenty of water and fresh fruit and vegetable juices, particularly those rich in vitamin C.

• Your child should get lots of rest to help throw off the infection.

• Avoid dairy produce and foods that are difficult to digest, until the illness has cleared.

• Sucking a zinc lozenge should help symptoms to clear and relieve a sore throat.

Coughs

There are many types of coughs, some of which accompany a cold. Others are caused by chemicals, infections such as ear and tonsil infections, excess catarrh, inflammation of the airways, and many other things.

! CAUTION

- If a cough is accompanied by a high fever, and your child has difficulty breathing, he or she may have pneumonia. See your physician immediately.
- If a cough does not improve within a few days, see your physician.

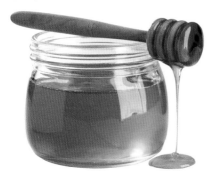

BELOW *A spoonful of warmed honey will help the medicine go down. Mix it with tincture of coltsfoot or comfrey for an expectorant effect. Honey on its own has an antibacterial action.*

 HERBALISM

- There are many herbs that encourage the body to fight off infections, and they can be taken daily, for as long as your child is suffering from the cough. They include echinacea and thyme.
- If the cough is accompanied by a fever, try infusions of chamomile and yarrow.
- Comfrey and coltsfoot are useful expectorants, which will help to expel the mucus from the lungs and airways—use about 10 drops of each tincture and mix with some warmed honey and serve by the teaspoonful as necessary.
- Thyme can be infused and used to treat a wet cough.
- When the mucus is tough to shift, try strong infusions of ginger and fennel or thyme.

 HOMEOPATHY

- Belladonna can be taken when the cough is accompanied by a fever and the child has bright red cheeks and neck.
- Try Aconite if the symptoms come on suddenly.
- Chamomilla will soothe a child who is inconsolable, but better for being held.
- Pulsatilla may be useful if there is a thick yellow discharge and your child is clingy and tearful.
- Antimonium tart. is useful for a cough that causes the chest to rattle and makes breathing painful.
- Bryonia is for a painful, dry cough, which is made worse with movement.
- Spongia is excellent for croup (*see page 122*), and for a loud, crowing cough.
- Use Drosera for a tickling cough that is worse for lying down.

 FLOWER ESSENCES

- Use Rescue Remedy when your child experiences distress, or panics because breathing is difficult. Rescue Remedy will also help your child to sleep. A few drops can be taken internally, or applied to pulse points, and Rescue Remedy

cream can be rubbed into the chest.

 AROMATHERAPY

- Add a few drops of eucalyptus and sandalwood to a carrier oil, or some petroleum jelly, and rub into the chest and upper back.
- Myrrh can be massaged in the same way to reduce mucus. Use a few drops on a cloth tied to the crib or bed.
- Lavender oil on a cloth or pillow will encourage sleep and aid the healing process.
- Use lavender, myrrh, eucalyptus, or thyme in a vaporizer.
- A few drops of essential oil of thyme, pine, cinnamon, clove, or eucalyptus can be used in combination or singly in a footbath to ease congestion.

 FROM THE LARDER

- Give your child lots of honey, which has antibacterial action and will also soothe a sore throat.
- Fresh garlic should be eaten as often as possible

to cleanse the blood, improve the immune response, and encourage healing.

- Lemon and honey will soothe a sore throat and ease a tickly cough.
- Blackcurrant tea will ease the pain of a sore throat and help to reduce catarrh.
- Ginger, added to meals, will help to get rid of any lingering catarrh.
- Pineapples are traditionally used for expelling excess catarrh.

 SELF-HELP

- Plenty of fluids and bed rest will make it easier for your child to shift a cough. Offer only fluids for the first couple of days, and then just light meals, avoiding dairy produce altogether until the catarrh has shifted.
- Take steps to boost the immune system (*see page 70*).
- Try not to use proprietary cough medicines, which will suppress symptoms but not rid the body of the catarrh, which may become infected.
- Cool a fever by bathing with tepid water.

Croup

Croup occurs when the larynx (voice box) become inflamed and swollen. It can be the result of a bacterial or viral infection, or even simply a cold. Because the larynx swells and blocks the passage of air, breathing can be very difficult, which can panic a child (and the parents). The cough is a loud bark or whistle, caused by inflammation of the vocal cords.

> CAUTION
>
> If your child turns blue in the face, call a physician immediately.

ABOVE *Aconite is the source of the homeopathic remedy of the same name, which is extremely beneficial for any complaint that is accompanied by sudden fear and panic.*

 HERBALISM

• Try infusing lavender flowers or chamomile in a bowl of hot water, and then placing your child's head over the bowl covered by a towel.

• Infuse some chamomile and give your child small sips before bedtime and during an attack.

 HOMEOPATHY

• Spongia is the traditional treatment for croup and can be taken every twenty minutes during an attack.

• Aconite can be taken at the same time.

 FLOWER ESSENCES

• Rescue Remedy will help to calm the child, which will make breathing easier. Parents may also benefit from a few drops! Alternatively, rub a little Rescue Remedy cream into your child's chest and upper back.

• Rock Rose will help if your child is frightened.

• Olive can be taken after an attack if your child is exhausted.

 AROMATHERAPY

• Essential oils of eucalyptus, lavender, pine, chamomile, cinnamon, and thyme can be added together, or separately, to a vaporizer, or a footbath.

• A few drops of eucalyptus or lavender can be placed on a handkerchief by the child's crib or bed to ease breathing and encourage the child to relax.

• Rub a few drops of lavender oil mixed with petroleum jelly into your child's chest and upper back.

• A footbath with some thyme or eucalyptus oil should help.

 FROM THE LARDER

• Olive oil is a good carrier oil for aromatherapy essential oils and has a therapeutic effect when rubbed into the chest and body.

• Offer a hot honey and lemon drink to ease the symptoms. Honey has strong antibacterial properties and will be useful if the cause of the croup is bacterial infection.

• A little bit of cider vinegar mixed with a mug of warm water can be sipped to ease symptoms.

• Blackcurrant tea is helpful and restorative.

 SELF-HELP

• Steam will help to open the airways and reduce spasm of the larynx. Sit with your child in a bathroom or shower room with the door shut and the hot water running, or fill a bowl with boiling water and gently place your child's head over it, covered by a towel.

• Raise the upper end of the crib or bed so that breathing is easier.

• Provide lots of reassurance and comfort and try not to panic.

• Serve only light meals for the first few days after an attack, until your child is entirely clear of symptoms.

Earache and Infections

The most common ear infections in children are middle ear infections. These are usually caused by the transmission of infection from the nose or throat by the Eustachian tube. Because this tube is short and small in babies and young children, it is easily blocked, and so infection does not have far to travel to the middle ear.

 CAUTION

An untreated ear infection may scar the eardrum and cause permanent hearing damage. Infection may also spread from the ear to other parts of the head, which may be life-threatening.

 HERBALISM

• A few drops of tincture of myrrh or golden seal in a light oil, warmed, can be dropped into the ear canal.

• Place a cotton ball with a few drops of warmed garlic oil gently into the ear canal.

• Apply a hot compress to the neck and ears using mullein or St. John's wort.

• Give chamomile tea to soothe pain and distress.

 HOMEOPATHY

• Use Aconite early on, if symptoms set in suddenly.

• Use Belladonna, when the affected ear is red and hot and the child is feverish.

• Use Chamomilla when the child is inconsolable.

 FLOWER ESSENCES

• Rescue Remedy or rock rose will ease panic.

• Use olive while recuperating.

 AROMATHERAPY

• Place drops of lavender oil in the ear on a cotton ball, or ease in with a Q-tip.

 FROM THE LARDER

• Gently massage the neck and head with mullein or lavender oil in a carrier oil.

• Tea tree or lavender oil can be used in a vaporizer.

• A few drops of lavender oil on a cloth by the bed will help your child stay calm.

• Mix fresh garlic with honey to fight off infection.

• Get your child to drink honey and lemon, or a little cider vinegar, in warm water to get rid of catarrh.

• Blackcurrant tea helps to boost the immune system.

 SELF-HELP

• Bed rest and plenty of fluids are suggested.

• Avoid dairy produce.

• Make sure your child's diet is rich in foods containing vitamin C and zinc.

• Smoking near your child can exacerbate ear infection.

LEFT *Avoid dairy products while your child has an earache or infection.*

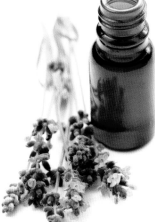

LEFT *Gently massage the neck and head with lavender oil in a carrier oil.*

Glue Ear

Glue ear is a chronic condition affecting a large number of children. It is characterized by a thick, often smelly mucus that builds up in the middle ear, impairing hearing and causing the eardrum to perforate to allow the mucus to be discharged. Glue ear is common in children who have frequent colds or other infections, which block the Eustachian tube.

BELOW *Echinacea can be taken internally or added to a footbath to reduce infection and relieve symptoms.*

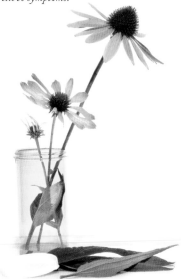

 HERBALISM

• Herbs to reduce catarrh include chamomile, elderflower, and eyebright, and they can be blended or taken separately in a variety of forms to clear congestion.

• Chamomile and echinacea can be taken internally or added to a foot—or handbath to reduce infection and relieve symptoms.

 HOMEOPATHY

• Use Kali bich. if there is mucus in the throat and pain in the sinuses.

• Use Graphites if there is a yellow discharge.

• Use Sulfur if there is a thick, yellow, smelly discharge from the ear.

• Use Calc. carb. if there is discharge with swollen glands and night sweat.

 FLOWER ESSENCES

• Rescue Remedy cream can be rubbed in around the ear canal, or Rescue Remedy can be taken internally to relieve pain and discomfort.

 AROMATHERAPY

• Massage the ear area with a few drops of essential oil of lavender in a light carrier oil.

• A steam inhalation of eucalyptus, chamomile, or lavender can help to reduce catarrh and ease symptoms.

• Apply a hot compress to the nose, ears, and throat using diluted essential oils of lavender, rosewood, or chamomile.

 FROM THE LARDER

• Garlic is excellent at shifting catarrh and cleansing the blood. Offer as perles, or chop fresh garlic and serve with a teaspoon of honey.

• Honey and lemon drinks are restorative, will soothe a sore throat, and are also antibacterial.

• A little cider vinegar with honey in hot water will help to clear infection and boost the immune system.

• Blackcurrant tea is excellent for catarrh and will encourage healing.

 SELF-HELP

• Avoid foods that cause mucus to be produced—dairy produce, refined sugars, and wheat are the main culprits.

• Offer foods rich in vitamin C and zinc, (*see Earache and Infections page 123*).

• Ensure that your child is not in contact with cigarette smoke or dust.

• Treat for ear infections accordingly (*see page 123*).

• Improve the immunesystem (*see page 70*).

 CAUTION

Glue ear should be treated to avoid later hearing problems caused by scarring of the eardrum.

Childhood Illnesses

*T*his section covers the most common childhood illnesses. Natural remedies can help to relieve many symptoms and to support the immune system. Clear illustration helps you identify the rashes that characterize chickenpox, measles, and rubella; and natural remedies to help combat the side-effects of immunization are given.

Chickenpox

Chickenpox is a contagious, common viral infection characterized by fluid-filled blisters that appear first on the trunk and then spread to the rest of the body. There is headache, fever, and fatigue. As the spots progress, they become very itchy and then dry up and form a scab. The incubation period is ten to fourteen days, and sufferers are contagious from just before the spots appear.

BELOW *Chickenpox (varicella) is the most infectious of the common viral diseases of childhood. Keep young sufferers away from elderly people since the same virus can cause shingles (Herpes zoster).*

Headache and fever
▼
Spots appear on trunk of the body first
▼
Spots appear later on the face and limbs

 HERBALISM

• Tincture of comfrey or elderflower can be applied directly to the spots to encourage healing and to relieve the itching.

• Add burdock tea to your child's bath.

• Crush peppermint leaves and apply directly to spots to relieve symptoms.

 HOMEOPATHY

• The nosode Variolinum can be taken once in an epidemic of chickenpox, before your child acquires the illness, and symptoms should be less severe.

• Rhus tox. can be taken for a few days after contact with an infected child, and then again as soon as the first spots appear.

• Aconite is useful in the early stages of the illness.

• Belladonna is useful for fever.

 FLOWER ESSENCES

• Chicory, Hornbeam, and Cherry Plum are usually suggested to help relieve some of the discomfort.

• Impatiens can ease irritability.

• Crab apple may be diluted and applied directly to the spots to encourage healing.

 AROMATHERAPY

• Essential oil of lavender can be dabbed directly on spots to ease the itching and encourage healing. Lavender also has an antibacterial action, which will help prevent a secondary infection.

• A few drops of Roman chamomile can be used in the bath to soothe.

 FROM THE LARDER

• Eat plenty of fruit and vegetables and drink raw vegetable juices in order to help cleanse the body, which will reduce the severity of the condition.

 SELF-HELP

• Cool the itchy spots with cold compresses and make your child comfortable.

• Try to encourage your child not to scratch the spots, which can lead to bacterial infection and scarring.

• Cotton garments should be worn next to the skin.

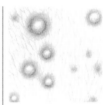

ABOVE *Chickenpox rash is characterized by small, raised spots, which develop into inflamed blisters. They appear over several days.*

 CAUTION

When fever lasts for more than a couple of days, or there is an obvious chest infection accompanying the rash, see your physician. Very rarely, chickenpox pneumonia can occur as a secondary infection.

German Measles (Rubella)

Rubella is a viral infection characterized by symptoms that mimic a cold, and go on to include loss of appetite, sore throat, mild fever, and swelling of the lymph nodes in the neck. There is an accompanying rash, made up of pale pink dots that usually cause only mild discomfort. Incubation period is fourteen to twenty-one days. The condition itself only lasts three to five days.

> Slight headache
> ▼
> There may be swelling behind the ear
> ▼
> Rash spreads from the face downward

ABOVE *German measles (rubella) has mild symptoms of fever, swollen lymph nodes behind the ears and a rash. Young girls who do not contract it should be encouraged to be immunized before puberty to protect their future babies from possible damage in the womb.*

BELOW *The German measles rash is a wash of pale pink spots that spread from the face; they may not be itchy.*

 HERBALISM

• Hot yarrow tea, cooled and drunk several times daily, will relieve symptoms.

• An infusion of elderflower combined with peppermint will help cool a fever and calm your child.

• Very high fever can be treated with an infusion of catmint, taken as required.

• Use Pulsatilla, when there is thick, yellow discharge and hot, red eyes.

 HOMEOPATHY

• Use Belladonna, for fever, a bright red rash and hot face.

• Use Phytolacca for painful ears and swollen glands, better on taking cool drinks.

• Use Aconite if there is a high fever and not too much mucus.

• Use Mercurius sol. where there is yellow discharge and a fever.

 FLOWER ESSENCES

• Rescue Remedy will ease any distress and calm the child.

• Chicory, Hornbeam, and Cherry Plum are useful for all childhood illnesses.

 AROMATHERAPY

• A few drops of lavender oil on the bedclothes or on a handkerchief near the bed will help ease symptoms and calm the child.

• If there is a buildup of phlegm, use a few drops of tea tree or eucalyptus oil in a vaporizer to encourage easier breathing.

 FROM THE LARDER

• Fresh fruit and vegetable juices will encourage recovery.

• Pound some anise seeds and allow them to steep in boiling water for about thirty minutes, and then offer by the teaspoonful to relieve symptoms.

• Borage stimulates the kidneys and can help when there is fever present.

• Honey and lemon in a little hot water can be drunk to reduce discomfort of the cold-like symptoms.

 SELF-HELP

• Frequent cool baths will relieve any itchiness and bring down a fever.

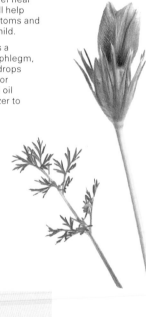

LEFT *Pulsatilla is a useful homeopathic remedy if the symptom picture fits.*

 CAUTION

If you suspect your child is suffering from German measles, keep her at home, even if she seems well. If a pregnant woman who is not immune to the condition contracts it, there is a serious risk of birth defects and miscarriage.

Measles

Measles is a viral illness that can be very serious, particularly in children (and adults) with reduced immune activity. It is characterized by white spots on the lining of the cheeks, and a very high fever as the rash comes out. The rash itself is brownish red, and the spots may join together. There may be diarrhea, vomiting, pain in the neck (around the lymph nodes), and there may be symptoms of a cold, including a cough and occasionally conjunctivitis. Incubation period is between eight and fourteen days, and the illness itself can last up to two or three weeks. Thankfully the spots are not itchy.

▼ Running eyes
▼ Running nose
▼ Small spots inside mouth
▼ Sore throat
▼ Rash starts on face and spreads downward

ABOVE *Measles (rubeola; morbilli) is potentially the most dangerous of childhood diseases. This is because it weakens the immune system and leaves the sufferer open to secondary infections. Major measles outbreaks are predictable, occurring regularly every three or four years.*

 HERBALISM

• Garlic and echinacea can be taken to improve the immune system (*see page 70*).

• Yarrow can be sipped as a tea to bring down fever and ease discomfort.

• Elderflower tea is also useful.

• Add chamomile or to the bathwater to calm your child, and soothe.

• A compress of ginger may be used to help encourage the toxins to be released from the body.

 HOMEOPATHY

• The nosode Morbillinum can be taken for three days if you child has been in contact with a sufferer; this will help to reduce the severity of the symptoms.

• Aconite and Belladonna can be taken for high fever;

• Use Pulsatilla when there is diarrhea, yellow discharge, and a cough.

• Use Bryonia when there is a hard, painful cough, and a high temperature accompanied by thirst.

• Use Stramonium when there is a high fever, a red face, and convulsions.

 FLOWER ESSENCES

• Rescue Remedy can be used to ease distress and discomfort.

• Cherry Plum, Hornbeam, and Chicory are suggested for all childhood illnesses.

 AROMATHERAPY

• A few drops of Roman chamomile in the bath will ease symptoms and help encourage sleep.

• Lavender oil can be dropped on the bedclothes or on a handkerchief by the bed to calm. It can also be applied neat to spots, to encourage healing.

• When there is a build-up of phlegm, and other symptoms of a cold, a gentle chest massage with a few drops of tea tree oil in a light carrier oil base will help.

• Essential oil of eucalyptus or chamomile can be used in a vaporizer.

 FROM THE LARDER

• Garlic will encourage the spots to "come out," which means that the body is expelling toxins.

• Ginger can be used as a compress directly on the spots.

• Eat foods rich in vitamin C to encourage the immune system (*see page 70*).

• Hot honey and lemon drinks are soothing and will encourage healing.

 SELF-HELP

• Avoid all solid foods until the fever has gone. Offer plenty of fresh, cool water—fever can lead to dehydration.

• Bed rest is recommended until symptoms are completely clear.

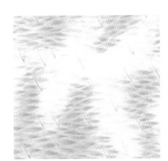

LEFT *The measles rash is a blotchy brownish red, the spots running together. It spreads down from the face. It is preceded by distinctive small red spots with white centers, which appear inside the mouth on the linings of the cheeks.*

 CAUTION

Watch your child carefully as he recovers from measles. There is a risk of complications, including pneumonia, ear infection, bronchitis, and, very rarely, encephalitis. If fever recurs several days after the spots have begun to heal, see your physician.

Mumps

Mumps are caused by a viral infection that attacks the saliva and parotid glands. The incubation period is fourteen to twenty-one days, and the illness lasts about a week. Symptoms include fever, headache, and pains in the neck area. Swelling occurs on the sides of the face, and there will be pain on swallowing. Any acidic foods, such as tomatoes or oranges, which stimulate the salivary glands will be very painful to eat.

 CAUTION

Complications can develop in teenage boys who contract mumps. If the illness is followed by severe headache, stiffness, or fever, see your physician immediately.

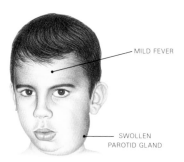

ABOVE *Mumps (epidemic parotitis) is characterized by a painful swelling of the parotid salivary glands on the side of the neck. In adult males, mumps may cause sterility because the infection can spread to the testes.*

MILD FEVER

SWOLLEN PAROTID GLAND

 HERBALISM

• Marigold can help to reduce the inflammation and swelling; drink as a lukewarm infusion.

• A warm compress with can be applied to the swelling to ease pain.

• Boost immunity and encourage healing with garlic, peppermint, and echinacea, taken internally.

 HOMEOPATHY

• If your child has not had mumps, Phytolacca or Parotidium can be taken during an epidemic to reduce severity of symptoms.

• Use Rhus tox. when the left glands are more severely affected than the right.

• Use Belladonna when there is high fever, shooting pains, and a bright red face and throat.

• Mercurius sol. is useful when there is heavy sweating and a coated tongue.

• Pulsatilla may help to prevent orchitis and is useful if fever continues.

 FLOWER ESSENCES

• Rescue Remedy can be used to ease distress and discomfort.

• Cherry Plum, Hornbeam, and Chicory are suggested for all childhood illnesses.

 AROMATHERAPY

• Massage the neck area with chamomile or lavender oil, diluted in a little grapeseed oil. Take care to do so gently.

• Eucalyptus and thyme can be used for steam inhalations and in the bath (use sparingly).

 FROM THE LARDER

• Chop fresh ginger and apply as a compress directly to the swollen glands to provide relief.

• Fruit (not citrus) and vegetable juices can be liquidized and then diluted with fresh, cool water, to encourage a speedy recovery. This will also relieve constipation, which is a common symptom of mumps.

• Cayenne powder mixed with vinegar can be warmed and applied to the affected area.

 SELF-HELP

• Bed rest is suggested until symptoms have disappeared.

• A hot-water bottle, wrapped in a towel and pressed on the affected area, will provide some relief.

• If fever becomes high, sponge your child, or place him or her in a lukewarm bath to cool.

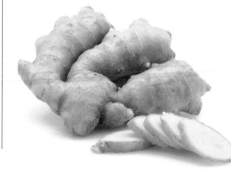

LEFT *For mumps relief, chop fresh ginger and apply as a compress directly to the swollen glands.*

Whooping Cough (Pertussis)

Whooping cough is an acute illness caused by a bacterial infection. It occurs most often in preschool children and is characterized by the symptoms of the common cold, which lead to a severe, spasmodic cough. The bacteria irritates the airways, which become swollen making breathing difficult. There will be a build-up of mucus that is difficult to shift, and there may also be vomiting—particularly while coughing. The "whoop" sound of the cough is unmistakable, and the feeling of being unable to draw breath may cause panic. The incubation period is between seven to ten days, and the condition may last for as long as two months, if left untreated.

 CAUTION

- There is a risk of secondary infection, in particular pneumonia and bronchitis. All cases of whooping cough should be seen by a physician. If the cough is accompanied by vomiting, make sure there is adequate intake of fluid to prevent dehydration.

- Call your physician immediately if your child becomes blue around the lips.

 HERBALISM

- Coltsfoot can be used to loosen the cough and help to expel the mucus.

- Wild cherry bark has a profound effect on the cough reflex.

- A few drops of tincture of thyme should be taken to loosen and expel the mucus. Thyme also works as an antiseptic.

- Massage comfrey ointment into the chest and back to relax the lungs.

- Elecampane is commonly used for children's coughs, and can be purchased in easy-to-use syrup form.

 HOMEOPATHY

- Aconite can be taken during an attack, or at the beginning of the illness.

- Drosera is useful when the cough is made worse by lying down, and there are pains below the ribs.

- Use Bryonia when there is a dry, painful cough and vomiting.

- Use Antimonium tart. when there is a rattling cough with gasping.

- Use Sanguinaria for a harsh, dry cough.

- Arnica is useful when there is bleeding, or the child is distressed before she coughs.

- Pertussin may be given in one dose toward the end of the disease to prevent an "echo" effect.

 FLOWER ESSENCES

- Rescue Remedy is excellent for calming a child who has difficulty drawing breath, and who is frightened by the condition. A few drops on pulse points, or sipped in a glass of cool water, will help.

- Cherry Plum will help if there is serious spasmodic coughing.

- Mimulus and Olive are good in the later stages of the condition.

 AROMATHERAPY

- Mix a few drops of lavender and chamomile oils in a light carrier oil and massage into the chest and back area to calm and to relax tensed muscles.

- Tea tree, lavender, chamomile, and eucalyptus can be used in a vaporizer to help open up the lungs and reduce spasm.

- A few drops of oil of thyme, in the bath, will soothe and reduce the severity of the cough.

 FROM THE LARDER

- Honey and licorice can be diluted with a little hot water and drunk to relieve the cough.

- A garlic poultice, placed on the chest and back area, is recommended to help expel the phlegm.

- Offer plenty of foods rich in vitamin C to help the body fight what can be a very long and debilitating illness.

- Fresh fruit and vegetable juices should be diluted and drunk for the first few days, but try to avoid citrus juices, which may induce vomiting.

- Avoid mucus-producing foods, such as dairy produce.

 SELF-HELP

- Plenty of bed rest and comfort are essential to a speedy recovery.

- Try to keep the air clean from smoke, dust, and chemicals, and raise the bed slightly at one end to make breathing easier.

SOOTHING RELIEF
A gentle massage of comfrey ointment on the chest and back can help soothe spasmodic coughing.

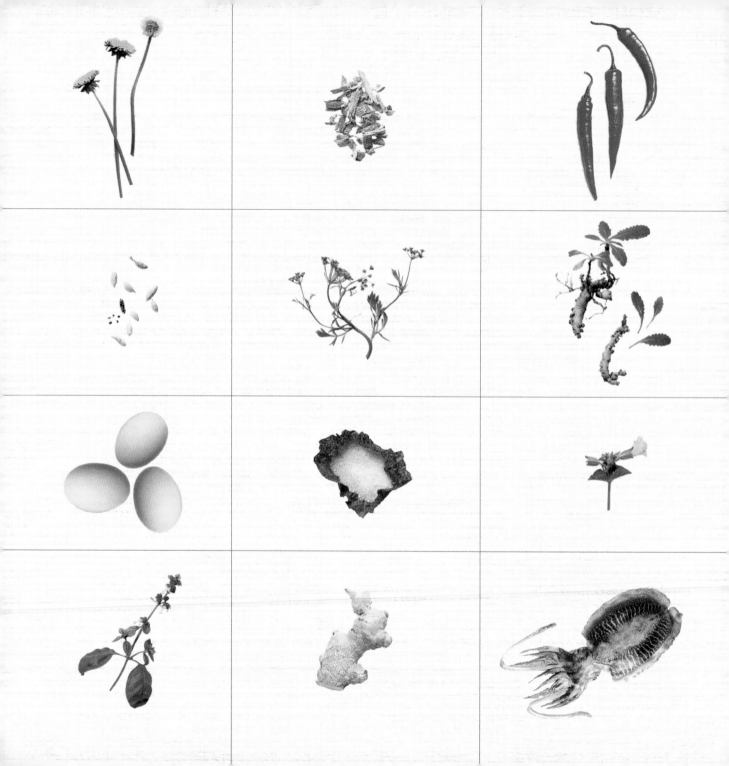

PART THREE

The Remedy Sources

This section is devoted to the sources that provide natural home remedies. It is subdivided into three parts: the first covers plant and animal sources; the second covers element, compound, and mineral sources; and the third covers food sources from the larder. In the plant and animal section, sources are arranged alphabetically according to their Latin name; in the chemical and mineral section and the food section, the sources are ordered into thematic groups.

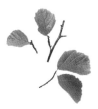

Plant and Animal Sources

Yarrow Achillea millefolium, millfoil

 HERBALISM

Yarrow tea can be used in the early stages of fevers or with elderflowers to break a fever. Use it with elderflowers and peppermint for colds and as a long-term remedy for people prone to runny noses, catarrh, sinusitis, hay fever, and dust allergies. Use it as a tea or tincture to disinfect wounds and stop bleeding and nosebleeds. It can be used internally or externally for varicose veins and spontaneous bruising. Mixed with hawthorn and linden, it is useful in cases of high blood pressure and, because it balances circulation, it is useful for overheating in otherwise healthy people. For cold feet and hands, blend with hawthorn and a little ginger. It can also be useful in cases of diarrhea, colicky pains, liverishness, and weak digestion. For women, it is useful in cases of pelvic congestion, heavy menstrual bleeding, period pains, stopped periods, and vaginal discharge. It improves pelvic circulation and may be added with benefit to teas used for any womb or pelvic problems. Yarrow is supportive for people undergoing radiotherapy. Infused yarrow oil as in the bath or added to creams brings relief to eczema sufferers. For toothache, chew the fresh leaves or root, or apply fresh plant tincture on a compress.

 CHILDREN

Yarrow is a good, safe remedy for colds and fevers as tea tincture or in the bath. Cream and lotion helps to soothe itchy rashes of all kinds.

 FLOWER ESSENCE

Yarrow is a Californian essence not widely available elsewhere but easily made. Follow the Sun Method described on *page 32*. Yarrow essence is used for protection against negative influences.

PROPERTIES
- Diaphoretic
- Anti-inflammatory
- Antiseptic
- Antispasmodic
- Diuretic
- Stops bleeding
- Gentle bitter tonic

Notes and Dosages
- Taken freely in acute complaints.
- One cup of tea or one teaspoon of tincture three times daily for long-standing complaints.

Contraindications
Some people develop an allergic rash on handling the fresh plant.

CAUTION
Do not use Yarrow during pregnancy

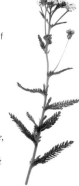

RIGHT *Yarrow, called millfoil by some, is a common wild plant with feathery leaves and a flat head of white or pink flowers, often found on lawns. The whole plant is picked in full flower.*

Aconite (Acon.) Aconitum napellus, monkshood

 HOMEOPATHIC

Aconite is used for illnesses that come on suddenly after being chilled by a dry, cold wind, or overheated by extreme summer heat, or following a sudden shock or fright. Use it at the beginning of illness, in the first twenty-four to forty-eight hours; after that time, if the person has not recovered, the symptoms will have changed to show another remedy picture.

 SYMPTOM PICTURE

Mental and Emotional Symptoms
Sudden unreasonable fear, afraid of the unknown, of dying.

Physical Symptoms
Colds and influenza:
- Burning heat alternating with chills at night.
- Hard, fast pulse and hot hands and cold feet, throbbing, bursting hot headache, worse on rising.

Earache: After exposure to dry, cold wind, unbearable pain, external ear hot, red, swollen. Very sensitive to noise.

Sore throat: Red, dry, tight throat, tonsils swollen and dry. May follow exposure to cold or after a shock.

Cough: For babies with croup that comes on after being out in a dry, cold wind. Hoarse, dry, cough with shortness of breath.

Vomiting: Due to fear with a profuse sweat and intense thirst.

Remedy Picture
- The Aconite person is robust and falls ill and recovers quickly.
- Sudden onset of fever, pains are hot and intolerable, face is hot, red, and swollen, or one cheek red, the other pale.
- Eyes are red and glassy.
- Dislike light, restless, better for open air, uncovering, worse in a warm room, and night-time.

Dosage 6c
Antidotes: Belladonna, Coffee, Nux vom., Sulfur

Red Chestnut Aesculus x carnea

 FLOWER ESSENCE

Red Chestnut is for those who suffer great fear and anxiety for others. They may have given up worrying about themselves but project their fear onto their loved ones. They often anticipate that some unfortunate accident or illness will befall those they and ceaselessly worry about the welfare of friends and relations. They want to protect loved ones and may cosset them. This fear limits both the Red Chestnut person and those close to them.

 FLOWER ESSENCES

The Boiling Method (see page 43)
The flowers blossom in the late spring. Pick about 6in. (15cm.) of twig, including the flowers and young leaves. Gather from many trees and from vaious parts of the tree.

Lesson
Sesitiviy to others
Each person has their own strengths and fears. Red Chestnut helps us realize that the anxiety we feel is a projection of personal fear. It helps us to be sensitive to the real fears and concerns of our loved ones so that we can offer appropriate support.

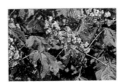

ABOVE *The red chestnut is often grown in public gardens for its large, decorative pink flower spikes. The tree is slightly smaller and less robust than its relative, the white or horse chestnut, which is also used to make Bach Flower Remedies.*

Chestnut Bud and White Chestnut Aesculus hippocastanum

 HERBALISM

White Chestnut is used for edema and pain associated with varicose veins. Make a cream by mixing the tincture into any suitable base cream or take 20 drops of tincture in a cup of yarrow tea, two or three times daily. Do not eat the nuts ("conkers").

 FLOWER ESSENCE

Chestnut Bud and white chestnut are remedies for those not sufficiently interested in present circumstances. Chestnut Bud is useful for people who are slow to learn, even from repeated experience, who find themselves struck in the same repeating pattern. White Chestnut is useful when the mind is full of unwanted thoughts, ideas, or persistent and worrying mental arguments.

 AROMATHERAPY

The Essential oil is used for rheumatism, gastiritis, constipation, and hemorrhoids. It should be used only by adults, in a bath with lavender and/or geranium.

 FLOWER ESSENCES

The Boiling Method for Chestnut Bud
(see page 43)
Pick the opening bud and about 6in. (15cm.) of twig from many trees. Try to pick from all parts of the tree, even the top.

The Sun Method for White Chestnut
(see page 42)
Pick male and female flowers

Lessons
Chestnut Bud – Vision
Chestnut bud helps move us into the present so that we can see with greater objectivity and learn from life's lessons. Chesnut bud is a useful additional remedy for the Cerato and Larch types.

White Chestnut – Clarity
White Chestnut helps us switch off and find peace and quiet within ourselves. If some thoughts persist, even after taking White Chestnut, other remedies should be taken to address the root cause of the problem, for example, Red Chestnut for worry over others or Walnut if picking up other's opinions.

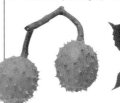

ABOVE *The white or horse chestnut is a large, strong, deciduous tree, growing up to 100ft. (30m.) high, with wide-spreading arched branches. When the leaves fall in the autumn they leave small horseshoe-shaped marks on the young wood. Chestnut Bud flower essence is made from the leaf buds of the white chestnut tree. The flowers are used for the remedy White Chestnut.*

Agrimony Agrimonia eupatoria

 HERBALISM

Agrimony can be taken as a tea or tincture for indigestion, heartburn, diarrhea, and liverish feelings. It is especially helpful for people suffering from food allergies—taken on a long-term basis. Use with St. John's wort and horsetail for bed wetting, chronic cystitis, and urinary incontinence. Use as a lotion to cleanse wounds and sores and an eyewash for sore and inflamed eyes. Agrimony can be taken freely and is a good substitute for ordinary tea.

 FLOWER ESSENCE

Agrimony flower essence is one of the Twelve Healers and Peace, and a remedy for those oversensitive to influences and ideas. Agrimony people hide their problems and inner selves behind humor and joyfulness. This masks real feelings of unhappiness and unworthiness, a reluctance to burden others love peace and pursue it at all costs. This leads to inner restlessness and discomfort, which is sometimes masked by alcohol and drugs.

 PROPERTIES

- Astringent and tonic
- Tones and strengthens the digestive system and liver
- A wound herb

 METHOD

The Sun Method (see page 42)
Agrimony flowers throughout the summer. Choose young plants where there are only a few unopened buds on the spike above the currently open flowers. Pick the whole spike above any dead or faded flowers.

Lesson
Self-acceptance and pure joy
True peace and joy come from acceptance and expression. Agrimony helps us love ourselves as we are, allowing the Agrimony type to use their humor and bravery to express and not repress themselves.

 CAUTION

Avoir agrimony in chronic constipation

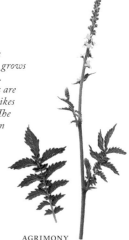

RIGHT *A deep-green perennial plant that grows up to 3ft. (1m.) high. Small yellow flowers are borne on tapering spikes like church steeples. The whole plant is used in herbalism.*

AGRIMONY

Lady's Mantle Alchemilla vulgaris

 HERBALISM

Lady's mantle is used as a tea or tincture for heavy menstrual bleeding, either alone or with an equal part of shepherd's purse or yarrow. It is also used for bleeding between periods and irregular periods. It may be combined with agnus castus berries. To prevent period pains, taken with marigold flowers on a regular basis. Use with uva ursi or shepherd's purse, as a tea or douche, for thrush and other vaginal discharges. Lady's mantle is a traditional treatment for infertility in women with no obvious cause.

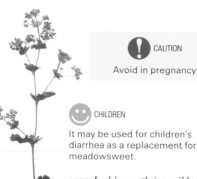

 CAUTION

Avoid in pregnancy

CHILDREN

It may be used for children's diarrhea as a replacement for meadowsweet.

LEFT *Lady's mantle is a wild plant of waysides and meadows, more common on hills. It is popular in shady gardens. The whole herb is used.*

PROPERTIES

- Astringent
- Tones and strengthens the womb

Notes and Dosages
- The tea is probably the most useful form. Use one or two teaspoons per cup. It is a pleasant drinking tea.

- Alternatively take one or two teaspoons of the tincture three times daily.

- In Sweden a sprig of the herb is put under the pillow of restless children to bring quiet sleep.

- Always seek medical assessment of bleeding between periods before starting home treatment.

Garlic Allium sativum

 HERBALISM

Garlic can be eaten daily or taken as pills as a preventive treatment for diseases of the circulation and as a supportive remedy in high blood pressure, high cholesterol, and hardening of the arteries. It strengthens the system against recurrent infections and is especially useful for children with continual coughs and colds. Given regularly it will dramatically reduce the need for antibiotic drugs. Use garlic syrup or tablets for bronchitis, lung infections in general, sinusitis, and intestinal worms. It is helpful in allergic asthma and hay fever. The infused oil is used as a chest rub for these conditions and as drops for earache. The fresh juice is used as an application to fungal infections.

 CHILDREN

Use the infused oil for ear infections for children past the toddler age; use tablets for children over three to prevent lung infections.

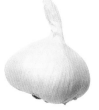

GARLIC BULB

ABOVE *Garlic belongs to the onion family. It has a very pungent odor and flavor, which some people find off-putting. This herb has a wide variety of uses, both medicinal and culinary. Supplements are available in capsule form for those who dislike eating garlic or want to take it in large therapeutic doses.*

 FOOD USES

Garlic is used to treat coughs, catarrh, sinusitis, and other infections of the mouth, throat, and digestive tract. It has a cleansing effect on the blood and helps to maintain a healthy flora in the intestines. It may have a role to play in the prevention of cancer, particularly stomach cancer. A poultice made with finely chopped garlic helps in the treatment of infected bites. Cut a garlic clove in half and rub the cut edge over a mosquito bite to relieve itching.

 PROPERTIES

• Garlic is an antiseptic with antibiotic and antifungal actions. Its antibiotic properties are a result of the presence of allicin. It is also an expectorant, lowers blood pressure, reduces cholesterol, reduces blood clotting, clears fatty deposits in the blood vessels.

• Garlic contains good amounts of Vitamin C, thiamine, and potassium and is an antioxidant.

Notes and Dosages

• Coated tablets made of garlic powder are the most user-friendly form. As a preventive treatment, follow the dosage on the package.

• For acute diseases, double the dose for a week or so.

• For children, give half the adult dose, usually two or three tablets daily.

• Make the syrup by putting finely chopped garlic in a jar, cover with honey, and let stand for four days. Strain off and give one or two teaspoons daily to children and 4 teaspoons daily to adults.

• Make the infused oil by covering finely chopped garlic with olive oil. Let it stand overnight to macerate. Strain off in the morning.

• Deodorized preparations are weak and not very useful.

• Eating fresh parsley will reduce the smell.

• Garlic used regularly in cooking is beneficial in circulatory disorders. Whole cloves roasted in their skin are especially good.

Special Notes

A chemical called disulfide that is present in garlic is excreted in sweat and through air expelled from the lungs. It is this that causes the odor given off after eating garlic. Some people believe that eating garlic in large amounts minimizes the odor. Certainly taking garlic supplements that contain odor suppressants may avoid this problem.

Contraindications

• Some people cannot take garlic for long periods because it irritates their stomachs.

• Enteric coated tablets are less irritating to the stomach.

> ⚠ CAUTION
>
> Not suitable for children under three.

GARLIC AS FOLK MEDICINE

Garlic grows wild almost everywhere in the world, and every culture has recognized its enormous repertory of healing powers. To the Greek physician Galen (c. a. d. 130-200) it was known as "the great panacea"; to the gangs who worked on the great pyramids of Egypt, it was a daily ration given to them to keep their strength up and prevent disease. Perhaps its supremacy in strengthening immunity, cleansing the blood, and driving out infection is why it was championed by the people of central Europe as one of the weapons of choice used to combat the depredations of the legendary blood-drinking vampires.

Aloe Vera Aloe vera

 HERBALISM

The fresh gel or cream made from aloe vera is a useful first-aid treatment for burns, radiation burns and sunburn, ringworm and other fungal infections, infected cuts, acne, shingles, eczema, wrinkles, stretch marks, and dry itchy skins in general. Use as a mouthwash for sore gums. Use as an internal medicine for indigestion and stomach acidity. A tincture of the whole leaves is excellent for chronic and stubborn constipation.

> **!** CAUTION
>
> Do not take Aloe internally during pregnancy.

 PROPERTIES

• The gel is soothing, cooling, antibacterial, antifungal and healing.
• The whole leaves are a strong laxative.

Notes and Dosages

• Aloes are easily grown as a houseplant—just remember not to overwater them. Cut the leaf and apply the fresh gel directly to the skin or take one tablespoon, twice daily, as an internal medicine. The cut leaves will keep for several months and can be used over and over again. You can buy many excellent preparations (creams, shampoos, preserved gel, etc.) of aloe; follow the instructions on the packages.
• The whole leaf tincture can be made at home or bought in herb shops. Take one teaspoon two or three times daily for constipation.

Contraindications
Many people are allergic to aloe vera.

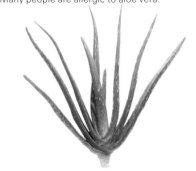

ABOVE *Aloe Vera is a tropical, succulent plant with thin, yellow banded leaves. The gel is squeezed from the leaves.*

Marshmallow Root and Leaf Althaea officinalis

 HERBALISM

Use marshmallow tea, tincture, or syrup with comfrey and meadowsweet for acid stomach, heartburn, ulcers, hiatus hernia, and colitis. Use the syrup, tea, or tincture for nonproductive coughs to encourage the expulsion of phlegm. Marshmallow leaves can be added to any tea for kidney and bladder problems for extra soothing. Leaf tea or tincture taken for some months will gradually soften dry skin. Use powdered root mixed into a cream or added to water to make a paste for insect bites and weeping eczema. Use as a poultice with marigold or chamomile for treating boils.

 CHILDREN

Marshmallow is the ideal children's remedy for irritable coughs and digestive problems.

It is very soothing and safe to use. Use with saw palmetto for failure to thrive. Use equal parts of the tinctures, 10 to 15 drops three times daily in pure fruit juice.

 PROPERTIES

• Soothing, mucilaginous
Notes and Dosages
• Marshmallow can be taken freely. For best results do not boil. Use as a tea or soak 1oz. (25g.) cut root or leaf in 1 pt. (500ml.) cold water overnight. In the morning strain and drink three cups daily.

• To make syrup, add 2.21b. (1kg.) sugar and stir until dissolved. This will keep for a few days.

• Leaves of the garden hollyhock have the same properties.

• Candied marshmallow roots were originally used for coughs.

• Modern-day candies and cookies known as "marshmallows" do not contain any of the herb.

MARSHMALLOW
FLOWERS AND
LEAVES

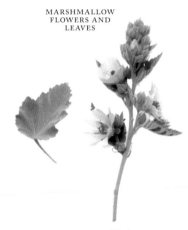

ABOVE *The leaves or roots of this wild plant are easily grown in herb gardens.*

Angelica and Chinese Angelica Angelica Archangelica and Angelica sinensis

 HERBALISM

Angelica can be used as a tincture, tea, or decoction for convalescence, persistent fevers, indigestion and weak digestion in general, colic and cramping pains, coughs, poor circulation, and general weakness with feelings of cold. Chinese angelica is used for period pains, anemia, and general debility in women and as a gentle laxative for constipation in elderly people. An infused oil made from the leaves or seeds of angelica and fennel is a useful, relaxing rub for tightness and feelings of cold in the chest.

 CHILDREN

Angelica leaf and chamomile flower tea is a good drink for tight, dry, irritable coughs in children.

 PROPERTIES

• Warming and restorative.

• Antiseptic, diuretic, diaphoretic, and expectorant; relaxes spasm and strengthens digestion.

• Angelica root is an excellent general tonic for those run down by prolonged stress or chronic disease.

• Chinese angelica root (dang gui or Angelica sinensis) is an especially good tonic for women.

• In China it is called the women's ginseng.

Notes and Dosages

• The leaves are better suited for children's medicine. They may be added to green salads.

• The leaf stems, picked before flowering, are candied for decorating cakes or as a sweet for children with weak chests.

• Angelica archangelica is the garden angelica. Wild angelica has the same properties, but always get expert identification before picking herbs in the wild.

• Some people can get a rash from handling fresh angelica in daylight.

 CAUTION

Do not use any Angelica in pregnancy without expert advice

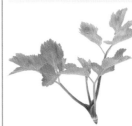

LEFT *Angelica is a tall, stately plant with flat masses of small green flowers; it is popular in large gardens. Both the root and leaves are used in herbalism.*

Apis Mellifica Apis mellifera

 HOMEOPATHIC

Use apis mellifica for complaints that have puffiness and swellings. Your patient may be thirstless, hot, bright red, shiny, swollen, and retaining water. Allergic reaction (anaphylactic shock) may occur after bee or wasp stings; the linings of the respiratory system plus the tongue and uvula can become so swollen that breathing becomes difficult. Get help immediately, and use apis as a first-aid remedy.

 SYMPTOM PICTURE

Mental and Emotional Symptoms
Changeable, tearful, irritable, jealous, childish, and spiteful.

Physical Symptoms
Eyes: Hay fever or infections that cause swollen, red, puffy lids; bright red, stinging eyes; tears feel hot; recurrent sties.

Throat: Bright red, swollen, sore throat, worse for swallowing; dry but thirstless; tonsils swollen.

Fever: Burning heat, thirsty during afternoon chill, sleepy.

Women's complaints: Right-sided ovarian cysts with stinging pains.

Urinary complaints: Scanty urination, but frequent urge to urinate. Last drops may *sting*.

Rheumatism: Joints hot, red, shiny and swollen with burning pains and a tired, bruised feeling.

Skin: Sore, stinging, itching, red, and swollen with hives especially after insect bites and stings.

Rheumatism: Joints hot, red, shiny and swollen with burning pains and a tired, bruised feeling.

Skin: Sore, stinging, itching, red, and swollen with hives especially after insect bites and stings.

Remedy Picture
• Burning hot, stinging pains or excessively itchy, like nettle stings, worse for heat, touch, tight clothing, afternoon, nights.

• Better for cold, cold drinks.

• Right-sided symptoms or moves from right to left.

Dosage: 6c
Antidotes: Cantharis, Ipecac, Lachesis, Natrum mur.

Complementary Remedies: None

BELOW *Apis mellifera is the honey bee. The Apis mellifica remedy is made from the entire insect, including the venom sac.*

Burdock Arctium lappa, Arctium minus

 HERBALISM

Burdock root is useful when taken as a tea or decoction and used as a lotion or poultice for "eruptive" skin conditions, especially hot and inflamed conditions, such as acne, spots, boils, and rashes in general. Use a decoction or tincture for all kinds of stubborn skin diseases, including psoriasis and fungal infections, rheumatism, gout, and arthritis. It is often used with dandelion root for skin and liver problems. It makes a soothing diuretic tea for kidney stones and chronic cystitis and a gargle for sore throats.

 FOOD USES

Use in cases of appetite loss.

 CHILDREN

The leaf stems and roots of burdock can be eaten to help treat skin conditions such as eczema, psoriasis, and boils. Boil or steam the leaf stems and roots; eat the roots raw in salads or stir-fry with other vegetables. Burdock root is a popular vegetable in the East, considered to be strengthening to the sex organs and immune system.

 PROPERTIES

• Blood cleanser and alterative.
• Gentle laxative, diuretic, lymphatic cleanser.
• Soothing and nourishing.
• Stimulates the appetite and soothes troubled spirits.
• Locally antiseptic.

Notes and Dosages

• Burdock is a common wayside weed; wash it well and be sure of your identification if you gather your own.

• Burdock root works best on stubborn conditions when taken in low doses for some months. Use 2 teaspoons of dried root by decoction daily or 1 teaspoon of the tincture twice daily for several months.

• For lack of appetite, take the tincture three times daily, before meals, in a little water or fruit juice. The recommended dose is 5 to 10 drops for children and 20 drops for adults.

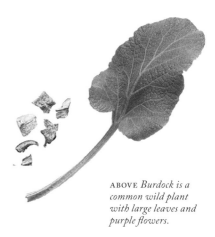

ABOVE *Burdock is a common wild plant with large leaves and purple flowers.*

Uva Ursi or Bearberry Leaves Arctostaphylos uva-ursi

 HERBALISM

Use uva ursi tea or tincture for cystitis, painful urination, and water retention. It is best combined with soothing remedies such as marshmallow or plantain. Use it with horsetail and nettle for irritable bladder with persistent urgency and frequency. Use it with lady's mantle and shepherd's purse for vaginal discharges, especially chronic, thick, white discharge; use with saw palmetto and echinacea or marigold for prostatitis. Use with agrimony for diarrhea.

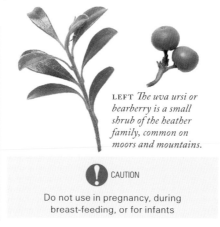

LEFT *The uva ursi or bearberry is a small shrub of the heather family, common on moors and mountains.*

⚠ CAUTION

Do not use in pregnancy, during breast-feeding, or for infants

PROPERTIES

• Diuretic, urinary antiseptic, astringent.

Notes and Dosages

• To make uva ursi tea, use one teaspoon to a cup, infuse for ten minutes.

• For cystitis, use one cup of tea or one teaspoon of tincture two or three times daily. Excellent remedy for acute cystitis but consult a herbalist if you do not get results in a week.

• Take in combination with the suggested herbs for long-term use.

• Works best for chronic cystitis and frequency of urination if combined with a diet high in green vegetables.

• Avoid in cases of kidney infections or weakness.

Arnica (Arn.) Arnica montana, mountain daisy, leopard's bane

 HERBALISM

Arnica is an irritant poison and best used at homeopathic dilutions internally. The herbal tincture can be used externally in place of the homeopathic mother tincture. It is usually cheaper to buy.

 HOMEOPATHIC

Arnica, essential for the first-aid box, is given after accidents that result in bruises and shock. The important symptom to prescribe on is the bruised feeling. Arnica soothes the pain and stimulates the body to heal the bruised tissues. Arnica may be appropriate for someone who is bruised and shocked, and who may also have soreness, tenderness, throbbing, or stinging pains.

 AROMATHERAPY

Arnica is used in the same way as when applying homeopathic methods.

 SYMPTOM PICTURE

Mental and Emotional Symptoms
• Shocked from an accident, says there is nothing wrong, wants to be left alone.

• If concussed, may slip in and out of consciousness.

• The bed feels too hard so tosses and turns at night.

• Fears sudden death, has nightmares of death and mutilated bodies.

• Is absent-minded, easily distracted, cannot concentrate.

Physical Symptoms
• M ay have a fever from the shock or injury, hot head, cold body.

• Head injuries with or without loss of consciousness.

• Black eyes *(see Ledum).*

Fractures: Arnica helps to heal the bruising and swelling around the break and allays the pain. After exercise: Muscles that have been worked too hard and ache. Before and after operations.

Childbirth: Uterus is working hard and the baby is pressing against the perineum—helps to heal the tissues, take away bruising and soreness and prevent septicemia; after-pains are too strong and leave the woman feeling bruised. Breast-feeding: Nipples feel sore and bruised. Mastitis, after a blow to the breast.

Remedy Picture
• Worse for touch or movement—afraid it will hurt—for rest and damp and cold.

• Better for lying down.

• May crave vinegar and dislike milk and meat.

Dosage
• For bumps and bruises take 6c three or four times a day as needed.

• For severe knocks take 30c and repeat as necessary.

• During labor take 30c in first stage, at transition, during second stage and after the birth, then take twice a day for a few days until the perineum is healed.

• Before and after an operation take 200c.

• Apply Arnica ointment or cream or compresses of Arnica tincture over bruises two or three times a day. Do not apply if the skin is broken because it may result in a severe inflammation or rash.

Antidotes: None.
Complementary Remedies: None.

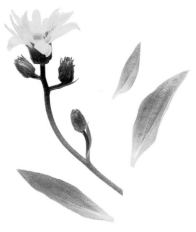

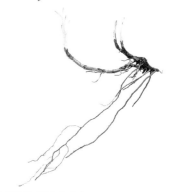

ABOVE & BELOW *Arnica montana is a hardy perennial that grows between 1 and 2ft. (30-60cm.) tall. Its yellow, scented flowers bloom in the summer.*

THE ENGLISH ARNICA
The source for Arnica, Arnica, Montana, grows prolifically in mountains; its usefulness was discovered by locals who used arnica infusion to soothe the bruises and bumps that resulted from climbing accidents. In England, the common daisy (*Bellis perennis*) plays the same role. One of its old names is woundwort, and daisy cream is an excellent cure for external bruising and sprains.

 CAUTION

Do not take internally unless using homeopathic remedy

Astragalus Root Astragalus membranaceus

 HERBALISM

Use a decoction or tincture for chronic fatigue, persistent infections, multiple allergies, and infectious mononucleosis. Modern research shows that the herb helps to counteract tiredness and lack of appetite in patients undergoing chemotherapy and radiotherapy for cancer. Soothing and healing for stomach ulcers.

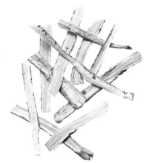

ABOVE *Astragalus is an herbaceous perennial plant related to licorice.*

 CAUTION

Always tell the hospital if you are taking herbal medicine in conjunction with their treatment.

 PROPERTIES

• Astragalus is one of the most famous Chinese tonic herbs. It boosts the immune system.

Notes

Astragalus is also called "huang qi." The root can be bought in Chinese herb shops and may be used in tonic soups, with nourishing vegetables, for severe immune deficiencies.

Contraindications

This is a safe herb for home use, but severely debilitated patients should always be seen by a professional herbalist who will prescribe according to the individual's condition and circumstances.

Belladonna (Bell.) Atropa belladnna, deadly nightshade

 HOMEOPATHIC

Belladonna is suited to robust people full of vitality, especially children who suddenly fall violently ill. Choose it when pains are violent and throbbing, and come and go suddenly. They are usually felt on the right side of the body.

 SYMPTOM PICTURE

Mental and Emotional Symptoms
• The person is in a turmoil, very hot, has throbbing pains, is restless and agitated, angry, screams with pain, may be delirious with fever.

Physical Symptoms
Fever:
• High fever, face flushed deep red, dilated pupils, glassy eyes.
• Hot to touch, can feel the heat coming off the person.
• Thirstless with fever.
• Wants to be covered, head hot, feet icy cold.

• Children may have febrile convulsions.
Headache: Sudden, severe headache in temples, eyes, forehead, whole head. Throbbing, bursting pains start and stop suddenly. Comes on from hot sunshine, cold air, chilled from wet hair.
• Worse for stooping, menstruation, movement, light, sunshine, noise.
• Better for lying propped up, head on pillows in a quiet, dark room.
Sore throat: Tonsillitis, quinsy. Dry, tight, hot, swollen, fiery red throat. Worse on right side, stitching pains into ear on swallowing.
Earache: Middle-ear infections -the ear-drum deep red, bulging. Throbbing, teasing, stitching, bursting pains in ear, cries out with pain. Right ear worse.
Sunstroke: Flushed, hot face, violent throbbing headache. Thirsty for cold water, may vomit, must lie with head propped up. Shivery despite the heat. Wants to be covered.

Remedy Picture
• Sudden onset of violent, throbbing pains which come and go quickly.

• Inflamed parts deep, bright red, hot to touch and swollen.
• Usually right-sided pains; throbbing, bursting, stitching, hot.
• Very thirsty for cold drinks except thirstless with a fever.
• Hot head and feet.
• Worse for movement, drafts, stooping, noise, night, lying down.
• Better for keeping still, sitting propped up, head resting back.

Dosage 6c or 30c
Antidotes: Coffee, Merc, Pulsatilla
Complementary Remedies: None

 CAUTION

Belladonna is a poisonous plant. Do not touch.

BELOW *Belladonna is a perennial that grows up to 2ft. (60cm.) high. Its lustrous but poisonous black berries are known a "the devil's cherries in folk medicine.*

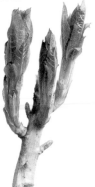

Wild Oats Avena futua

HERBALISM

Use the tea or tincture for weakness with anxiety or depression or following severe illness and for nervous exhaustion. This is a good remedy to help us "keep going during periods of mental or physical strain." Use with valerian or vervain for chronic anxiety; for sleeplessness and restless sleep; and for shingles and neuralgia. Wild oats aids withdrawal from tranquilizers, alcohol, stimulants, and narcotic drugs and is a useful adjunct to major tranquilizers and anti-epileptic drugs. It is also supportive in heart diseases. Use it with saw palmetto for impotence in men, wet dreams, and premature ejaculation. It is also useful for PMS with scanty periods and cramps; for exhaustion after childbirth and when breast-feeding; and for lack of sexual interest in women. Use with horsetail to strengthen bones in children and in elderly people. In the bath and as a lotion it is very soothing for eczema and dry skin and relieves tension in the body.

CHILDREN

Use for hyperactivity and failure to thrive.

PROPERTIES

• Nourishing
• Restoring to nerves and reproductive organs
• Gentle stimulant

Notes and Dosages
Tea: 1 or 2 teaspoons per cup of boiling water, allow to infuse fifteen minutes, drink freely.

Tincture: 40 drops three times daily or 20 drops every two hours when you need to keep going.

• Eating porridge made from oats is also strengthening.

Baths: Infuse 6oz. (150g.) oat straw in 3pt. (1. 51.) water and add to the bath or hang a bag of oat bran under the hot water faucet, so that the water flows through it.

• Wrap some porridge oats in a piece of light cloth and use instead of soap. Commercial preparations of oats, for making baths, can be bought at pharmacies.

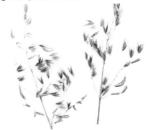

ABOVE *Avena futua, a wild grass, is the origin of cultivated oats* (Avena sativa), *which may be substituted. The whole plant is picked while still green.*

Frankincense Boswellia carteri

AROMATHERAPY

Used as a massage oil, frankincense is wonderfully calming and relaxing for the nervous system, helping anxiety and tension. It helps you to breathe more deeply and evenly, and so encourages relaxation. It improves the skin, has anti-aging properties, and assists the healing of scars, ulcers, and wounds. It combines well with other oils, such as myrrh, geranium, neroli, basil, pine, and sandalwood. It is excellent when added to the bath or burned in a room in an oil or ring burner. Use for asthma, bronchitis, coughs, and laryngitis. It also helps to treat diarrhea, cystitis, and menstrual problems of all kinds.

PROPERTIES

• Anti-inflammatory
• Respiratory system
• Nervous system
• Meditative
• Excretory system
• Regenerative

Cautions and Contraindications
Use at half the measure while pregnant.

 CAUTION

Do not use directly on babies or infants, but do burn the oil in the room. Do not overuse.

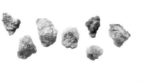

ABOVE *Frankincense essential oil is produced by steam distillation from gum resin that has been extracted from the bark of the frankincense tree. Frankincense has a long history of use, beginning in Ancient Egypt, where it was an element of perfumes, and in the Far East in meditation and prayer. The trees are found in North Africa and Arabia.*

Wild Oat Bromus ramosus, hairy brome, wood brome

 FLOWER ESSENCE

Wild oat is one of the remedies for those who suffer uncertainty. It is useful for capable people who have ambition to do something meaningful in their lives but have not yet found their true calling. They may have several choices or directions and may be working hard on a given path but basically they are dissatisfied and frustrated. They are scattered and seek to know what particular thing they should do with their life.

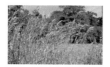

 METHOD

The Sun Method *(see page 42)*
Wild oats bloom in summer with loose, nodding flowers on thin leafless stems. The stems and leaves are very hairy. Pick the whole spike when the flowers are full of pollen. Float on top of the water in a thick layer.

LEFT *This elegant grass of damp woods, wasteland, and waysides grows from 2 to 5ft. (60cm. to 1.5m.) high. The common name is Hairy or Wood Brome grass because the long, finely pointed leaves are soft and hairy.*

• Although Bromus is an English version of the Greek word for oat, the plant does not look much like an oat. Accurate identification is essential.

Lesson
Meaningful purpose
We all have many roles to play and different parts according to our talents. Wild Oat helps us listen for our calling, tune in to the constant self, and find our true meaning. It helps us express this and make choices that bring purposeful harmony between inner and outer calling, spirituality, and making a living.

Bryonia Bryonia alba, wild hops, white bryony

 HOMEOPATHIC

Bryonia is used for a robust dark-haired person with lean, firm muscles, and irritable nature. There is usually a slow onset of complaints brought on by a cold, dry east wind or by getting chilled when hot. Bryonia is a very important homeopathic remedy, and has applications in many conditions. It is often chosen for remedy pictures that include lung problems, arthritis, and digestive complaints.

 SYMPTOM PICTURE

Mental and Emotional Symptoms
• The person is irritable with everything, dislikes being disturbed, anxious for the future, worries about work and financial security, dreams of work.

• Delirious—"wants to go home" although he or she is there.

Physical Symptoms
Headache: Bursting occipital headache, frontal headache with sinusitis, bursting and stitching. Pressing pain behind the eyes. Worse for stooping, motion, and opening eyes.

Throat: Dry, rough, hoarse, stitching pain. Worse for swallowing.

Chest infections: Colds and flu go to the chest, dry, sore, chesty cough, very little

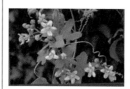

ABOVE *White bryony is a member of the gourd family. It is a climbing plant with white flowers that blossom in the summer.*

⚠ CAUTION
White bryony root is extremely poisonous.

sputum, hurts to cough. Better for holding his or her sides. Pleurisy, stitching pains, better for lying on affected side and for pressure. Gastrointestinal tract: Lips and mouth dry, bitter taste. Thirsty for long drinks of cold water. Nausea and vomiting on rising, tender aching stomach. Large, dry, hard, crumbly stools or diarrhea like muddy water.

Rheumatism and arthritis: Stitching pains in swollen pale or red joints. Better for affected part being kept still and pressure applied. Worse for cold and movement.

Remedy Picture
• Hot and dry people, heat and dryness runs through their symptoms.

• Thirsty for long drink of cold water—gulps.

• White-coated tongue.

• Severe stitching pains worse for slightest movement, better lying down on affected side, for pressure.

Dosage: 6c
Antidotes: Chamomilla, Coffee, Nux vom., Pulsatilla, Rhus tox. *Complementary Remedies:* None.

Marigold Flowers or Calendula (Arn.) Calendula officinalis, Calendula, pot marigold

 HERBALISM

Marigold tea or tincture and compress are useful for boils, spots, inflamed wounds, inflamed and painful varicose veins, and sore eyes. Drink the tea for colic and colicky pains; use with meadowsweet, comfrey leaf, and chamomile for stomach ulcers; use with lady's mantle—on a regular basis—for period pains. Infertility in women due to blocked Fallopian tubes or cystic ovaries may respond well: persist with treatment for best results. Use for depression, especially for women at the menopause. Use with sage as a tea or tincture and compress for painful, lumpy breasts. Sage and marigold tea will stave off infections. Use as a mouthwash and gargle for sore throats, tonsillitis, chronic ear infections, mouth sores, and ulcers. Use calendula lotion or cream for itchy skin rashes, grazes, cuts, eczema, and fungal infections. The ointment or infused oil is good for chapped skin and a lip balm.

 CHILDREN

Use the infused oil for cradle cap and add two or four teaspoons to the bath for dry skins. The cream is applicable for all inflamed and sore skin problems.

 HOMEOPATHIC

Calendula is a wonderful healing remedy for cuts and wounds. It is antiseptic and promotes quick healing of wounds so make sure that you cleanse the wound thoroughly first with 10 drops of Calendula tincture diluted in 8fl. oz. (250ml.) of cool, boiled water. Then apply a compress soaked in the Calendula water over the wound to stem bleeding or apply Calendula cream. Taking Calendula internally also helps the wound to heal.

 FOOD USES

Essential oil of Marigold, which is dark green in color, is useful for skin problems such as eczema, rashes and inflammation, for greasy skin, and for first-aid attention to wounds, cuts, and burns.

 AROMATHERAPY

Use the flower petals of calendula (pot marigold) as a substitute for saffron to color rice dishes or to decorate salads. In such small quantities calendula will have little medicinal benefit and is safe to use.

 PROPERTIES

Marigold lifts the spirits, relaxes spasm, is healing and anti-inflammatory. It is especially helpful for skin and eye problems.

Physical Symptoms
• Cuts from injuries, operation wounds, cuts and tears to the perineum during childbirth.
• Insect bites and stings.

Dosage: 6c potency three times a day until better. 5 drops (Q) mother tincture diluted in water, three times a day until better.

Antidotes: None
Complementary remedies: Hepar sulf.

NOTES AND USAGES
• Normal dosages throughout.
• Marigold cream may be sold under the botanical name Calendula.
• Hyperical cream, made from marigold flowers and St. John's wort, has the same uses.
• Marigold infused oil can be made at home or bought in specialist herb shops.
• Add a good pinch of the petals to salads and soups.
• Marigolds are easily grown but make sure you have Calendula.

• Do not use tagetes, also called French, African, or Mexican marigolds, for medicine.

Contraindications
Always have breast lumps medically assessed before relying on home treatment.

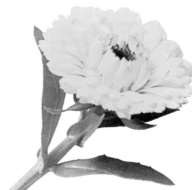

ABOVE *Marigold is a popular garden plant with orange or yellow flowers. An annual herb, it grows up to 2.5ft. (70cm.) high.*

Heather Calluna vulgaris

 FLOWER ESSENCE

Heather is one of the remedies for those who suffer loneliness. Heather people are filled with self-centered concerns and will talk to anyone available. They dominate the conversation and company with accounts of their own affairs and experiences. They are poor listeners and do not like to be alone. To avoid loneliness they may be concentrating on fulfilling personal needs. Heather helps move from the narrow obsession with immediate personality needs, making it possible to experience the wider love and companionable nurturing that comes from considering and sharing with others.

 METHOD

The Sun Method *(see page 42)*
White and pink flowers bloom from the late summer onward. Pick small freshly flowering sprays with their small leaves. Avoid spent or faded flowers. Gather from a wide growing area and from all parts of the plant, especially the heart of the bush and the spreading outside branches.

• Do not confuse with Erica cinerea, the bell heather.

Lesson
Love; space to share

We should love and nurture ourselves. This is the rock of self-knowing from which we move out and relate to others with empathy. Heather people are stuck and have not made that step. When they do, they can love with empathy.

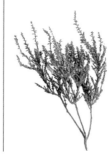

LEFT *Heather is a tough, rough, scrubby plant of dry moors and open heaths. The stems are wiry and much branched, growing and spreading to 2ft. (60cm.) high.*

Ylang Ylang Cananga odorata

 AROMATHERAPY

The exotic, sensual qualities of ylang ylang when used in massage, in a bath, or burned in a room have a calming and balancing effect on the nervous system. It helps to prevent hyperventilation and palpitations and to slow down a racing heartbeat, aids anxiety and depression, and helps to lower a fever. Used in a vaporizer, it has an antiseptic effect on the skin—in particular, on skin that is dry or oily, or affected by acne. Abdominal and lower—back massage with ylang ylang may reduce symptoms associated with the menopause, including hot flushes and vaginal dryness. It is a valued oil for sexual problems, frigidity, and impotence in men. Burned in the room, it has a pleasantly aphrodisiac effect. It has an invigorating effect on the elderly. A few drops in the final rinse improves the condition of the hair. It combines well with other oils, such as jasmine, sandalwood, rose, lemon, vetivert, and cedarwood.

 PROPERTIES

• Antiseptic
• Regulator of the nervous system
• Antispasmodic
• Sexual tonic
• Hypertension reliever
• Emotional balancer
• Febrifuge—lowers fevers

Contraindications
Use at half the measured amount while pregnant, and on babies and infants.

BELOW *Ylang ylang essential oil is extracted by water, or water and steam distillation from flowers that have been picked in the early morning. Ylang ylang is a small tropical tree that grows in Madagascar, Indonesia, and the Philippines. The oil is a pale yellow color, is oily in its consistency, and has a wonderful, exotic, sweet, flowery aroma. Called the "flower of flowers," ylang ylang is often known as the poor man's Jasmine because of its powerful aroma and affordability.*

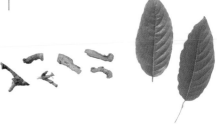

Cantharis (Canth.) Cantharis vesicatoria, Lytta vesicatoria, Spanish fly, blister beetle

 HOMEOPATHIC

Cantharis is one of the most frequently required remedies for burns and for urinary tract infections. It is particularly useful for extreme cases of cystitis that come on violently and suddenly.

 SYMPTOM PICTURE

Mental and Emotional Symptoms
• Irritability and anger from the pain.

Physical Symptoms
• Burns, scalds, and sunburn with or without blisters, stinging, burning pains. Alleviates the pain and aids healing.

Cystitis: Frequent urge to urinate. Urine is passed drop by drop, may be bloody, with scalding, stinging, spasmodic pains throughout urination. Worse for cold drinks.

Remedy Picture
• Cantharis is useful for sudden, intense onset of inflammations with restlessness and burning, scalding pains.

• Great thirst from heat yet worse for cold drinks and coffee.

• Better for rubbing and warmth.

Dosage: 6c
Antidotes: Apis met, Camphor, Pulsatilla
Complementary Remedies: None.

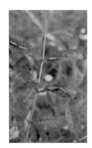

LEFT *Cantharis vesicatoria, also known as Spanish Fly or Blister Beetle, is a native of southern Europe and western Asia. It lives on olive trees and honeysuckle. The whole insect is ground up to make the remedy.*

Hornbeam Carpinus betulus

 FLOWER ESSENCE

Hornbeam is one of the remedies for those who suffer uncertainty. It is useful for those who feel that they do not possess enough strength to fulfill the responsibilities of daily life. Everything seems too much effort, and they have to expend much will-power just to survive. This feeling often comes from boredom or some basic dissatisfaction with the work they are doing. Elm and Hornbeam both deal with fatigue and temporary feelings of inadequacy but there are important differences. The Elm person loves his work and calling and is temporarily overcome with responsibility. The Hornbeam type lacks strength for the mundane nine-to-five aspects of life.

 METHOD

The Boiling Method *(see page 43)*
The flowers bloom in spring. Pick young twigs about 6in. (15cm.) long with leaves and male and female flowers. Hornbeam is sometimes coppiced and used in hedging. Try to gather twigs from a selection of coppices and naturally growing wood.

Lesson
Strength to carry out daily tasks

• If the weakness characteristic of Hornbeam is a regular occurrence, the person may be exhausting himself or herself in the wrong direction. Wild Oat will help in finding a path more in harmony with inner purpose and talents.

• Scleranthus will help those indecisive about change.

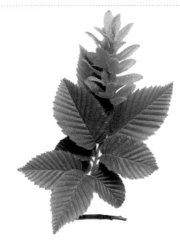

ABOVE *Hornbeam is a deciduous tree growing to 70ft. (21m.) high. When young, the tree grows in a tight, erect pyramid shape; but when mature, it opens out and the branch tips start to hang down. The heart-shaped leaves are alternate and grow on short stalks.*

Sweet Chestnut Castanea sativa

 FLOWER ESSENCE

Sweet chestnut is one of the remedies for those who suffer despondency and despair. It is useful for those moments that happen to some people when the anguish is so great as to seem unbearable, when they have "come to the end of their rope," reached their limit and are being stretched beyond endurance, when it feels as if the mind or body will give way and all that is left is annihilation.

 HERBALISM

Sweet chestnuts are used for their nourishing quality. The leaves are used as a tea for asthma, whooping cough, and paroxysmal coughs of any kind.

 FOOD USES

The fruit, or seeds, of sweet chestnut can be roasted or boiled as a vegetable to help in the treatment of rheumatic pains and coughs. They are also used in stuffings for poultry and in desserts.

 METHOD

The Boiling Method *(see page 43)*
The flowers blossom in the late summer after the leaves have appeared. The male and female flowers are found on the same tree. The male catkins are long and slender. The female flowers are fewer in number and grow in clusters at the base of the catkins. Gather when the male catkins are thick with their heavy, sweet pollen. Pick about 6in. (15cm.) of twig with male flowers, some female flowers and a few leaves.

Lesson
Transformation, widening the boundaries
There are several remedies for those in the throes of despair, and each is subtly different. It is important to remember their general category. Gorse is for uncertainty, and Cherry Plum is for fear. The root of

Sweet Chestnut is for despondency. Sweet Chestnut types frequently have "more rope" and hidden reserves; the stress they are experiencing is the result of too rapid expansion—events are pushing too hard at their current boundaries. Sweet Chestnut helps open boundaries and expand limits, giving the strength to grow.

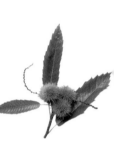

RIGHT *The edible chestnut is a deciduous tree growing to 80ft. (24m.). The bark is covered with deep longitudinal furrows. These are straight when the tree is young, but as it matures they twist and spiral around the trunk.*

Cedarwood Cedrus atlantica

 AROMATHERAPY

Cedarwood is used in essential oil massage or as an astringent. It is a powerful antiseptic and contains regenerative properties. It is useful in arthritic conditions, bronchial and urinary tract infections. Its regenerative properties make it suitable for treating eczema, acne, oily skin and hair, dandruff, alopecia, and nervous tension. It is also effective for athlete's foot and fungal infections. It combines well with other essential oils such as jasmine, neroli, and bergamot and is excellent for arthritic conditions. Used as an inhalation or compress, it helps bronchial and respiratory conditions. When used in the bath or as a douche, its antiseptic properties aid venereal infections, leucorrhea, cystitis, and diarrhea.

When used in a vaporizer or burned in a room, Cedarwood acts as a balancer of anxiety and nervous tension and has aphrodisiac properties.

 PROPERTIES

- Antiseptic
- Regenerative
- Diuretic
- Wound-healing
- Antifungal
- Lymphotonic

Contraindications
Use half the usual stated amount on children with care.

 CAUTION

- Do not use while pregnant: can be abortive
- Do not use on babies and infants

BELOW *Cedarwood essential oil is extracted by steam distillation from the wood and sawdust of the cedarwood tree. It was one of the earliest known essential oils, widely used in Ancient Egypt in embalming, cosmetics, and perfumes, and also used in ancient civilizations for medicine and perfumery. It is still used today by the Tibetans in their temples and medicine. The essential oil is a yellowish color and provides a woody, warm aroma.*

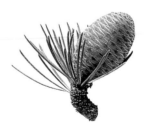

Centaury Centaurium erythraea

HERBALISM

In herbal medicine, centaury is used as a bitter tonic with the same applications as its more famous relative, gentian. The tea is drunk for weak digestion, lack of appetite, jaundice, rheumatism, and low-grade, persistent fevers. It is antiseptic and often included in ointments for wounds.

FLOWER ESSENCE

Centaury is one of the twelve healers, relating to weakness and strength. It is one of the remedies for those oversensitive to influences and ideas. Centaury people can become doormats. Their will to help others is so strong that it undermines their individuality and they find it hard to say "no." They can become servants rather than helpers and end up giving more than their fair share. They can become exploited, overtaxing their strength and resources so that life becomes a drudgery or even stoically borne self-martyrdom.

METHOD

The Sun Method *(see page 42)*
Pick small clusters of the salmon-pink flowers, which bloom throughout the summer, from many plants. Float on the water as soon as possible, covering the entire surface area.

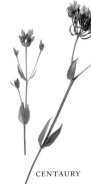

LEFT *Centaury is a small annual, varying greatly in height depending on habitat. It likes chalk soil and is abundant in chalky areas. It has an erect, square stem and small sessile leaves.*

CENTAURY

Lesson
Service in the widest sense
Centaury helps balance the desire to serve by strengthening our appreciation of the self, and the responsibility we have to our path. It allows us to be able to say "yes" or "no" from the heart.

Cerato Ceratostigma willmottianum

FLOWER ESSENCE

Cerato is one of the twelve healers, relating to ignorance and wisdom. It is one of the remedies for those who suffer uncertainty. Cerato people are intelligent and curious, but they lack confidence in themselves and doubt their abilities and opinions. They constantly seek advice and approval from others and can exhaust friends with a ceaseless stream of questions. They admire those who seem together, like the Agrimony type, and can be motivated by what others are thinking. They will follow advice, sometimes quite misguidedly. The unsure Cerato people like approval and try to do and be seen to do the right thing; it is important that they are perceived to be politically correct.

METHOD

The Sun Method *(see page 42)*
This beautiful plant is a native of Tibet and is grown for its blue flowers in the late summer. Choose plants in a country garden where there has been no spraying. Pick the flowers singly, just below the calyx, and float them quickly on the water until it is entirely covered. Try to gather flowers from several plants.

Lesson
The strength of inner knowing Cerato teaches us to listen to advice from within and strengthen our trust in ourselves; it also teaches us to follow our path, even if it runs contrary to others. When balanced, Cerato is capable of great wisdom.

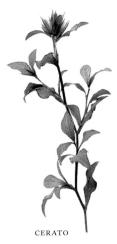

LEFT *Cerato is a small deciduous shrub, often grown in gardens, reaching 3–4ft. (1–1.2m.) high. It is a native of the Himalayas.*

CERATO

Roman Chamomile *Chamaemelum nobile*

 HERBALISM

The uses and properties of this herb are the same as for the German Chamomile, but Roman Chamomile is stronger and best avoided in early pregnancy. Roman Chamomile is sold in the double-flowered form, whereas the German is a simple daisy.

 AROMATHERAPY

Chamomile essential oil, because of its low toxicity, is safe to use in low doses on babies, infants, and children, and is safe during pregnancy. Used in massage or in a bath, Roman Chamomile has a calming effect on the nervous system. It is helpful for insomnia and anxiety and neuralgia caused by anxiety and stress. It is also helpful for anemia. It is used in treating anorexia because it assists digestive problems, dyspepsia, vomiting, nausea.

When massaged over the solar plexus and abdomen, it helps intestinal ulcers and gastric problems. Used on the skin as a massage oil, or in a vaporizer or bath, it helps dermatitis, eczema, psoriasis, burns, sores, herpes, and wounds generally. In a shampoo, it will give highlights to the hair. It is essential for menopausal problems, helping with profuse sweating, hot flushes, fluid retention, and general aches and pains.

 PROPERTIES

- Anti-inflammatory
- Antispasmodic
- Antiparasitic
- Pre-anesthetic
- Calming to the central nervous system
- Febrifuge—reduces fever
- Diuretic

Contraindications
Overuse will counteract its calming qualities. Overuse will stimulate bowel action.

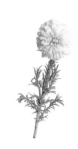
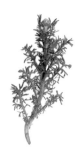

BELOW Chamomile essential oil is extracted by steam distillation from the dried flowers of the plant. Roman Chamomile has been well known for its medicinal qualities since ancient times. The oil starts out as pale blue, but becomes a greenish-yellow color over time. It has a herbaceous, warm, fruity aroma.

Chicory *Cichorium intybus*

 FLOWER ESSENCE

Chicory is one of the twelve healers, relating to fussiness, emotional congestion, and love. It is used for those who overcare for the welfare of others. Chicory types need to be loved, but they see love as a transactional exchange of energy, with costs. They fuss and worry and are overanxious to please others. This fussiness is exhausting rather than pleasing to others and can inhibit them from expressing love to the Chicory type. The Chicory types will care publicly, even melodramatically, but love still does not flow their way. This is giving love in order to receive it. The Chicory type fears obscurity. The Chicory archetype is the "stage mother." Eating chicory has beneficial effects on

the liver and may help in the treatment of liver ailments. It is also recommended for the treatment of rheumatism, gout, and hemorrhoids.

 FOOD USES

The Sun Method *(see page 42)*
The beautiful blue flowers, which appear in the late summer, are very delicate and fade quickly when picked. It is recommended that they are gathered in small groups and floated on the water immediately.

Lesson
Love, interpersonal, free and without strings
Chicory is one of the three remedies that deal with the quality of love. See also Heather and Holly.

 PROPERTIES

Chicory is a cooling herb. It has a laxative and diuretic action when eaten, with a strengthening effect on the gall bladder and liver.

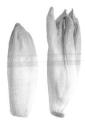

RIGHT The heart of the chicory plant, known as the chicon, is the white, closed-leaf vegetable much used in French cooking. Like its relative the dandelion, chicory has a bitter taste that stimulates digestion, and it is blanched for use in salads. Both the leaves and the long tap root are used for therapeutic purposes.

CHICORY
(CHICONS)

Actaea Racemosa (Actaea rac.) Cimicifuga racemosa, black cohosh, black snake root, bugbane

 HERBALISM

Herbalists use black cohosh as a relaxing analgesic and antispasmodic for sciatica, low back pain, neck pain, painful menstruation, intercostal neuralgia, and melancholia. It is a strong herb and should only be taken in small doses. For decoctions use half a teaspoon per cup of water twice daily, or take 2ml. of tincture three times daily. Do not use in pregnancy or when breast-feeding.

 HOMEOPATHIC

Actaea rac. is primarily a female remedy, used mostly for menstrual disorders, depression, and rheumatism.

 SYMPTOM PICTURE

Mental and Emotional Symptoms
• Depressed, overwhelmingly gloomy, feels as if a black cloud has settled over her head.
• Agitated and anxious, afraid of death, sits sighing quietly to herself.

Physical Symptoms
Rheumatism: Sore, bruised pains come on after being out in cold weather. Pains afflict opposite sides of the body, for example, a crick in the neck on one side and opposite shoulder is sore, or pain in one shoulder and opposite knee.

Headache: Pains press up and out from the top and back of her head, or from forehead to back of head. Brain feels too large. Headache is better for fresh air.

Women's complaints: Irregular, painful heavy periods. The pain starts just before the period; the more the flow of blood the greater the pain. Pains fly across the pelvis from hip to hip, the blood is profuse, dark and clotted.

Remedy Picture
• Better for fresh air, warmth, continued motion.
• Worse for cold, wet weather and at night.

Dosage: 6c
Antidote: Aconite
Complementary Remedies: None.

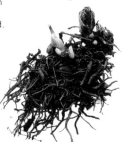

BELOW *Actaea racemosa is a perennial herb from North America. Its root was used by Native North Americans to cure snakebite and women's problems.*

BLACK COHOSH

Neroli Citrus aurantium amara

 AROMATHERAPY

Neroli is safe to use on babies and infants but avoid while pregnant. It helps hyperactive children, insomnia, and balances the nervous system when used in massage or in a bath. Burned in a room, it creates a warm and relaxing atmosphere and helps treat exhaustion and depression. It is good for heart problems, and massaged over limbs it assists varicose veins and other circulatory disorders such as palpitations, and to a lesser extent, hemorrhoids. Keep in the medicine cabinet with Dr. Bach's Rescue Remedy for treating shock and hysteria. Massaged over abdomen it will ease tummy upsets associated with stress (for example, diarrhea). A natural skin rejuvenator, it helps aging skin, broken capillaries, dry skin, and stretch marks. It combines well with other oils such as lavender, jasmine, benzoin, geranium, and clary sage.

 PROPERTIES

• Antibacterial
• Antidepressant
• Anti-infectious
• Antihypersensitive
• Antiparasitic
• Digestive tonic
• Balances the nervous system
• Regenerative

BITTER ORANGE FRUIT

 CAUTION

Avoid while pregnant

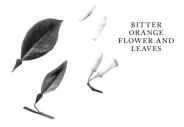

BITTER ORANGE FLOWER AND LEAVES

ABOVE *Neroli essential oil is extracted by water distillation from the freshly picked flowers. The flowers bloom on the Seville bitter orange tree, which is found in France, Italy, Morocco, Tunisia, Algeria, and the Comoro Islands. The oil is a pale yellowy color that gets darker with age. It has the most exquisite sweet, floral, exotic, light smell and is used extensively in perfumery.*

Petitgrain or Seville Bitter Orange Citrus aurantium amara

 AROMATHERAPY

Petitgrain used in massage or in a bath has a refreshing and uplifting effect on tiredness, anxiety, and stress. Massaged into the limbs it relieves the symptoms of juvenile rheumatism and osteoarthritis and soothes disorders of the nervous system. It is good for palpitations and respiratory tract infections, asthma, and panic attacks. Petitgrain is another oil that is good to keep in the medicine cabinet and to use in combination with Dr. Bach's Rescue Remedy. Petitgrain enhances hair after shampooing if used in the final rinse. It combines well with other oils such as neroli, bergamot, lavender, geranium, and rosemary.Used in a vaporizer, it helps acne and open pores. As a foot bath or massaged into swollen ankles, or calves, it can help edema. Its uplifting aroma is lovely burned in a room.

 FOOD USES

The bitter-tasting Seville orange is used to make marmalade, and its flowers to produce orange-flower water, used to flavor cakes and puddings. Eaten in these forms, in the small quantities usually consumed, Seville oranges have little medicinal benefit and are safe for general use. Those on a sucrose-restricted diet should avoid eating marmalade since it is full of sugar.

RIGHT *Petitgrain essential oil is extracted by steam distillation from the leaves and twigs of the Seville bitter orange tree, the same tree that produces the flowers for neroli oil. This tree is found in France, Italy, Morocco, Tunisia, Algeria, and the Comoro Islands. The essential oil is pale to dark yellowy color and exudes a warm, woody, flowery aroma, similar to neroli, but lighter.*

 PROPERTIES

• Antispasmodic
• Anti-infectious
• Anti-inflammatory
• Fortifies and soothes the nervous system

Contraindications
Use half the measured amount after four months of pregnancy. It is best used during pregnancy in a vaporizer or burned in the room.

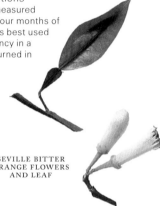

SEVILLE BITTER
ORANGE FLOWERS
AND LEAF

Bergamot Citrus bergamia

 AROMATHERAPY

Bergamot essential oil when used in massage is excellent for uplifting depression and general fatigue. It has a lovely, refreshing, sweet citrus smell. It acts as a tonic and assists the central nervous system. It restores appetite and combats colic and intestinal problems, and is good for the treatment of hemorrhoids. It can lower fever and help with bronchitis and indigestion.Bergamot acts as an antiseptic and is particularly helpful for skin conditions such as psoriasis, acne, general wounds, ulcers, scars, herpes, and seborrhea of the scalp. It has a refreshing and calming effect when used in a vaporizer or

room spray and is used extensively in eau de cologne, creams, soaps, and perfumes. It is also used in confectionery and gives Earl Grey tea its distinct flavor. Bergamot combines well with other oils such as neroli, cypress, and juniper.

 PROPERTIES

• Antiseptic
• Antispasmodic
• Analgesic
• Antidepressant
• Anti-infectious
• Antibacterial
• Relaxant

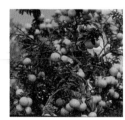

BERGAMOT

Contraindications
Care must be taken in the sun. It is better not to apply bergamot while sunbathing or in sunny climates because the essential oil increases the photosensitivity of the skin and can cause skin pigmentation.

LEFT *The bergamot tree is found in Morocco, West Africa, and in southern Italy; it produces a bitter bergamot orange fruit. The oil, which is emerald green in color, is extracted from the peel of the almost ripe fruit by cold expression.*

 CAUTION

Avoid while pregnant. Not for babies, infants, or young children.

Lemon Citrus limon

AROMATHERAPY

The essential oil is good as an inhalant or a massage for greasy skin and spots. Rub directly on to affected area for skin bites. Lemon oil can be used on the skin to treat acne and greasy skin, cold sores, spots, warts, and varicose veins. As a massage oil it can help rheumatism, arthritis, and poor circulation. Diluted with carrier oil and rubbed on the chest, or added to a steam inhalation, it can help catarrh, throat infections, asthma, and bronchitis.For colds and flu, rub lemon oil on throat and chest as a decongestant. A few drops added to the bath will reduce mental fatigue and stimulate concentration. Lemon oil can also be used in pot pourri.

FOOD USES

Lemon has many uses—culinary, therapeutic, and cosmetic—and is often regarded as something of a cure-all. It is rich in vitamin C.
The leaves and fruit of the lemon tree are used.Drink lemon juice in hot or warm water first thing in the morning as a liver tonic. Lemon juice taken in hot water will ease stomach acidity; when drunk before going to bed it may help to relieve cramp and "restless legs" syndrome. Lemons protect blood capillaries and strengthen the body's cell membranes.
Taking lemon juice with iron supplements, or foods rich in iron, increases the absorption of iron in the body. Lemon strengthens the immune system and helps relieve the symptoms of colds and flu. It can also be beneficial in the treatment of other infections. Use pure lemon juice on wasp stings in order to relieve the pain.
Lemons may be of use in treating hemorrhoids, kidney stones, and varicose veins. Lemon juice mixed with olive oil and taken internally may help to dissolve gallstones. To help cure cold sores, put a few drops of undiluted lemon juice on them several times a day. A drop of lemon juice may also benefit ulcers on the tongue and in the mouth; some people may be sensitive, so test first.

PROPERTIES

- Lemons are rich in Vitamin C (50mg. in 100g. of lemon juice) and potassium, and contain good amounts of calcium and B vitamins. They are low in sugar and sodium. Lemons are cleansing, refreshing, antiseptic, astringent, and an antioxidant.
- They have anti-inflammatory properties and aid peripheral circulation.

PROPERTIES

- Antiseptic
- Astringent
- Diuretic
- Insecticidal
- Tonic

Contraindications

- The essential oil may irritate the skin of sensitive people when the skin is exposed to sunlight (see phototoxicity, page 52).
- Lemon juice may cause mouth ulcers in sensitive people.

THE VERSATILE LEMON

The lemon is possibly the most versatile fruit we have. Its dried peel can be used to flavor cakes or as an ingredient in pot pourri. Fresh lemon juice is known as "the poor man's wine" because it can be used in place of wine in sauces and marinades. It also doubles up as a stain-remover, brightening up brass, silver, and marble and removing rust. It can also be used as a cosmetic; a lemon juice rinse will bring out the highlights in blonde hair; neat juice may diminish nicotine stains on teeth and nails, and fade freckles. A cut lemon rubbed on the hands can neutralize the smell of garlic and onions.

LEMON

LEMON SLICE

RIGHT *The lemon tree is evergreen, with serrated oval leaves and stiff thorns. It grows up to 20ft. (6m.) high and is found in southern Europe, western Asia and the southern United States. Its flowers are very fragrant. Lemon oil is extracted by cold expression from fresh peel.*

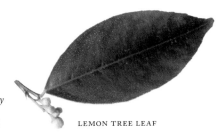

LEMON TREE LEAF

Grapefruit Citrus x paradisi

 AROMATHERAPY

In massage oil or in the bath, grapefruit oil acts as a wonderful pick-me-up and is used to treat mood swings, anger, and stress. It acts as a detoxifier to the liver—so it is great for a hangover. It acts upon the lymphatic system. It is good as a diuretic. It acts in a cleansing way, cooling down the heat of the skin, and is particularly useful for acne and cellulite. Used in steam inhalation or burned in a room, grapefruit is good for treating colds, flu, and general respiratory problems. It combines well with other oils, such as eucalyptus or pine, neroli, palmarose, lavender, and other citrus oils.

 FOOD USES

Grapefruit can be beneficial to health when eaten regularly as part of the normal diet. Drinking grapefruit juice can help promote healthy skin; it is particularly beneficial for acne, oily skin and open pores. Regular drinks of grapefruit juice help to relieve the symptoms of colds and flu and flush out the kidneys. Grapefruit as part of the daily diet may help in the treatment of osteoarthritis. Grapefrui—oil, whole fruit, and juice—may help the healing process in any complaint. Drinking grapefruit juice with iron supplements, or foods rich in iron, increases the absorption of iron in the body. Eating grapefruit is helpful for those who want to lose weight. The bitter-tasting Seville orange is used to make marmalade, and its flowers to produce orange-flower water, used to flavor cakes and puddings. Eaten in these forms, in the small quantities usually consumed, Seville oranges have little medicinal benefit and are safe for general use. Those on a sucrose-restricted diet should avoid eating marmalade since it is full of sugar.

 PROPERTIES

- Astringent
- Digestive tonic
- Balances nervous system
- Relaxant
- Detoxifier

 PROPERTIES

Grapefruit contains excellent supplies of vitamin C (about 40mg. in an average-sized fruit) and potassium. It is cleansing, refreshing and invigorating. It stimulates the circulatory system, cleanses the digestive and urinary systems, and benefits the respiratory tract.

 CONTRAINDICATIONS

- Phototoxic - take care to use half the measure if going into the sun within twelve hours of application.
- Use with care.
- Use at half measure for babies, infants, and children.
- Use at half the normal measure while pregnant.

GRAPEFRUIT AND THE LIVER

Grapefruit is particularly useful for cleansing a congested liver and curing constipation. For a homemade remedy try boiling a few thick pieces of peel and a little pulp in enough water to cover for five minutes. Strain and cool, add lemon juice and honey to taste. You can also use grapefruit oil, diluted by a carrier base, rubbed into the abdomen to help the liver.

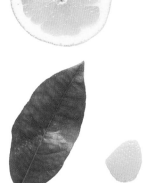

GRAPEFRUIT LEAF, PEEL, AND FRUIT

ABOVE *Grapefruit is grown extensively in the United States, South America, the Caribbean, and Israel. Grapefruit essential oil is extracted by machine expression from the peel of the ripe grapefruit. Grapefruits used vary in color, so the essential oil could be a pale yellowy-green or pale orange in color. It has a wonderful mellow, rich, fruity aroma.*

Mandarin/Tangerine Citrus reticulata

 AROMATHERAPY

It is safe to use mandarin or tangerine on babies and infants, even in massage or in a bath. The lack of toxicity means that children's tummy upsets, burps, and hiccups can be treated by massage to the tummy. Mandarine/tangerine is helpful in treating indigestion in adults and colic in children. It is also good for insomnia, hyperactivity, and stress. It reduces cellulite and acts as an excellent diuretic. Mandarin/tangerine used in a vaporizer is helpful for skin conditions such as acne and oily skin. Burned in the room it is a very relaxing and calming oil. In massage or in a bath it is a natural relaxant, calming the nervous system, especially for pregnant women and hyperactive children. It treats aches and pains well including rheumatism and is suitable for the weak and the elderly. Mandarin and tangerine combine well with oils such as lavender, geranium, neroli, and other citrus oils (lemon, grapefruit, orange, petitgrain).

 FOOD USES

Fresh mandarins and tangerines are a good source of vitamin C and as part of the daily diet may contribute to a healthy immune system.

 PROPERTIES

- Antifungal
- Antispasmodic
- Antiseptic
- Tonic
- Relaxant of central nervous system
- Dyspeptic
- Aids digestion

Contraindications
- Can cause skin irritation because of sprays used during growing, which can be transferred during extraction.

- Safe, but may trigger mouth ulcers in those who are sensitive to acid foods.

> **! CAUTION**
> Photosensitive; do not use before sunbathing.

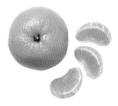

MANDARIN

ABOVE *Mandarin essential oil is extracted by machine expression from the peel of the ripe fruit. It has been used since ancient times in China and the Far East and the fruit was traditionally offered as a gift to the Mandarins. Mandarin has been grown in Europe since the early nineteenth century. The oil is an amber or orangy color and has a marvelous, uplifting, mellow, rich, orangy aroma. Tangerine is the American variety of Eastern mandarin and it is grown mainly in Florida and California. Tangerine essential oil is extracted by steam distillation from the peel of the ripe fruit. The oil is orangy in color and has a zesty, fresh, uplifting aroma.*

Sweet Orange Citrus sinensis

 AROMATHERAPY

Massaged over the stomach area, orange oil is good for constipation and flatulence. Orange is a known regulator of the digestive system, helps enhance a diet to lose weight, and can reduce cellulite. It strengthens the muscles if used in massage. It helps prevent travel sickness. Burned in a room, or used in a bath, its natural uplifting aroma helps relieve stress, anxiety, and depression and soothes nervous headaches. Used in a vaporizer, orange refreshes. As a mouthwash, it can be used to treat gum disease and mouth ulcers.

 CHILDREN

Orange oil is safe to use on babies and children. When used in massage, orange will help a colicky baby and is good for the skin. Helps reduce fever and headaches.

 FOOD USES

Oranges are an excellent source of vitamin C, and as a regular part of the diet can help boost the body's immune system.

 PROPERTIES

- Mild sedative
- Febrifuge—reduces fever
- Antispasmodic
- Antidepressant
- Stomachic
- Reinforces the immune system

SWEET ORANGE

RIGHT *Orange essential oil is extracted by machine expression from the orange peel. The orange tree originally came from China, but can now be found widely across the world, particularly in Spain, Portugal, Cyprus, Brazil, and the United States. The oil is a pale yellow or pale brown color and gives off a zesty, fresh, uplifting aroma.*

Clematis Clematis vitalba

 FLOWER ESSENCE

Clematis, one of the twelve healers, relates to indifference and gentleness, and is for those who are not sufficiently interested in present circumstances—who are dreamy, drowsy, and not fully awake. Sometimes they daydream or fantasize about a utopian future. Clematis people prefer to live in the mind, or the spirit, rather than deal with contemporary issues and everyday life. Airy and impractical individuals, sometimes pale and lacking in vitality and ambition, they are sensitive and sometimes need lots of sleep.

 METHOD

The Sun Method *(see page 42)*
Clematis flowers in summer and early fall. Gather separate flowers by their stalks. Pick from many different plants, and from different parts of the plants.

Lesson
Being present, awake, and fully grounded
• The positive Clematis brings lightness into everyday reality.
• Clematis is also useful for those suffering from boredom.
• Honeysuckle is the other remedy that deals with time.

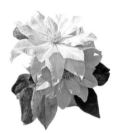

ABOVE *Clematis is a rambling, deciduous, perennial climber of woods, waysides, and country hedges. The common name is "old man's beard" because of the wispy seed heads. Clematis is a popular garden plant for a sunny wall.*

Cocculus (Cocc.) Cocculus indicus, Anaminta cocculus, Indian cockle seed, Levant nut, fish berry

 HOMEOPATHIC

Cocculus is very useful for travel sickness and extreme states of exhaustion. It can be used for people who need their sleep, become wornout and exhausted from late nights or disturbed sleep-patterns and then suffer insomnia—a vicious cycle. Cocculus is also a good choice when food or the thought of food stimulates nausea and vomiting, where there is vertigo, blurred vision, and heavy, painful and stiff limbs.

 SYMPTOM PICTURE

Mental and Emotional Symptoms
• Very stressed and irritable due to loss of sleep or from grief or anger, mind goes blank, cannot remember things. May be trembly with stress.
• Time passes too quickly.

Physical Symptoms
Exhaustion: Wornout, weak, and trembly, through lack of sleep, hard work or emotional stress. Back feels weak and stiff, head feels too heavy, and legs tremble when walking. Arms and legs go to sleep easily causing numbness or pins and needles. Worse sitting-up; need to lie down in bed to gather strength.

Travel sickness: Car-sick, sea-sick—sights flashing before the eyes brings on nausea, which is felt in the mouth and head. Has to turn head to look, not move his or her eyes. May vomit and have a sick headache in the forehead or back of head. Has to lie down. Worse for the thought or smell of food.

Headache: From lack of sleep, exhaustion, headache felt in forehead, back of head with sensation of opening and shutting, or nape of neck. Feels empty-headed, has to lie down but cannot rest on back of head—head too tender.

Remedy Picture
• Cocculus people are worse for loss of sleep, movement, talking, fresh air. They sweat easily all over their body from exertion—a slight sweat. They tremble from exhaustion.

• Worse for sight and smell of food, coffee, tobacco smoke.

• Better for lying still in bed, for adequate sleep.

Dosage: 6c
Antidotes: Coffee, Nux vom

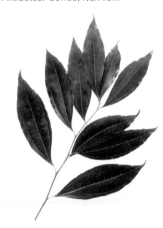

ABOVE *Cocculus indicus, also known as Anaminta cocculus, is a native plant of India and Sri Lanka. Its berries contain a powerful anesthetic agent.*

Codonopsis Root Codonopsis pilosula, dang shen

 HERBALISM

For general debility, exhaustion, weakness, lack of appetite, chronic diarrhea, excessive perspiration, acidity, chronic coughs, asthma, and shortness of breath. It can be used as a decoction, tincture, or a powder sprinkled on food.

 PROPERTIES

• Soothing and strengthening

• An immune system tonic

Codonopsis is also called Dang shen in Chinese herb shops. It is often referred to as the poor man's ginseng.

Contraindications
• Safe but best used for long-term debility.
• Use other herbs in acute conditions.

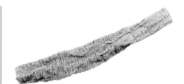

ABOVE *Codonopsis is a sprawling herb with yellow, bell-shaped flowers; it is grown in China.*

Coffea Cruda (Coff.) Coffea arabica, coffee

 HOMEOPATHIC

Coffee is stimulating and causes insomnia in many people. Homeopathically Coffea is used to treat insomnia in people who are sensitive to emotion, overjoyed by good news, cannot unwind and go to sleep—the mind is wide awake and active, despite being physically tired. It may help to settle overexcited, sleepless children and nervous, excited, overstimulated people. It is also useful for PMS, but persistent PMS needs professional assessment. Think of Coffea as a remedy when looking at a person who lives on their nerves, is a workaholic, and heading for "burn-out."

 SYMPTOM PICTURE

Mental and Emotional Symptoms
Insomnia: Wakes at 3 a.m. and cannot get back to sleep. Agitated and restless.

Physical Symptoms
Headache: From overstimulation or exhaustion from insomnia. Tight pain as if a nail is driven into the head. Sensitive hearing, aware of every little noise.

• Coffee (and Coffea the remedy) is thought to antidote and stop or even reverse the action of many homeopathic remedies, so if you are sensitive to coffee you should not drink it while being treated homeopathically. If you have had a bad aggravation from a remedy, or if you have tried with little effect to treat yourself with several remedies, drinking a cup of strong black coffee can antidote them and clear your symptom picture.

Women's symptoms: Menstrual periods start too early and last too long. Large black clots, stabbing, flitting, cramping pains.

Remedy Picture
• Worse for extreme joy and elation, strong smells, noise, night, outdoors.
• Better for warmth, lying down.

Dosage: 6c
Antidotes: Aconite, Merc., Pulsatilla, Chamomilla, Nux vom., Sulfur
Complementary Remedy: Aconite; give before Coffea if well indicated.

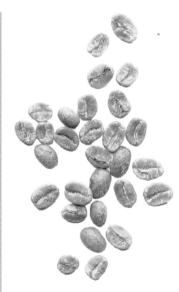

ABOVE *Berries from the coffee tree Coffea arabica are the source of the homeopathic remedy Coffea. They are left unroasted.*

Myrrh Commiphora myrrha

 HERBALISM

In herbalism, myrrh tincture is used as a powerful antiseptic and astringent. Tinctures are weaker than essential oils and may be applied directly to infected cuts or mouth ulcers —it stings but heals very quickly. Use 10 to 15 drops in a little water for infections, especially of the digestive tract. Avoid in pregnancy.

 AROMATHERAPY

Myrrh oil used in massage or in a bath is strengthening, balancing, and antiseptic. It is good for treating athlete's foot, gangrene, fungal infections, and ringworm and combines well with other oils such as lavender, frankincense, sandalwood, sage, and citrus oils. It has a good effect on the digestive system, and if massaged over the abdomen, helps chills, diarrhea, and dysentery. Used in a vaporizer, it is excellent for chronic lung conditions, bronchitis, and laryngitis. Although bitter to the taste, it is an excellent mouthwash for mouth ulcers, bleeding gums, pyorrhea, bad breath, and sore throats. As a vaginal douche, myrrh helps thrush and is also helpful in the treatment of viral hepatitis. Used on a wound in the form of a compress or as a lotion, it will help aging skin and skin infections.

 PROPERTIES

- Anti-inflammatory
- Antiviral
- Anti-infectious
- Antiseptic
- Regenerative
- Aphrodisiac
- Decongestant
- Parasiticide
- Moderator of thyroid action

Contraindication
Use at half measure externally only or burned in the room while pregnant.

> ⚠ CAUTION
> Not for babies and infants

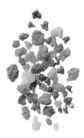

MYRRH

ABOVE Myrrh essential oil is extracted by steam distillation from the resin that exudes from cracks and incisions made in the bark of the myrrh tree. The tree is small, tough and spiny and grows in Libya, Iran, and by the Red Sea. Since ancient times, it has been used by the Egyptians for its rejuvenating properties and in embalming. It has been used by the Chinese in medicine for arthritic and dermatological problems. The sticky oil is a dark amber to dark red color and has a warm, smoky, bittersweet aroma.

Hawthorn Crataegus oxyacantha, Crataegus monogyna

 HERBALISM

Hawthorn is the herb for the heart. Use the tea, tincture, or tablets for heart failure (weak heart with poor circulation and breath—lessness, usually in elderly people). Persist for at least six months. Restorative after heart attacks. Settles irregular heartbeats. It is helpful for angina and high blood pressure, as part of an overall strategy. It may safely be used with orthodox drugs (except digoxin) and taken over some months will usually reduce the need for drugs. It is especially helpful taken with yarrow and linden flowers or used with nervine herbs such as valerian and linden flowers for anxiety with palpitations. Hawthorn helps to mend a "broken heart."

 PROPERTIES

- Strengthens the heart, lowers blood pressure, relaxes arteries, calming.

Notes and dosages
- Flowering tops and berries are commercially available as tea, tincture, or tablets.
- For tablets follow the directions on the box. For tincture take one teaspoon in a little water twice daily.
- For heart disease take this dosage for at least six months. For stress affecting the heart, carry a dropper bottle of the tincture with you and take ten drops when needed.

Contraindications
It may make allopathic heart drugs such as digoxin or digitoxin overpowerful but is otherwise safe to use with orthodox drugs.

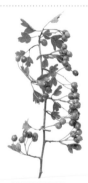

HAWTHORN BERRIES

LEFT The hawthorn or May is a small tree very common in the wild and much grown in parks and gardens. It flowers in May (hence the country name). The berries or flowering tops are used in herbalism.

> CAUTION
> Do not reduce drugs for heart problems or blood pressure without telling your physician.

Colocynthis (Coloc.) Cucumis colocynthis, Citrullus colocynthis, bitter cucumber

HOMEOPATHIC

Use for nerve pains brought about by anger with indignation. The pains are severe and give rise to paroxysms. There may be extremely violent cramping pains in the abdomen, which feel better for hard pressure.

SYMPTOM PICTURE

Mental and Emotional Symptoms
• Quick-tempered, haughty people who suffer ill-effects of anger.

Physical Symptoms
Gastrointestinal tract: Severe colic, cutting bruised pain, as if stones are being ground together in abdomen. Pain makes the person restless and writhe around. Vomit and diarrhea from pain. Wants to press hands hard into abdomen. For colicky babies who draw their knees up to their chest and scream with pain. *Headache:* One-sided headache, boring pain, sore scalp, pain behind eye and in forehead.

• Better for pressure and warmth. Worse for stooping.

Women's symptoms: Ovarian pain: Boring pain, restless, causes her to bend double. Better for hard pressure. Neuralgia: Severe sharp, boring pains that follow a nerve and come on after indignant anger. Great restlessness, scream with pain, better for warmth and hard pressure.

Remedy Picture
• Better for strong pressure, warmth.
• Worse for rest.

Dosage: 6c
Antidotes: Camphor, Coffea Complementary *Remedies:*Bryonia, Merc., Nux vom., Pulsatilla follow well.

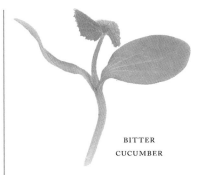

BITTER CUCUMBER

ABOVE *Leaves from the bitter cucumber, a member of the gourd family. A native of the eastern Mediterranean area, it is also known as the bitter apple, and its fruit is poisonous.*

Cypress Cupressus sempervirens

AROMATHERAPY

When used as a massage oil, in steam inhalations, or burning in a room, cypress acts on the nervous system and aids tension and stress. It is excellent for menopausal problems. Massaged over the limbs, it assists varicose veins and broken capillaries. It acts as a diuretic and assists with problems of the bladder, diarrhea, and hemorrhages. It can be used effectively in treating hay fever, asthma, coughs, and bronchitis. Used in a bath, it acts as a relaxant and an astringent. Cypress is one of the safest oils to use.

PROPERTIES
• Antirheumatic
• Antispasmodic (coughs)
• Diuretic
• Menopausal
• Circulatory (varicose veins)
• Detoxifying

Contraindications
For infants and children, use with care (dotted on a pillow perhaps) to relieve breathing problems.

CAUTION

• Do not use on very young babies
• Avoid during pregnancy

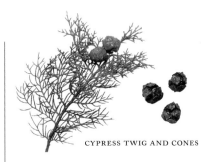

CYPRESS TWIG AND CONES

ABOVE *The evergreen cypress tree is found in France, Italy, Corsica, Portugal, Spain, and North Africa. In Ancient Egypt it was known for its medicinal properties, and in Tibet cypress is still used in incense. The essential oil is extracted by steam distillation from the leaves, twigs, and needles, and the oil is a pale yellow or green color that has a marvelous fresh pine aroma.*

Lemongrass Cymbopogon citratus

 AROMATHERAPY

Lemongrass is the oil for sportsmen and women. In massage or in a bath it aids aching muscles and strains and is a deodorizer and cooler. Burned in a room, it is an excellent remedy for nervous exhaustion and stress. Massaged over the abdomen, it helps to soothe gastric infections, colitis, and enteritis. Lemongrass combines well with other oils, such as eucalyptus, rosemary, vetivert, geranium and lavender.Used in a vaporizer, it opens pores, and treats acne and blackheads. Lemongrass, like its cousin citronella, is widely used as an insect repellent against mosquitoes and fleas, it helps to eliminate lice, scabies, and ticks, and works wonders by keeping spraying cats at bay.

 FOOD USES

Lemongrass leaves can be infused to make a tea. The leaf stems are used in Asian cooking, particularly Thai recipes, to flavor food. Children with digestive problems will benefit from drinking the tea.

 PROPERTIES

- Digestive suggestion
- Antidepressant
- Tonic
- Antiseptic
- Prasiticide

Contraindication
Avoid on damaged or very sensitive skin.

(!) CAUTION

- Do not overuse
- Do not use while pregnant
- Not for babies, infants, or small children

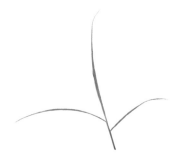

ABOVE *Lemongrass essential oil is obtained by steam distillation from the chopped grass. Two types of grass are used—West and East Indian—and the oil is either an amber or pale yellow color. It has a refreshing, pungent, lemony aroma.*

Palmarosa Cymbopogon martinii var. martini

 AROMATHERAPY

Palmarosa is a natural balancer; in a bath it helps to calm the nervous system and it is enjoyable and soothing if burned in a room. In massage, it has been used to assist both ME and anorexia nervosa sufferers. It aids digestion. Massaged over the stomach, it can relieve symptoms of gastroenteritis, diarrhea, and dysentery. It works well in conjunction with antibiotics in treating fungal conditions in the intestine. Used in a vaporizer or as a compress, it helps skin problems, opens pores, treats acne, acts as an astringent for oily skin, and has natural rejuvenating properties for aging and wrinkled skin. It is good for stretch marks. Palmarosa combines well with other oils such as bergamot, rose, cedarwood, geranium, citrus oils, ylang ylang, and other floral oils.

PROPERTIES

- Antibacterial
- Antiviral
- Aphrodisiac
- Antifungal
- Regenerative
- Aids the nervous system
- Tonic

(!) CAUTION

- Not for babies
- Avoid while pregnant

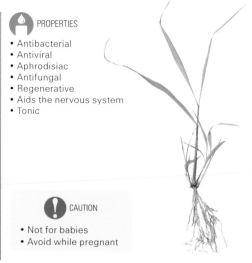

LEFT *Palmarosa essential oil is extracted by steam or water distillation. It is a member of the grass family, a cousin of citronella and lemongrass, and the whole plant is used. Found originally in India, it is also grown today in Indonesia, Africa, and Brazil. The oil is either a pale green or pale yellow color and has a soft, soothing, cozy aroma. Palmarosa is much used in the perfume industry.*

Wild Yam Dioscorea villosa

 HERBALISM

A decoction or tincture is useful for stomach cramps, nausea, vomiting, hiccups, recurrent colicky pains, pain of diverticulitis, and gallbladder pains. Use with a little ginger for a quicker action. Wild Yam is useful for period pain, pain on ovulation, menopausal symptoms, and vaginal dryness. Use it with willow bark and cramp bark for rheumatoid arthritis.

 HOMEOPATHIC

The homeopathic Dioscorea is used for abdominal and renal colic and severe period pains.

 CAUTION

Do not use in pregnancy except under professional guidance for specific problems

 PROPERTIES

• Anti-inflammatory
• Antispasmodic
• Relaxes tension

Notes and Dosages
• Standard doses *(see pages 22-23)*.

• Works especially well on persistent and recurrent problems.

• Wild yam is the starting point for synthesization of hormones for the contraceptive pill and for "natural progesterone," used in a prescription cream for the menopause.

• Wild yam itself is a safe, gentle remedy without side effects.

• A good example of the herbalist's maxim that the whole plant is safer than any extracts. It is used as a contraceptive,

although it is not as reliable as conventional methods.

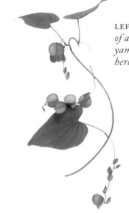

LEFT *The rhizome of a Mexican wild yam is used in herbalism.*

Drosera (Dros.) Drosera rotundifolia, round- leaved sundew

 HERBALISM

Drosera is called sundew in herbal medicine and its uses are the same as in homeopathy. It is considered especially good for whooping cough. Use 1 teaspoon of dried herb to a cup of water and take half a cup three times daily or as needed.

 HOMEOPATHIC

Drosera is used homeopathically for rheumatism, bronchitis, and whooping cough.

 SYMPTOM PICTURE

Mental and Emotional Symptoms
• Restless, uneasy, sad and anxious, frightened.

Physical Symptoms
Rheumatism: Drawing, shooting pains felt in the bones ending in stitching joint pains. The bed feels too hard.

• Severe night sweats all over, yet shivering at rest.

Coughs: Tickling deep in the throat leads to coughing fit. Deep, dry, hacking spasmodic coughs that follow each other rapidly (in paroxysms) and may end with a whoop and vomiting.

• The coughs may follow each other so closely the child cannot breathe and becomes blue in the face during the attack.

Remedy Picture
Worse after midnight, for talking, laughing, eating and drinking, and lying down.

Dosage
For whooping cough (pertussis) give one dose of Drosera 30c if indicated and wait

seven to nine days, by which time they should be better.

Antidotes: Drosera is antidoted by camphor so do not use ointments, chest-rubs, or inhalations that contain camphor.

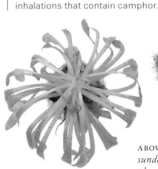

ROUND-LEAVED SUNDEW

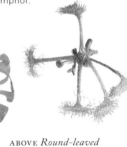

ABOVE *Round-leaved sundew is an insectivorous plant that thrives in a boggy habitat. The whole plant is used for both herbal and homeopathic remedies.*

Echinacea Echinacea purpurea

 HERBALISM

Echinacea is a versatile remedy, very useful for a weak immune system with chronic tiredness and susceptibility to minor infections.

Decoction or tincture for boils, acne, food poisoning, duodenal ulcers, flu, tonsillitis, shingles, herpes, and persistent infections of all kinds. Combine with sage for chronic infections in the mouth and throat and to combat the fatigue following viral infections. Use echinacea with milk thistle seed for chronic hepatitis and tiredness following glandular fever; with marigold or burdock root for boils, and skin and pelvic infections; with damiana for herpes, prostatitis, and chronic cystitis; with garlic for persistent colds and minor infections. It makes a good gargle and mouthwash for oral infections such as sore throats, tonsillitis, mouth ulcers, gum infections, and tooth abscesses. Use it as wash for infected wounds and rashes, purulent spots, and pimples.

 HOMEOPATHIC

Traditionally echinacea is used in homeopathy for blood-poisonings; severe infections from snake-bites to gangrene when there is pus and rotting flesh. Choose it if there is depressed immunity with depressed spirits; weakness, tiredness, and aching; fevers with chills and nausea. It is useful for boils, pustular acne, infected cuts, ulcerated tonsillitis, colds, and influenza.

 PROPERTIES

• Antiseptic
• Anti-inflammatory
• Stimulates the immune system

Notes and Dosages
• Echinacea may be taken by itself for acute conditions but is best combined with other herbs for long-standing conditions.

• For acute conditions take large doses, a quarter of a cup of the decoction or one teaspoon of the tincture every two hours for up to ten days.

• For food poisoning double this dosage.

• For chronic conditions use in combinations and take ½ a cup of the combined decoction or 1 teaspoon of the combined tincture, three times daily.

• Echinacea tablets and combination tablets are available, follow the instructions.

• Echinacea and garlic tablets are especially useful.

 DOSAGE

10-30 drops mother tincture three to six times a day.

Contraindications
Severe immune weakness should be treated by a professional.

RIGHT *A beautiful, purple daisy, native to America and sometimes grown in English gardens. The root is used in herbalism. Echinacea is also known as purple cone flower.*

Siberian Ginseng Eleutherococcus senticosus

 HERBALISM

Esiberian ginseng is similar to Chinese ginseng but less likely to be overstimulating. The decoction, tablets, or tincture are useful for dealing with prolonged stress. Use for digestive weakness, especially with diarrhea and lack of appetite; it is also helpful for rheumatism and rheumatoid arthritis.

 CHILDREN

Over five: It is suitable as a tonic for persistent infections and classroom stress. Use half the adult dose. Ten drops of tincture, in pure fruit juice twice daily, is suitable.

 PROPERTIES

• Replenishes vital energy
• Strengthens the immune system
• An adaptogen
• Improves appetite
• Antirheumatic

Notes and Dosages
• This remedy was popularized by the Russians who use it during cosmonaut training. It is cheaper than Chinese ginseng and just as good a tonic in stress and prolonged illness.
• Dosage as for Chinese ginseng *(see page 186)*
• Tablets are easily available; follow the instructions on the box.

Contraindications
Best not taken continuously. A two-week break every two months is recommended.

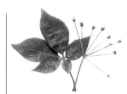

LEFT *Siberian ginseng is a shrubby member of the ginseng family, found in China, Japan, and Siberia.*

 CAUTION

• Do not take in pregnancy except with expert advice
• Do not take with tea or coffee
• Avoid in high blood pressure

Horsetail Equisetum arvense

 HERBALISM

Use a decoction, tincture, or hip bath for chronic bladder infections, irritable bladder with urgent or constant desire to pass water; blood in the urine (consult your physician); incontinence of urine. Horsetail, taken as a decoction, strengthens nails and hair and speeds healing of deep wounds and surgical wounds. Use a decoction with equal part of crushed saw palmetto berries for prostatitis and bladder problems associated with a swollen prostate. Use as a compress for infected and weepy skin conditions.

 CHILDREN

Use for bedwetting, with equal parts of cramp bark or St. John's wort.

 PROPERTIES

- Styptic
- Diuretic
- Strengthens the bladder
- Rich source of minerals
- Restores elasticity to tissue

Notes and Dosages

The healing and restorative properties of horsetail are due to its high content of silica, selenium, and zinc. To extract a sufficient quantity of the minerals, make a slow decoction by simmering 1 teaspoon in 2 cups of water for at least half an hour. Drink this amount twice daily for one month. Make up a pitcherful at a time and keep it in the refrigerator.

Contraindications

Always seek medical advice before starting home treatment if you have blood in the urine.

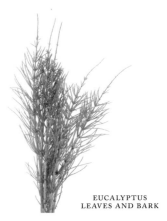

EUCALYPTUS LEAVES AND BARK

ABOVE *Horsetail is a common weed found on damp ground. The dried stems and branches are used in herbalism.*

Eucalyptus Eucalyptus globulus

 HERBALISM

Eucalyptus leaves may be used as a tea for coughs, colds, and fevers. Historically, herbalists considered it specific for malaria and other fevers endemic to swampy areas. A strong decoction of the leaves can be used for cleaning sores. Crush the leaves from the garden eucalyptus and inhale the vapor as a quick treatment for colds and sinus problems.

 AROMATHERAPY

Eucalyptus is a very antiseptic oil and is excellent when used as an inhalation for pneumonia, bronchitis, asthma, colds, flu, mucous congestion, sinusitis, and tuberculosis. Also effective as a room spray, on a burner, or in a bath. Eucalyptus combines well with other oils such as pine, lemon, marjoram, and cedarwood. When used in massage, eucalyptus is good for

rheumatic conditions, in diabetes, and in cases of cystitis. The antibiotic properties are helpful in the treatment of skin infections, herpes, and dabbed on with a Q-tip will help stop the irritation of insect bites and stings. Is helpful in the treatment of ulcers and herpes. Eucalyptus will also help the treatment of lice, athlete's foot, and other fungal infections of the skin.

 PROPERTIES

- Antiseptic
- Antirheumatic
- Antineuralgic
- Vermifuge—gets rid of worms
- Febrifuge—lowers temperature
- Balsamic expectorant

Contraindications

- Use in a room for babies and infants in assisting breathing problems.

- Safe to use at half the amount for babies, infants, and children.

- Use at half the amount while pregnant.

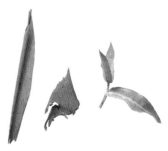

ABOVE *The eucalyptus tree is also known as gum tree, and there are more than three hundred varieties. Only fifteen varieties are used in the steam distillation of this pale yellow, woody, camphor-smelling essential oil; both the leaves and older branches are used. Eucalyptus is one of the most important essential oils available.*

 CAUTION

Do not use the essential oil internally; it is toxic.

Euphrasia (Euphr) Euphrasia officinalis, eyebright

 HERBALISM

In herbal medicine, euphrasia is known as eyebright and is used for much the same conditions as in homeopathy. Eyebright tea, well strained, makes an especially useful eyewash. Drunk regularly it is said to strengthen eyesight. Capsules of powdered eyebright are a very effective remedy for hay fever. Carry them with you and take two whenever needed.

 HOMEOPATHIC

Use for the eyes and nose where there are acrid tears and eye discharge, bland nasal discharge. It is also very effective for catarrh and the headaches brought on by excess catarrh, if the rest of the remedy picture fits.

 PROPERTIES

- Anticatarrhal
- Anti-inflammatory
- Astringent
- Tonic

Notes and Dosages
- Infusion—three times a day
- Tincture—three times a day

 SYMPTOM PICTURE

Physical Symptoms
Conjunctivitis: Eyelids puffy with red margins. Eyes red, burn and sting, feel gritty. Watery eyes, yellow pus. Tears and discharge burn and irritate the skin around the eyes.
Hay fever and colds: Bland nasal discharge, sneezes, eyes hot, and irritated with burning tears.
Measles: At onset of illness, before or just as rash appears with above eye and nose symptoms.
Tired eyes: Refreshes and brightens the eyes and strengthens the eye muscles.

Remedy Picture
- Worse—evening, indoors, warmth, light
- Better—in the dark
- They cannot get warm and suffer from catarrhal headaches

Dosage: 6c
Antidotes: Camphor, Pulsatilla
Complementary Remedies: None

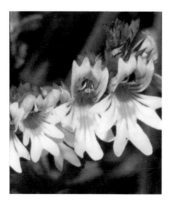

ABOVE *Eyebright is an annual plant that grows 2–8in. (5–20cm.) high and produces small white flowers dappled with yellow and purple in the late summer. It is semiparasitic on grass.*

EUPHRASIA EYE COMPRESS
Mix one teaspoonful dried Euphrasia into 1pt. water and boil for ten minutes. Let the liquid cool to hand heat, then soak a compress of gauze or absorbent cotton in it. Wring out excess fluid and place the compress over the eyes. Leave for fifteen minutes and repeat three or four times a day.

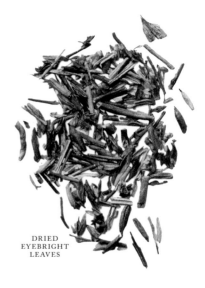

DRIED EYEBRIGHT LEAVES

CULPEPER'S EYEBRIGHT
Euphrasia, known commonly as eyebright, was familiar to the great herbalist Nicholas Culpeper. In his *Complete Herbal*, he points out that it is ruled by the sun, comes under the zodiac sign of Leo, and "helps all infirmities of the eyes that cause dimness of sight... it has restored sight to them that have been blind a long time before." The juice could be dropped into the eyes, or taken in wine or soup, or the flowers could be made into jam, all with the same powerful effect.

Beech Fagus sylvatica

 HERBALISM

Beech is one of the remedies for those who over-care for the welfare of others. Dr. Bach says that this remedy is for "those who feel the need to see more good and beauty in all that surrounds them." It is for people who judge and criticize. Beech is overdependent on the environment, which never matches the Beech type's inner perfection. They feel unsupported and unappreciated, which leads to dissatisfaction, criticism, and intolerance. Beech is especially useful for Impatiens and Chicory types. It can also be used to lighten the arrogance found with Vervain.

 METHOD

The Boiling Method *(see page 43)*
• Male and female flowers are found on the same tree. They bloom in spring. Male flowers hang in silky clusters below the new leaf growth.

• Female flowers are covered with scales that later develop into the covering for the beech nut. Pick young shoots, 6in. (15cm.) long, with newly opened leaves and male and female flowers. Gather from as many trees as possible.

Lesson
Empathy and tolerance

Beauty is not a static perfection but a celebration of uniqueness. Beauty surrounds us. Beech fills hearts with empathy and opens eyes to see beauty without judgment—to accept the self and appreciate that we are all individuals with different attitudes and methods for dealing with the world.

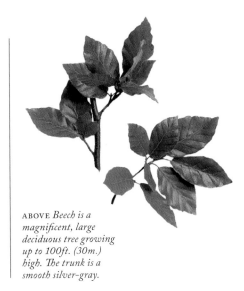

ABOVE *Beech is a magnificent, large deciduous tree growing up to 100ft. (30m.) high. The trunk is a smooth silver-gray.*

Meadowsweet Filipendula ulmaria

 HERBALISM

Use the tea for an acid stomach, heartburn, and ulcers. It combines well with comfrey, marshmallow, and chamomile. Persist. Use the tea or tincture with peppermint or chamomile for indigestion and wind. Meadowsweet is helpful for rheumatism and arthritis. It clears sandy deposits in the urine.

 CHILDREN

Excellent for summer diarrhea and summer fevers with an upset stomach.

 PROPERTIES

• Antacid
• Astringent
• Anti-inflammatory
• Diuretic
• Calming for overactive digestive systems

Notes and Dosages
• Half dosages for children and elderly people.

• Will give quick relief for stomach pains but best results come from long-term use.

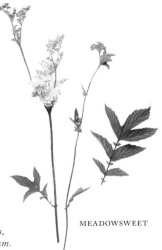

RIGHT *Meadowsweet is a wild plant common in damp meadows. The leaves, stalks, and flowers are used in herbalism.*

MEADOWSWEET

Fennel Foeniculum vulgare

 HERBALISM USES FOR SEEDS

Use the tea or tincture for colic, wind, and irritable bowel conditions. Fennel is very effective at increasing milk. It passes into the milk, winding the baby at the same time. Use fennel and sage tea or tincture to soothe premenstrual breast pain. It is soothing for anxiety and. disturbed spirits in general. Fennel is a diuretic and cleansing herb, helpful for people with arthritis and water retention. Chewing the seeds is a quick way to settle a rumbly stomach. Traditionally they were eaten during fasts or to help people lose weight. Fennel tea makes a good eyewash for conjunctivitis.

 CHILDREN

Suitable for colic in infants; give the tea in teaspoon doses, as much as they will take, or add 2 teaspoons to milk formulas.

 FOOD USES

Fennel is beneficial for ailments of the respiratory systems, particularly for coughs and colds, fennel tea is a useful remedy for flatulence. It is particularly effective when made with equal quantities of caraway and aniseed. Fennel improves the function of the liver. The root is used as a diuretic.

 ESSENTIAL OIL/AROMATHERAPY

The oil is used in the manufacture of toothpaste, soap, and gripe water, and is recommended for the relief of bronchial congestion.

 PROPERTIES

• A gentle warming herb for digestive problems
• Carminative
• Antispasmodic
• Clears wind
• Promotes milk flow in nursing mothers
• Lifts the spirits

Notes and Dosages
• Fennel seed tea bags are easily available – remember to cover the cup to avoid losing any goodness in the steam.

• Fennel seeds and leaf are used in sauces for fish and mushrooms.

• Florence fennel bulbs (Foeniculum vulgare var. dulce), eaten as a vegetable or in salads, are helpful as part of a regime for arthritis.

Contraindications
• The small amounts used in cooking and Florence fennel are quite safe.

• Fennel oil can produce an adverse reaction in certain circumstances.

 CAUTION

• Do not take large amounts in early pregnancy
• Do not take the fennel and sage combination during pregnancy
• Avoid fennel if you suffer from chronic gastrointestinal ailments

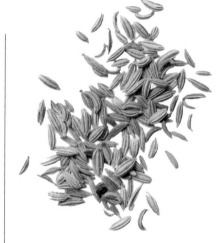

FENNEL SEEDS

ABOVE & BELOW *Fennel is an aromatic herb with culinary, cosmetic, and medicinal uses. It is a pretty border plant with feathery leaves. The seeds and leaves are used to flavor food; the white and green leaf base is eaten as a vegetable.*

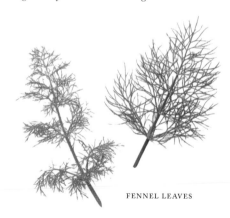

FENNEL LEAVES

Bladderwrack Fucus vesiculosus, kelp

HERBALISM

Use the powder, capsules, or tablets for obesity with tiredness and dry skin, low thyroxine levels, and simple goiter. Use as a nourishing tonic especially in cases of poor absorption due to digestive problems and for people who are not eating properly. It can also help cellulite, chronic dry skin conditions, chronically swollen lymph nodes, stubborn constipation, and pain in the groin and testicles. Regular use will often delay the progress of arthritis and hardening of the arteries. A good tonic for old age. Use in the bath for dry skin problems and rheumtism.

CHILDREN

Bladderwrack can help children with slow mental and physical development, and those who have a constitution weakness.

PROPERTIES

• Nourishing and soothing

• Stimulates the thyroid gland

• Contains iodine and many other useful minerals

Notes and dosages
• The familiar "popping" seaweed of childhood vacations, also called kelp. If you are gathering seaweed from the beach, make sure you have the identification correct and avoid dirty beaches and those near sewer outlets.

• For tablets take one three times a day, or follow the instructions on the package.

• For powder take one or two teaspoons daily, sprinkled onto cooked meals or stirred into soups.

• For tea drink one or two cups a day—allow a long infusion.

• Half doses for children.

• Bladderwrack contains iodine, sodium, calcium, iron, manganese, sulfur, silica, zinc, and copper.

Contraindications
Not recommended for children under five.at a time and keep it in the refrigerator.

CAUTION

• Do not use for overactive thyroid
• Avoid the baths in weepy skin conditions and fevers

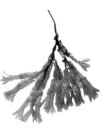

RIGHT *Bladderwrack is a black or lark brown seaweed common around coasts.*

Gelsemium (Gels.) Gelsemium sempervirens, false jasmine, yellow jasmine, Carolina jasmine

HOMEOPATHIC

Heaviness and weakness run through this remedy. It is a useful remedy for reactions following fear or embarrassment, delayed shock, and for anticipation of an unpleasant ordeal. Thick headaches often indicate a need for gelsemium.

SYMPTOM PICTURE

Mental and Emotional Symptoms
The person feels mentally dull and stupid, becomes paralyzed with fear, seizes up with anxiety before exams, driving tests, public speaking. May have diarrhea from fear and tremble with anxiety.

Physical Symptoms
Influenza: Feels heavy as if weighted down. Everything aches, eyeballs, head, limbs. Chills run up and down spine, shivery. Fever with heat and chills alternating. Thirstless. Trembles with exhaustion.

Headache: Heavy, tight headache, starts in the back of the head, spreads up into forehead. Better for copious urination.

Measles: Dark red mottled face, drowsy with above symptoms.

Remedy Picture
• Complaints come on slowly over a few days.

• Affected parts feel heavy and weak.

• Worse for warm, humid weather, exertion, afternoon, sun-heat, emotional stress.

• Better for rest, urinating.

• Thirstless

Dosages: 6c or 30c
Antidotes: Coffea
Complementary Remedies: None

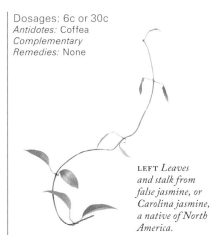

LEFT *Leaves and stalk from false jasmine, or Carolina jasmine, a native of North America.*

Gentian Gentiana lutea, Gentianella amarella

 HERBALISM

Gentian root is the best-known bitter tonic in herbal medicine. Usually the yellow gentian (Gentiana luted) is used, but all gentians have the same property. Often added to nervines for nervous exhaustion and used on its own for indigestion. It is especially good for low stomach acidity. Avoid in acid indigestion.

 HOMEOPATHIC

Gentian lutea is used in homeopathy as at tonic to restore appetite during illness or convalescence.

 FLOWER ESSENCE

Gentian, one of the twelve healers, relates to discouragement, doubt, and understanding. It is one of the remedies for those who suffer uncertainty. The source is Gentianella (*Gentianella amarella*). Gentian people are prone to negativity and are therefore easily discouraged. When everything is going well they are happy, but at the slightest problem they become disheartened and think "Is it worth it? Whatever I do I always lose." They lack heart and courage.

 METHOD

The Sun Method (see page 42)
• Gentian blooms as purplish-blue flowers in the fall. As with all delicate flowers, they should be handled as little as possible.

• Pick the flowers just below the calyx and float them on the water immediately. Pick from a wide area, and keep going until the surface of the water is completely covered.

Lesson
Courage to accept what is
To understand that life is not a competition and that there is no failure when trying our best. The positive Gentian types take responsibility for their own life and thoughts; they can be a solid rock of strength, their faith being a comfort and example to others.

 PROPERTIES

• Stimulates appetite
• Activates sluggish digestion
• Cleanses the liver
• Tonic for the system

Notes and Dosages
Herbal remedies are made from the dried, sliced root of Gentiana lutea. It combines well with ginger and cardamom.

Decoction
Make a decoction using teaspoon shredded root to one cup of water. Boil for 5 minutes. Drink 15 minutes before a meal, or whenever indigestion from overindulgence strikes.

Tincture
Take ½-1 teaspoon three times a day for sluggish indigestion.

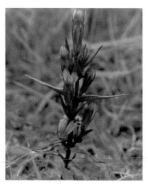

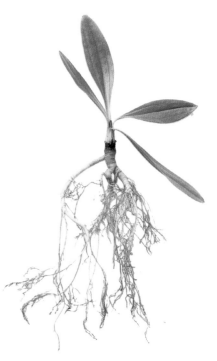

ABOVE & LEFT *Gentian is a small plant native to dry hills and dunes from 6 to 12in. (15–30cm.) in height. The stem is square and leafy. The numerous flowers grow on short stalks and are a wonderful purplish blue. It can be grown in rock gardens.*

Ginkgo Leaves Ginkgo biloba

 HERBALISM

The tea, tincture, and tablets are used for poor circulation, thrombosis, varicose veins, cramp that comes on walking, white fingers, and spontaneous bruising. Ginkgo is especially helpful for failing circulation to the brain in elderly people. Strengthens memory. Helps protect against strokes. Often improves deafness, tinnitis, vertigo, and early senile dementia. Also helpful for asthma, enabling people to reduce their dependence on drugs.

 PROPERTIES

• Improves blood flow
• Strengthens blood vessels
• Anti-inflammatory
• Relaxes the lungs

Notes and Dosages
• The tea is best taken in large doses—at least three cups a day for some months.
• It is a pleasant drinking tea.

Contraindications
None; it does not interfere with drug therapy.

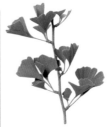

 CAUTION

Do not reduce drugs without telling your physician.

ABOVE *The ginkgo or maidenhair tree, originally from China, is often grown in parks.*

Licorice Glycyrrhiza glabra

 HERBALISM

Use decoction, tincture, or powdered herb for irritable, dry, and nonproductive coughs and bronchitis. Use for inflamed stomach, acidity, heartburn, ulcers, colitis, and intestinal infections, either alone or with comfrey and meadowsweet. Licorice strengthens the digestion and improves assimilation of foods in wasting conditions. Use with other strengthening herbs such as ginseng for exhaustion, or with dandelion. Licorice is usually mixed with other herbs for long-term use. Use in creams or pastes for inflamed psoriasis and hot and weepy skin conditions. Sticks of dried root are chewed for acid indigestion and to strengthen teeth and gums. A small amount is often added to make bitter medicines more palatable. Licorice is a sugar-free sweetener.

 CHILDREN

Suitable as a cough medicine for children of school age—use one-quarter to half of the adult dose. Larger doses tend to be laxative.

 FOOD USES

The roots are used to make the candy licorice, and licorice extract is a traditional ingredient in Yorkshire gingerbread. Pontefract cakes are made from pure licorice and are soothing for the stomach and lungs, but avoid prolonged use. Other forms of licorice confectionery have sugar added, which ruins their value as medicine. Chinese licorice (gan-cao, Glycyrrhiza uralensis) is used in the same way. Processed gan-cao, sliced and stir fried in honey, is sold in Chinese herb shops for strengthening the digestion.

 PROPERTIES

• Soothing
• Anti-inflammatory
• Expectorant
• Antiseptic

Notes and Dosages
• Large doses are laxative.
• Prolonged doses can cause water retention and exacerbate high blood pressure.
• For acute bronchitis and stomach acidity take 5g. of powdered root three times daily with a little water or in capsules for up to two weeks.
• For a decoction use half a teaspoon of chopped root in one cup of water—take three cups daily.
• Licorice is also available as a fluid extract—use one teaspoon, three times daily. For long-term use take a quarter of this dose.

Contraindications
It is contraindicated for patients taking drugs based on digoxin.

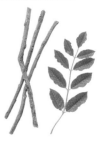

! CAUTION

Not to be taken in medicinal doses by pregnant and lactating women, people with high blood pressure or diseases of the kidneys.

RIGHT *Licorice is a sweet root grown widely for use in confectionery and medicine.*

Witch Hazel Hamamelis virginiana

 HERBALISM

The decoction, tincture, and creams are used externally for bruises, cuts, oily skin, spots and pimples, broken capillaries, hemorrhoids, and painful varicose veins. Use the compress for sprains, phlebitis, sunburn, and hot swollen joints. The compress and wash are useful for hot and tired eyes. The bath and compress are useful for tired and aching muscles. Use as a mouthwash for tender gums.

 PROPERTIES

- Astringent
- Anti-inflammatory
- Antiseptic
- Styptic

Notes and Dosages
- Distilled witch hazel, witch hazel water, and other preparations are easily available.
- The decoction and tincture are stronger but tend to stain clothes.
- Dilute the tincture with three parts of water to use as a compress or lotion.

Contraindications
Not to be used internally except under professional guidance.

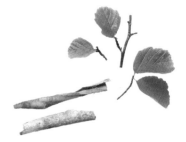

ABOVE *The bark and leaves of this small American tree are used in herbalism. The tree is often grown in gardens for its spring flowers.*

Devil's Claw Harpagophytum procumbens

 HERBALISM

The decoction or tincture is used for all types of arthritis, especially for inflamed joints and arthritis affecting a number of small joints, such as in the hands. It is good for flare-ups of chronic arthritis. Use for gout, lumbago, sciatica, rheumatism, gallbladder inflammation, hemorrhoids, phlebitis (internally), and itchy skin with no obvious cause. Devil's claw may be combined with white willow bark for long-term use.

 PROPERTIES

- Bitter tonic
- Anti-inflammatory
- Mild analgesic

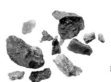 CAUTION

Avoid in pregnancy

Notes and Dosages
Decoction—½ a teaspoon to a cup of water, 2 cups a day.
Tincture—1 teaspoon twice daily.
- Tablets are available in most healthfood stores—follow the dosage on the box.
- For acute flare-ups, double the dosage for a week or two.

Contraindications
May exacerbate stomach acidity and ulcers.

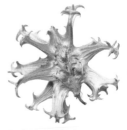

DRIED DEVIL'S CLAW

DEVIL'S CLAW TUBER

ABOVE *Devil's claw is the tuber from a South African plant.*

Rock Rose Helianthemum nummularium

 FLOWER ESSENCE

Rock rose, one of the twelve healers, relates to terror and courage. It is one of the remedies for those who suffer fear, and is especially helpful for children. Rock Rose is a mainstay of Dr. Bach's Rescue Remedy. It is to be taken in all cases of extreme fear, terror, panic, urgency, or danger; when there is danger to the mind, or threatened suicide or insanity; nervous breakdown; fear of death; or hopeless depression. The Rock Rose types feel intense fear and panic although they may not know why. The fear is a deep, unrecognized terror at the prospect of loss of life or personal identity. These phantoms can cause physiological disturbances, metabolic dysfunction, and exhaustion leading to neurosis, paranoia, and nightmares.

 METHOD

The Sun Method *(see page 42)*
• The yellow flowers appear from spring to late summer.

• Gather the open flowers a few at a time and immediately float them on the surface of the water. Pick from a wide area until the surface of the water is completely covered.

Lesson
Courage
Rock Rose gives courage to face death and the idea of death—to see the small everyday deaths, of ideas, flowers, seasons, etc. as transformations—part of the growing process of life.

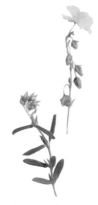

ABOVE *Rock rose is a low-growing perennial shrub of spreading habit, with short, much branched woody stems. It grows on chalky, limestone, and gravely soil. The varieties of rock rose cultivated in rock gardens are not suitable for the remedy.*

Water Violet Hottonia palustris

 FLOWER ESSENCE

Water violet is one of the twelve healers, relating to grief and joy. It is one of the remedies for those who suffer loneliness, and isolation. Water Violet is useful for self-reliant people, aloof with a live-and-let-live attitude. They are quiet and spend much time alone, keeping others at a distance. When ill they keep to themselves and do not wish to be any "trouble" to those around them. In their isolation they may feel special/different or chosen, a sensation that can distort their sense of belonging. This remedy is sometimes called the hermit's or monk's remedy.

 FLOWER ESSENCE

The Sun Method *(see page 42)*
The flowers bloom in the early summer. Gather the flowers by their long stalks. Pick from the widest possible area.

Lesson
Communication, sharing
It is good to meditate and be alone with the inner self, but this experience should be the settled starting point from which to reach out. By keeping themselves, to themselves, the Water Violet types miss the heart-to-heart communication possible between people. The remedy helps us realize that interaction with others is not "trouble" but one of the privileges of kinship. The positive Water Violet can share the skill of their stillness and their joy with others.

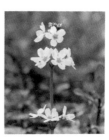

ABOVE *Water violet is a small water plant found in the shallows of ponds and slow-moving rivers. The submerged base leaves form a rosette-like anchor, from which the erect flower stem issues. It rises several inches above the water with whorls of small, pale mauve flowers at the top.*

St. John's Wort Or Hypericum (Hyp.) Hypericum perforatum

 HERBALISM

The tea or tincture is useful for nerve pains, including neuralgia, sciatica, pain in the coccyx (tail bone), pain with tingling in hands or feet. Use with cramp bark for back pain. Use for mild to moderate depression; depression from viral infections, including HIV; anxiety and depression of menopause. Use the tincture as a lotion for shingles, cold sores and herpes; add a few drops of a suitable essential oil such as myrrh or melissa for extra effect. Use the cream for sore skin and cuts. The infused oil can be used as base oil for aromatherapy back massage and with lavender essential oil for neuralgia.

 HOMEOPATHIC

Hypericum should be given after any accident or injury to parts of the body rich in nerve endings where there are shooting pains that dart upward, such as the coccyx (base of spine), a blow to the head, eyes, fingers, toes. It will ease the pain and heal the nerves.

 PROPERTIES

• Strengthens and speeds healing in the nervous system
• Relieves pain
• Antiviral
• Anti-inflammatory

Notes and Dosages
• Standard doses *(see pages 21-25)*.

• It may be a week or so before depression begins to lift.

• May be sold in the stores as hypericum.

• Hyperical is a mixture of St. John's wort with marigold.

• Make the infused oil by putting fresh tops in olive oil, in a clear glass jar in sunlight, until it turns deep red.

 SYMPTOM PICTURE

Mental and Emotional Symptoms
Melancholic, depressed, shocked, sensation as if he or she is lifted high in the air or will fall from a great height, as if the ground has been taken from beneath.

Physical Symptoms
• After an operation it soothes pain and promotes healing.

• For deep puncture wounds (e. g. stepped on a rusty nail) with pain that shoots upward from site of injury.

• Traditionally used to promote healing and prevent tetanus.

Postnatal: Where the woman has suffered injury to her perineum or coccyx and is left with shooting pains that dart up her spine or up her pelvis.

Remedy Picture
• Worse in cold, damp conditions, for touch.

• Better bending head backwards.

• Nerve pains that shoot upward especially following injury.

Dosages: 6c or 30c
Antidotes: Ars. alb., Chamomilla, Sulfur
Complementary Remedies: Ledum

Contraindications
Concentrated tablets are coming on to the market, high doses of which can bring on a rash in sunlight. This does not happen with standard doses.

 CAUTION

Avoid in severe depression

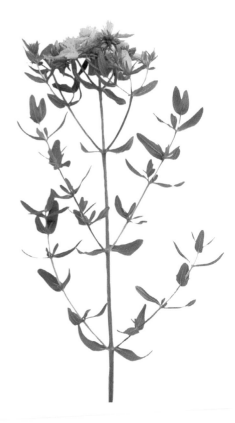

ABOVE *St. John's wort is a common European wild plant, now a weed in many parts of the world. The tops of the plant are picked in full flower.*

Hyssop Hyssopus officinalis

HERBALISM

Hyssop is used primarily for the respiratory system. Hyssop tea with honey is an excellent treatment for children's coughs and fevers, especially if the child is nervous or anxious.

HOMEOPATHIC

Make in the normal way and drink freely. Hyssop is one of the remedies used by homeopaths to treat epilepsy.

AROMATHERAPY

Hyssop is useful for skin problems such as dermatitis and inflammation and for minor injuries such as cuts and bruising. It can help in cases of rheumatism and high or low blood pressure. Asthma, bronchitis, catarrh, colds, flu, and throat problems respond well. Minor digestive upsets and menstrual problems can also be helped.

HERBALISM

Add a few leaves to red kidney beans and other pulses during the cooking. Add a few leaves to salads. Do not use too many because hyssop has a bitter flavor and astringent quality. Used in small amounts this herb has a negligible effect on ailments.

NOTES AND USAGES

- Anticatarrhal
- Antispasmodic
- Carminative
- Expectorant
- Diaphoretic
- Hepatic
- Sedative
- Tonic
- Vulnerary

! CAUTION

Do not use if pregnant or epileptic

Notes and Dosages
- Infusion: Three times a day
- Tincture: Three times a day

Contraindications
- Anyone with epilepsy should not self-prescribe but is advised to consult a qualified homeopath or medical herbalist.

- Hyssop essential oil is subject to legal restrictions in some countries because it can cause epileptic fits.

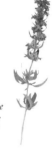

RIGHT *Hyssop is a hardy semi-evergreen shrub that grows to a height of 18in.–4ft. (45cm.–1.2m.). Its flowers appear in the late summer and are magnets to bees and butterflies.*

Holly Ilex aquifolium

FLOWER ESSENCE

Holly is one of the remedies for those who are oversensitive to influences and ideas. Holly is for those who are sometimes attacked by feelings of hatred, envy, jealousy, suspicion, and revenge. The Holly types have lots of intense feelings but they are too frightened to express their hearts fully, so the free flow of love is blocked or expressed unclearly. The tension of this leads to real or imagined vexations. Children of Holly types will say, "I know she loved me because she continually chastised me." Holly is one of the three remedies for aspects of love, along with Heather and Chicory.

METHOD

The Boiling Method *(see page 43)*
Holly flowers blossom in the spring. Pick flowering twigs about 6in. (15cm.) long. Pick female and/or male flowers. Pick from as many bushes and trees as possible, gathering the experience of different ages and positions.

Lesson
Love, unconditional expressions of affection and love

- Holly makes it possible to recognize that these feelings are the negative expression of our caring interaction with others. There is a choice in how the emotions of love are expressed.

- Holly gives us the strength to open the heart to the full flow of love.

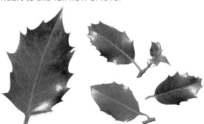

ABOVE *The spiky and glossy evergreen leaves and red berries of the holly tree are extremely striking and holly is well known for its decorative contribution to winter festivals. Although holly grows into a tree in woods, it is usually grown as a bush in gardens.*

Impatiens Impatiens glandulifera, touch-me-not, jewelweed

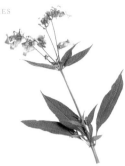

 FLOWER ESSENCE

Impatiens is one of the twelve healers and relates to impatience, pain, and forgiveness. It is also one of the remedies for those who suffer loneliness. Impatiens is for those who are quick in thought and action and who are always on the go. They know their mind and want things to be done with speed. They become irritable at hindrance, hesitation, and delay and impatiently blame others. They can alienate people by being brusque and unsympathetic. They refuse to slow down even when illness overtakes them.

 METHOD

Notes and dosages *(see page 42)*
Flowers bloom in the late summer. Protect the flowers from the heat of the hand by covering it with a broad leaf from the bottom of the plant. Only pick the pale mauve flowers. Pick each separately by its stalk.

Lesson
Patience
• Beech is acceptance of differences. Impatiens is for forgiveness of differences and forgiveness of the self. Impatiens makes it possible to accept the natural pace of life rather than trying to live at speed outside it.
• Positive Impatiens types are capable and decisive; they know how to get things done and turn the pace of life to their advantage.

ABOVE *Impatiens is an annual plant that grows to 6ft. (2m.) tall in damp places. It likes to grow on river banks and irrigation ditches. The seed pods which follow the flowers are over an inch (2.5cm.) long. As the seed pod ripens the inner tension becomes so great that a drop of water or a brush with an adjacent leaf is enough to release the spring and send seeds catapulting over a great distance.*

Jasmine Jasminum officinale

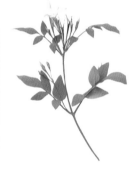

 AROMATHERAPY

In massage or in a bath, the aroma is an excellent relaxant for the nervous system, PMS, menopausal and menstrual problems. It treats mood swings and depression and promotes an increase in self-confidence. It helps postnatal recovery, and massaged over the lower back and stomach during labor, relieves pain and assists the expulsion of the placenta after delivery. Jasmine is also excellent for masculine problems, such as prostate problems, impotence, frigidity, and male menopause. It is a powerful aphrodisiac. Used in inhalation or burned in a room, it helps with colds, catarrh, coughs, and chest infections. Although rather costly, it combines well with bergamot, ylang ylang, clary sage, and citrus oils.

PROPERTIES

• Antidepressant
• Treats PMS and other feminine complaints
• Uterine tonic
• Aphrodisiac
• Relaxant
• Anticatarrhal

Contraindications
Use half the measure while pregnant.

ABOVE *Jasmine essential oil is produced by solvent extraction. The solvent is removed and the absolute is obtained from something called a "concrete," by separation with alcohol. Jasmine is one of the most costly essential oils since only the flowers are used. Known as the king of oils, jasmine also has the most feminine, exotic, rich aroma. The oil is a rich ruby color. Jasmine is found in France, Morocco, Egypt, China, and India.*

Walnut Juglans regia

 FLOWER ESSENCE

Walnut is one of the remedies for those who are oversensitive to influences and ideas. It is used for people who need to find constancy and protection from outside forces, and who need to move on and break links and old patterns with people and things. We are all maintained by the ideas and expectations of friends and acquaintances, but at some times in our lives these patterns can be limiting or distracting. Walnut is useful for people on the brink of some major decision or change, for example children leaving home, those undergoing the menopause, marriage, or having babies.

 FOOD USES

Walnut oil is popular as a salad oil and is used in cooking. It is rich in vitamin E and folic acid and may be helpful for menstrual problems and dry skin conditions. The nuts are eaten as sweetmeats and used in sauces, cakes, and desserts.

 METHOD

The Boiling Method (see page 43)
The flowers bloom in the spring, with or just before the leaves open. Both male and female flowers are found on the same tree. The male flowers are born on catkins. The few female flowers grow upright at the end of the shoot. Pick about 6in. (15cm.) of shoot, with new leaves and female flowers.

Lesson
Protection, sanctuary
Walnut gives protection to break inappropriate links and pursue personal freedom. It is also useful for those who become distracted by the enthusiasm, salesmanship, and strong opinions of others.

Contraindications
Generally safe, except for those people who are allergic to nuts.cause epileptic fits.

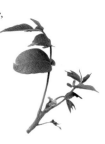

RIGHT *The large, handsome, deciduous walnut tree grows to 80ft. (24m.) in height. In mature trees the massive trunk is deeply furrowed, the top is huge and spreading. The nuts are edible, and an oil is extracted from them.*

! CAUTION

Do not give to children under two years of age

Juniper Juniperus communis

 AROMATHERAPY

Used in massage or in a bath, juniper is a stimulating and uplifting oil. It is good for aching limbs, rheumatism, arthritis, and reinforces the immune system. It encourages the elimination of uric acid and toxins, so is excellent for cellulite, fluid retention, obesity, and diabetes. Juniper's astringent properties help to treat skin conditions such as eczema, psoriasis, and sunburn. It is also useful for treating leucorrhea, hemorrhoids, and menstrual problems. Used in a vaporizer it will help unclog open pores and blackheads. As a compress on the lower back it will help to relieve kidney stones. It combines well with other oils, such as pine, rosemary, cypress, lavender, benzoin, and citrus oils. Burned in a room it has a cleansing and healing effect on both mind and body.

 FOOD USES

Use the berries to flavor vegetable dishes, game, pickles and pates. They may contribute to the treatment of cystitis, arthritis, and digestive problems.

 PROPERTIES

JUNIPER BERRIES

• Anticatarrhal
• Antiseptic
• Antirheumatic
• Diuretic
• Immune system fortifier: (useful for ME, MS, and HIV)
• Expectorant

Contraindications
Safe to use externally while pregnant.Generally safe, but not to be taken in medicinal doses by pregnant and lactating women, or people with diseases of the kidneys.

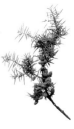

RIGHT *Juniper essential oil is extracted by steam distillation from the berries alone or from the berries, needles, and twigs of the juniper bush, which is found in Europe, Canada, and the United States. The oil is a pale yellowy color and has a lovely clean, warm, woody, pungent aroma. Juniper berries are also a well-known ingredient of gin.*

! CAUTION

Not for babies or infants

Lachesis (Lach.) Lachesis muta, surucuccu snake, bushmaster

HOMEOPATHIC

Lachesis affects the heart and circulation causing palpitations and dark, passive hemorrhages, bleeding into tissues, and a blueness to the complexion and wounds. Constitutional type: Trembling and bloated with a puffy, purplish face, red hair and freckles. Thirsty, enjoys socializing, very talkative, and enjoys alcohol.

SYMPTOM PICTURE

Mental and Emotional Symptoms
Very talkative, lively, and excitable. Stubborn and manipulative, suspicious, jealous, depressed.

Physical Symptoms
Headache: Wake from sleep with a headache, worse in the mornings.
• Pale, bluish face. Flickerings and dim sight. Pressure and burning on top or left side of head. Waves of pain as if head would burst. Vertigo. Pain is relieved by a discharge such as nasal catarrh, menstrual flow. Worse by moving, stooping. Caused by head-cold, sun-heat, menstruation, menopause, jealousy.
Throat: Left-sided pain that extends into the ear. Dry, intensely swollen, dark purple and inflamed. Sensation of a lump in throat. Chronic sore throat with thick mucus that is difficult to clear. Worse left side, pressure, touch, swallowing liquids or hot drinks.
Women's symptoms: Menstruation is too short, too feeble, dark blood, pains relieved by flow. Menopausal hot flushes to head, feet icy cold, hot sweats, palpitations, headache on top of head, fainting, worse pressure of clothes.
Skin: Bluish, purplish, insect bites, boils, wounds all have bluish or blue-black margin.

Remedy Picture
• Dislikes tight clothing especially around the throat.
• Very sensitive to touch.
• Worse in the morning, on walking, complaints are worse for sleep.
• Left-sided pain or may move from left to right side.
• Desire for coffee and alcohol.
• Worse for a warm bath, hot drinks, closing eyes, in the springtime, hot sun.
• Better for appearance of discharges, warm applications.
• Prostrated and trembly when unwell.

Dosage: 6c
Antidotes: Acid phos., Ars. alb., Belladonna, Calc. carb., Coffea
Complementary Remedies: Hepar Sulf., Lycopodium

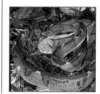

LEFT *The surucuccu snake, or bushmaster, is a deadly pit viper from South America. Its venom is used to make the Lachesis remedy.*

Larch Larix decidua

FLOWER ESSENCE

Larch is one of the remedies for despondency and despair. It is also useful for those who lack confidence in themselves and fear failure, who do not think that they are as good or as capable as those around them. This limits their actions, and at times lack of confidence may completely immobilize and prevent them from even trying. They do not think that they are capable of success.

METHOD

The Boiling Method *(see page 43)*
Flowers blossom in the spring. The male catkins are about ½in. (1.5cm.) long, the female catkins are conspicuous and bright, confident red. Pick twigs about 6in. (15cm.) long with male and female catkins and young leaf buds. Gather from as many trees as possible.

Lesson
Confidence
There is no such thing as success or failure in life, only experience. Each new morning demonstrates the skill of our survival stratagems. Larch helps us appreciate our real worth and value our personal contribution to the overall pattern of life. Also see Gentian, one of the twelve healers.

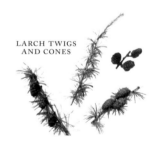

LARCH TWIGS
AND CONES

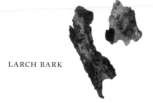

LARCH BARK

ABOVE *The larch is a tall, coniferous tree, growing to 100ft. (30m.) high. The bark is rough and covered with deep longitudinal cracks. The slender, needlelike leaves grow in large bunches and fall in the autumn. Larch is the only coniferous tree to do this.*

Lavender Lavandula angustifolia

 HERBALISM

Lavender flowers can be taken as a herbal tea for their calming and cheering action and to reduce the effects of stress on the system. They combine well with other nervines such as linden flowers and chamomile. Drink a tea of lavender, chamomile, and marigold flowers for a quick recovery after giving birth. Lavender is particularly effective for stress-related headaches.

 AROMATHERAPY

Lavender is a must for the first-aid cabinet and can be dabbed directly onto bites, stings, burns, wounds, bruises, sores, and scar tissue. It is known to have a strong balancing action on the solar plexus area, and used in massage can assist during labor. A compress over the abdomen can help with expulsion of the placenta after birth.It is helpful for high blood pressure, general stress, palpitations, faintness and dizziness and regulates scanty periods. In a bath it is also helpful for sciatica and muscular back pain. Used in a vaporizer or burned in the room, it balances, purifies, and acts as a natural insect repellent.Lavender combines well with other oils such as bergamot, marjoram, rosemary, and pine. This oil can be used in a lower dose on babies, infants, pregnant women, and children.

 CHILDREN

Good for diaper rash and snuffly babies.

 PROPERTIES

- Antiseptic
- Antispasmodic
- Analgesic
- Anti-inflammatory
- Disinfectant
- Anti-infectious
- Insecticide
- Regulates the nervous system
- Parasiticide
- Decongestant
- Regulates heart and circulatory system
- Adaptogenic

Notes and Dosages
- Infusion: Three times a day.
- Oil should not be taken internally but can be used in a liniment to ease the pain of rheumatism.

Contraindicationsns
Caution needed in cases of low blood pressure.

A VERSATILE ESSENCE

As well as being regarded as the most versatile essence, lavender has had a long-cherished place in the laundry and the bathroom. Indeed its name comes from the Latin word lavare, to wash. In warm climates, sheets and household linen are spread out to dry on lavender bushes; in colder places, they may be stored away interleaved with dry lavender or homemade lavender bags. Lavender scent stays sweet and fresh for a long time, and it doubles up as an insect repellent.

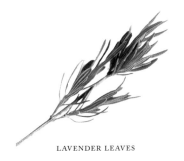

LAVENDER LEAVES

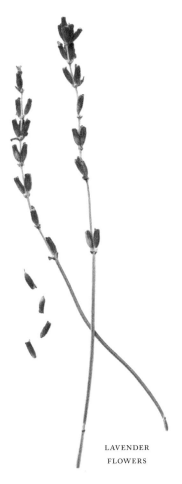

LAVENDER
FLOWERS

ABOVE *Lavender essential oil is extracted by steam distillation from the fresh flowering tops of the plant. Lavender is found extensively in the south of France, Italy, Corsica, and in the east of England. It has a long history of being used in medicine, perfumery, and household goods. The oil is a pale yellowy color and has a fresh, distinctive flowery smell. Lavender is often called the mother of all essential oils because of its subtle balancing qualities.*

Ledum (Led.) Ledum palustre, wild, rosemary

 HOMEOPATHIC

Ledum is a first-aid remedy for puncture wounds and black eyes—see physical symptoms.

 SYMPTOM PICTURE

Mental and Emotional Symptoms
Often not pronounced but may be anxious, timid, and morose.

Physical Symptoms
• Bites, stings, puncture wounds, and deep cuts, eg. knife cuts, splinters, trod on nail.

• The wound hardly bleeds.

• Skin is pale and cold to touch, may be puffy.

• May feel either hot or cold internally but is better for cold compresses, cold-bathing, even icy-cold water.

• Pricking, throbbing pains that radiate out from the injury.

• May be used for old injuries that have healed but are still painful.

• Traditionally used to prevent tetanus, may be given on its own or combined with Hypericum if it is in an area rich with nerve endings.

Black eyes: Where the orbit is very bruised following injury. If the eyeball is painful may need to follow Ledum with Symphytum.

Rheumatism: Cold, puffy, pale purplish joints that loosen up from cold bathing, cold compresses. The joints are cold to touch but may feel hot inside.

Throbbing pains: First small joints are affected then rheumatism moves up into large joints, may start in toes, move up to knees then right shoulder. Better for cold, rest. Worse for warmth.

Remedy Picture
• Chilly people who are better for cold applications, cold bathing, and rest.
• Worse for heat, warmth of bed, movement.

Dosage: 6c
Antidotes: Camphor
Complementary Remedies: Belladonna, Bryonia, Pulsatilla, Rhus tox., and Sulfur follow well.

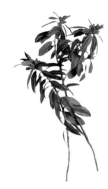

ABOVE *Wild rosemary is a small, shrubby plant native to Canada and northern Europe. Its tonic properties are recognized in its folk names of marsh tea and Labrador tea.*

Motherwort Leonurus cardiaca

 HERBALISM

Use the tea and tincture for anxiety with heart racing, palpitations, and tachycardia from overactive thyroid. Use it with skullcap and valerian to assist in tranquilizer withdrawal; with vervain for anxiety from stress and overwork; and with sage for menopausal hot flushes. For period pains, it will be effective to take Motherwort on a regular basis. Motherwort is an aid for childbirth, taken daily during the last two or three weeks of pregnancy.

 PROPERTIES

• Calms the heart
• Relaxes the womb
• Antispasmodic
• Emmenagogue

Notes and Dosages
• Normal doses—3 cups of tea or 3 teaspoons of tincture per day.
• May take a few weeks to work.
• Chinese motherwort has the same uses.

Contraindications
Always check heart problems with your medical practitioner.

RIGHT *Motherwort is a European wild plant with a tall spike of small pink flowers. It is easily grown in gardens where it will seed itself freely.*

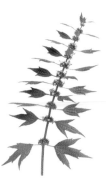

CAUTION

Do not take during pregnancy (until the last three weeks)

Honeysuckle Lonicera caprifolium

 FLOWER ESSENCE

Honeysuckle is one of the remedies for those not sufficiently interested in present circumstances. Use for nostalgia—for those who dwell too much on memories of the past, sometimes a period of great happiness: "It was much better then"; who experience a faraway sense of regret or loss and do not expect to experience such happiness and companionship again. They can become pessimistic. Honeysuckle is one of the two remedies that deal with Time. The Clematis type avoids the here-and-now by drifting away into daydreams; the Honeysuckle type lives in the past. Both are frightened by change and the speed of change.

 METHOD

The Boiling Method (*see page 43*)
Flowers blossom throughout the summer. Pick the flowering clusters with about 6in. (15cm.) of the stalk and leaves. Pick from various parts of the plant.

Lesson
Being completely centered
Honeysuckle integrates past experiences. It helps us realize that the past is the foundation of the present, giving strength to face the new challenges of the now.

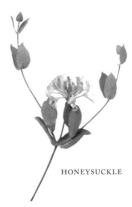

HONEYSUCKLE

ABOVE *Honeysuckle is a woody climber, growing by wrapping new shoots around adjacent plants for support. The flower has a strong and unique fragrance, which seems to trigger an undefined remembrance and melancholy longing.*

Lycium Lycium barbarum, Lycium chinense

 HERBALISM

Use the decoction or tincture for weakness with vertigo, tinnitus, headache, failing eyesight. Use for aches and pains, especially backache, in old age. Lycium is useful for impotence and premature ejaculation. During convalescence, use it with equal parts of schisandra to improve skin color and restore strength.

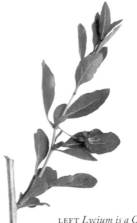

 PROPERTIES

Tonic for old age and weakness.

Notes and Dosages
• Also called wolfberry and the Duke of Argyle's tea plant.

• Chinese herbalists call the berries Gou-qi-zi. Tincture—1 tablespoon (15ml.) with a little water daily.

Dried fruit—½ oz (10g.) daily chewed or in decoction.

• Traditionally the berries are added to soup to strengthen the eyesight.

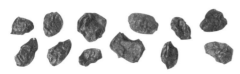

DRIED LYCIUM FRUIT

LEFT *Lycium is a Chinese shrub, grown in Europe as a hedging plant. The bright red fruit is used in herbalism.*

Lycopodium Lycopodium clavatum, club moss

HOMEOPATHIC

Lycopodium is a remedy often required to treat respiratory and digestive complaints when symptoms fit the picture. Constitutional type: Academic, intelligent individuals who appear older than their years, hair grays early, foreheads are furrowed from studying. Intellectually energetic but physically weak, thin, easily exhausted especially after mental work. Sedentary lifestyle. Chilly, better for fresh air.

SYMPTOM PICTURE

Mental and Emotional Symptoms
Anxiety from anticipation of exams, public speaking, etc. Lacks self-confidence. Dislikes being alone, does not want company. Worse for mental strain, causes poor concentration, sluggish. Children appear mature for their age. Wake up cross. Irritable.

Physical Symptoms
Colds and flu: Yellow catarrh, dry, blocked nose, mouth breather. Snuffly babies. Right-sided sinusitis with throbbing headache. Cold, clammy, sour sweat with feverish chills.

Coughs: Dry, tickly, and burning pains worse at night, thick phlegm. Rapid breathing, nostrils may flare. Better for hot drinks. Sore throat: Right-sided raw, dry, dusty sensation, thirstless but better for warm drinks.

Mumps: Start on the right and have general symptoms. Headaches: Right-sided, throbbing, tight pains in forehead, back or top of head. Worse for coughing, warmth; better for fresh air.

Indigestion: Hungry, desires sweet foods. Cramping pains in hard bloated abdomen from sour wind after eating cabbage, beans etc. Better for burping (hot and sour), loosening belts and clothing.

Abdominal complaints: Ache in small of back from weakness or kidney complaints. Stiff. May have red sand in urine. Worse for starting to move. Better for moving, passing wind, urinating.

Remedy Picture
• Worse between 4 and 8 p.m.

• Desire sweets, hot drinks, occasionally cold drinks.

• Acidity and wind, bloating.

• Yellow discharges. Right-sided pains, or start on the right and move to the left. Pains come and go suddenly. Better for fresh air.

Dosages: 6c or 30c
Antidotes: Aconite, Camphor, Chamomilla, Graphites, Pulsatilla Complementary
Remedies: Do not give Lycopodium after Sulfur.

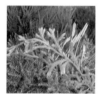

LEFT *This is a mossy plant that grows on mountain pastures and heaths. The fruits produce spores that are used to make the remedy.*

Crab Apple Malus Sylvestris

FLOWER ESSENCE

Crab apple is one of the remedies for those who suffer despondency and despair. It is useful for self-condemnation and disgust. Crab apple cleanses the mind and the body, so it is helpful for people who feel in need of cleaning or detoxification, or who are in a state of remorse over some act of which they are ashamed. It is good for people who are holding grudges.

FOOD USES

Crab apples are sour-tasting fruit that are used to make jelly. Although, like eating apples, they are a good source of vitamin C, the high temperatures needed to make jelly destroy this vitamin. Safe, but those on a sucrose-restricted diet should avoid eating crab apple jelly since it is full of sugar.

METHOD

The Boiling Method *(see page 43)*
Crab apple flowers blossom in spring. The pink flowers grow in clusters with the leaves at the top of short stems. Pick this spur, with the leaves and flower clusters, from as many trees as possible.

Lesson
Cleaning and purification

This remedy is a cleanser. It helps cleanse the body on all levels, physical, emotional, and spiritual.

• Crab Apple makes cleansing a positive experience and part of our growing process

preparatory to change. It is useful for the Scleranthus type and the Water Violet type. Many skin conditions benefit from Crab Apple; five drops can be added to the water in a bath, or two drops to a skin cream. For those who permanently yearn for deep cleaning and purging, Crab Apple should be taken with one of the love remedies: Heather, Chicory, or Holly.

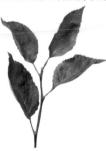

LEFT *The crab apple is a small, stout, deciduous tree growing to 30ft. (10m.). The trunk can look old and gnarled even on young trees. The apples are small and tart.*

German or Wild Chamomile, Chamomilla (Cham.) Matricaria recutita, Matricaria chamomilla

HERBALISM

Chamomile tea is used for anxiety, nervous tension, and headaches. Tea or tincture is used for insomnia and for any kind of digestive upset including acidity, ulcers, nausea, heartburn, wind, and colic. Use with linden, on a long-term basis, to strengthen the nervous system. Chamomile lotion or cream is used for itchy skin conditions including eczema. An infusion diluted with water makes a good mouthwash for sore and inflamed gums and an eyewash for conjunctivitis. The vinegar is soothing for genital irritations. Use a cupful in the bath or dilute it with six parts of water for a soothing lotion. It can also be used as a conditioner for fair hair. The infused oil makes an excellent base oil for aromatherapy. Add two teaspoons to the bath for dry, itchy skin.

CHILDREN

Tea is helpful for restless and overexcitable children and for most children's complaints including fevers and teething troubles. Homeopathic tablets and drops (see right) have the same uses and children will often take them in preference to the tea.

HOMEOPATHIC

Chamomilla is a valuable homeopathic remedy. It is useful for intolerable neuralgic pain and for ailments brought on by bad temper. It is good for those who are excessively sensitive to pain, which appears to be out of proportion to the ailment. Take Chamomilla when you cannot bear the ailment any longer.

SYMPTOM PICTURE

Mental and Emotional Symptoms
Oversensitive, irritable, cross, bad tempered, peevish, cannot bear to be looked at, fretful, crying, doesn't know what he or she wants, demands something then pushes it away.

Physical Symptoms
Hot, red, tender, sore, unbearable pains associated with numbness.

Joints and muscles: Unbearable aches and pains often with a sensation of numbness.

Women's complaints: Heavy menstrual periods with dark clots and unbearable pelvic cramps, irritability and restlessness often following a fit of anger.

Labor: Unbearably strong but ineffectual contractions with irritability, nervousness, and restlessness, possibly physically or verbally abusive, feels she cannot cope with the labor anymore. Chamomilla often helps with the transition from the first to second stage of labor—give 200c potency, repeat if necessary.

Breast-feeding: Unbearably painful with inflamed tender nipples.

• Think of Chamomilla for any ailment that follows a fit of anger, whether it is asthma, rheumatism, painful menstrual periods, insomnia, etc., and the person cannot bear the pain, is restless and irritable, hot and thirsty for cold drinks, and worse at night with a damp, sweaty head.

Babies and Children
Colic: Fretful, crying, demands to be carried, cannot be soothed, abdomen is full of wind yet burping and passing wind causes distress instead of relieving the pain.

Teething: One cheek red and hot, the other cool and pale. Gums swollen, red, and tender. May have a fever and green or yellow diarrhea looking like chopped egg or spinach with a sour or sulfurous (rotten egg) smell. Fretful and crying, soothed only by being carried and rocked.

Crying: For a fretful baby, inconsolable, nothing pleases it. Children who are irritable, cross, and peevish, whine, appear spoiled, want this-then-that, nothing pleases them.

Toothache: Worse from warm drinks or warm air in the mouth, better by cold water, there may be a sensation of the teeth being too long.

Remedy Picture
• Thirsty for cold drinks. Hot at night, uncovers, sticks feet out of covers, head hot and sweaty.

• Worse for warmth, coffee, warm drinks, evening and nighttime; better for being carried.

Dosages: 6c or 30c
Antidotes: Camphor, Nux vom., Pulsatilla
Complementary Remedies: None

PROPERTIES

• Calming, soothing, healing
• Anti-inflammatory
• Antiseptic
• Relaxes spasm
• Settles the digestion

Notes and Dosages
• For acute conditions in adults make a double-strength tea, using two teaspoons of flowers or two tea bags. For best results use a teapot or cover your cup with a saucer, so that the steam does not escape.

• For infants make an ordinary strength tea and give them two or three teaspoons to drink, either directly or in some pure fruit juice.

• Chamomile is perhaps the most popular herb in the world.

• Readily available as tobacco.

Contraindications
Some people find that the taste makes them nauseous.

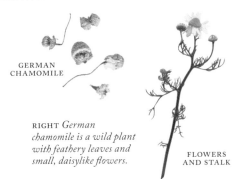

GERMAN CHAMOMILE

RIGHT *German chamomile is a wild plant with feathery leaves and small, daisylike flowers.*

FLOWERS AND STALK

Tea Tree *Melaleuca alternifolia*

 AROMATHERAPY

In massage or in a bath, tea tree is beneficial for depression and general debility. It is used in the treatment of HIV, AIDS, ME, and in X-ray treatment of breast cancer. Used gradually before and after any surgery, it will help shock, encourage healing of the wound, and minimize scarring. Used in a vaporizer, tea tree helps bronchitis, colds, and flu. As a gargle or mouthwash, tea tree can be used to treat sore throats, tooth abscesses, and gum infections. As a douche, it addresses genito-urinary infections, NSU (non-specific urethritis), and thrush. Soak a Q-tip in tea tree oil and dab on cold sores, blisters, chicken pox, shingles, plantar warts, and spots. As an astringent, tea tree helps skin problems such as acne, eczema, and dermatitis. Use as a footbath for chilblains, athlete's foot, corns, and other ailments affecting the feet. Use for the treatment of ringworm. Combines well with other oils such as peppermint, eucalyptus, bergamot, and lavender.

 CHILDREN

For babies, tea tree is an excellent treatment for diaper rash and cradle cap.

 PROPERTIES

- Antiseptic
- Antiviral
- Antibacterial
- Antifungal
- Antiparasitic
- Vein decongestant
- Neurotonic
- Wound-healing
- Immune system stimulant

Contraindications
- Can cause skin irritation. Do not use on people who have impaired kidney functions or kidney infections.
- Safe to use while pregnant, on babies, infants, and children.
- Check a small patch of skin first before using tea tree since it can be a skin irritant.

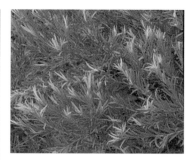

ABOVE *Tea tree essential oil is extracted by steam distillation from the leaves and small branches of the tea tree, which is native to Australia and grows up to 15ft. (5m.) in height. The oil is clear or a yellowy color and has a strong, clean, camphorous aroma. Produced in Australia, it is without a doubt one of the most remarkable oils and a must in any medicine cabinet.*

Cajeput *Melaleuca leucadendra*

 AROMATHERAPY

Cajeput is excellent as an inhalation for chronic pulmonary diseases such as tuberculosis, bronchitis, asthma, and also for the common cold and sinus trouble. Cajeput when used in a vaporizer acts as a purifier of the atmosphere in its surroundings. It is also very effective as a mouthwash, and in the event of toothache or tooth decay, one drop of essence on the troublesome area brings relief. For an earache, a piece of absorbent cotton soaked in the essence and placed gently in the ear will bring relief. As a massage oil, Cajeput is useful in cases of cystitis, urethritis, and dysentery. It is a healer for open wounds, acne, sores, and psoriasis and used in a bath assists aching limbs and rheumatic conditions and helps to relieve nervous tension, neuralgia and general fatigue. Cajeput combines well with other oils such as chamomile and rose.

 PROPERTIES

- Antiseptic
- Anti-infectious
- Tonic
- Decongestant—useful for respiratory system
- Antirheumatic

! CAUTION

Not for babies under eighteen months

Contraindications
- Cajeput is a powerful stimulant and is not helpful to use before bedtime unless mixed with a sedative oil.

- Use sparingly on the skin since it can act as an irritant.
- During pregnancy use half the usual stated amount; this also applies for young children.

A POWERFUL ANTISEPTIC
Cajeput essential oil is extracted by stream distillation from the leaves and buds of the tree Melaleuca leucadendra. The oil is a greenish yellow color and has a camphorous, strong, clear smell. It can be uplifting and purifying. Cajeput is a powerful antiseptic and acts on the respiratory system and digestive system and benefits the pulmonary, intestinal, and urinary tracts.

Niaouli Melaleuca viridiflora

 AROMATHERAPY

Niaouli, a natural antiseptic, is very effective in treating respiratory tract infections, colds, bronchitis, asthma, catarrh when used in a vaporizer or massaged around chest and lung areas. In a bath or massage it assists in treating skin conditions, including psoriasis, herpes, and acne. Niaouli is an oil for the medicine cabinet—it will work quickly if placed on a burn or a wound. Niaouli has been used in conjunction with chemotherapy cancer treatment. As a douche it will help cystitis and vaginal problems. In massage or in a bath it is helpful for rheumatism.

Massaged around the stomach area niaouli will help intestinal problems, such as diarrhea. It combines well with other oils such as bay, basil, citrus oils, lavender, and pine.

 PROPERTIES

- Anti-infectious
- Antibacterial
- Anticatarrhal
- Anti-inflammatory
- Antiseptic
- Antiparasitic
- Vein decongestant
- Controls high blood pressure
- Expectorant

Contraindications
Not for babies—and take care with young children.

NIAOULI ESSENTIAL OIL
Niaouli essential oil is extracted by steam distillation from the leaves of the niaouli tree that grows wild in Australia and the French West Indies. The oil ranges from clear to a greenish yellow and has an uplifting, strong, sharp camphorous aroma.

Melissa or Lemon Balm Melissa officinalis

 HERBALISM

Lemon balm herb tea is an excellent nervine and digestive, especially useful for nervous palpitations, children's restlessness and nightmares. Historically, herbalists considered that it "strengthened the brain." It adds to the depth of flavor of other herbal teas and combines well with peppermint or linden flowers and chamomile.

 AROMATHERAPY

Melissa is well known for its healing properties, and it is particularly useful for heart disorders and for treating depression. Used in massage or in a bath, melissa has a calming yet uplifting effect and is helpful in treating migraine, headaches, neuralgia, tension due to stress, and hysteria that is manifested around the neck and shoulders. It helps skin conditions such as eczema and shingles, and other stress-related skin problems. It can also regulate the menstrual cycle and assists ovulation in natural methods of birth control. As an inhalation it helps palpitations, asthma, and respiratory problems. Melissa is excellent when used in conjunction with Dr. Bach's Rescue Remedy for shock or sudden bereavement.

 FOOD USES

Use the fresh leaves to flavor soups and salads and wine-based drinks. In such small quantities the herb has little therapeutic value, but it may contribute to the treatment of digestive ailments in children. Iced tea made from the fresh leaves is a good cooling drink in hot weather.

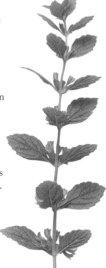

PROPERTIES

- Good for the digestive system
- Affects the menstrual cycle
- Neurotonic
- Antispasmodic
- Useful in treating heart conditions
- Works on the respiratory system

Contraindications
- In pregnancy use half the measured amount.
- Use with care, half the measured amount for babies, infants, and children.

LEFT *Melissa essential oil is extracted by steam distillation from the aromatic herb lemon balm. It was probably introduced to England by the Romans, and has been used across the centuries in medicine. The oil is a pale yellowy color and has a fresh, lemony, clean aroma.*

Peppermint Mentha x piperita

 HERBALISM

Use peppermint tea for indigestion, colic, wind, nausea, vomiting, depressed appetite, period pains, and to relieve abdominal and gallbladder pain. A couple of drops of the essential oil in hot water, or sucking a strong peppermint candy, is also effective. Use with meadowsweet for diverticulosis. Use with elderflower and yarrow for colds, sinus problems, and blocked nose. Inhale the steam as you drink. Add a couple of drops of the essential oil to creams for hot, itchy skin conditions. A strong tea used as a lotion is also effective.

 CHILDREN

A safe tea for tummy upsets. Only small amounts are needed—2 or 3 teaspoons. Fennel or chamomile are better for infants.

 AROMATHERAPY

Used in massage or in a bath, peppermint oil acts effectively on the digestive system, treating hiccups, flatulence, and bad digestion. When massaged over the stomach area, it will treat diarrhea. It helps sickness generally, including morning sickness and travel sickness. Used in a vaporizer it is excellent for colds, pneumonia, sinusitis, asthma, bronchitis, and laryngitis. It is also an effective diuretic and helps in the treatment of gallstones. Peppermint oil is an excellent insect repellent. It is good as a mouthwash for teeth and gums and as a footbath for aching feet. Combines well with other oils such as lavender, eucalyptus, benzoin, and rosemary. It soothes aching muscles and, burned in the room, has a stimulating, refreshing aroma.

 FOOD USES

Use peppermint leaves to flavor iced drinks and salads.

 PROPERTIES

- Digestive
- Carminative
- Antispasmodic
- Clears wind
- Mild stimulant
- Emmenagogue
- Cooling on the skin

Notes and Dosages
- Take freely. Widely available as tea bags.

- A small amount of peppermint may be added to most herb teas for flavor. Peppermint oil capsules are available for colicky pains and cramps. Some people may find them too strong, in which case use the tea.

- Garden mint (spearmint) has the same properties but is generally weaker. Peppermint tea was traditionally used as an aphrodisiac.

 PROPERTIES

- Anti-infectious
- Antiseptic
- Anticatarrhal
- Expectorant
- Antiviral
- Fungicide
- Affects the digestive system
- Antispasmodic
- Tonic

Contraindications
- Safe in pregnancy from the fourth month onwards, and is particularly effective when burned in the room.

- Nervous and overexcitable people may find it too stimulating.

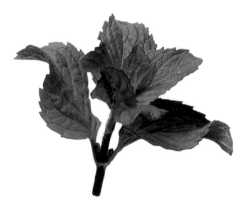

ABOVE *Peppermint is one of the most popular herb teas. It is easily grown in gardens and is found all over the world. Peppermint essential oil is extracted by steam distillation from the whole plant. The oil is colorless or pale yellow and has an invigorating, fresh minty smell. Peppermint has been renowned for its medicinal properties across the centuries.*

 CAUTION

Do not use with heart conditions. Not for babies.

Mimulus Mimulus guttatus

 FLOWER ESSENCE

Mimulus is one of the twelve healers, relating to fear and sympathy and for those who have fear. Dr. Bach has five remedies dealing with different aspects of fear. Mimulus is for the kind of fear that can be identified, of known, worldly things. Aspen is the opposite, dealing with gray, formless, undefined fear. Mimulus should be taken for the everyday fears of pain, accident, poverty, being alone, and misfortune. Fear dominates responses, either prodding into hasty action or freezing into inaction. These fears are easily identified and faced, but underneath they are fed by insecurity and a negative attitude toward past experience.

 METHOD

The Sun Method
Gather the flowers by their stalks throughout the summer. Mimulus, called monkey flower, is a popular garden flower. Cultivated monkey flowers should never be used for remedies.

Lesson
Freedom
The positive side of this remedy is not "being fearless" but "sympathy." Mimulus liberates us from fear and helps us understand the rhythms and balances of everyday life, so that we have the freedom to respond in all ways and not just through fear.

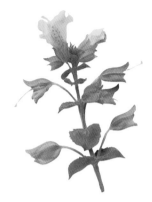

ABOVE *Mimulus is a perennial plant, growing to 12in. (30cm.) in damp places and near streams.*

Tabacum (Tab.) Nicotiana tabacum, tobacco

 HOMEOPATHIC

Tabacum is useful for sea-sickness, and may be beneficial for car and train sickness.

 SYMPTOM PICTURE

Mental and Emotional Symptoms
Mental and emotional symptoms Irritable, wretched, despondent, and forgetful.

Physical Symptoms
• Travel sickness and morning sickness in pregnancy with above general symptoms.

• Tightness, constriction, and cramping pains—can be useful for constipation or diarrhea with nausea and vomiting, wants abdomen uncovered.
Chest ailments: Tightness, difficult to breathe. Dry, tickling cough better for sips of cold water.

Angina: Pain radiates out from center of chest and down left arm or between shoulder-blades. Feeble pulse, fast or slow. Worse for exertion.

Remedy Picture
• Constant nausea and vomiting from motion of boats, cars, trains.

• Worse for opening their eyes, for tobacco, airless rooms, before breakfast.

• Better for fresh air, rest, uncovering.

Dosages: 6c or 30c
Antidotes: Ars. alb., Cocculus, Ipecac
Complementary Remedies: None

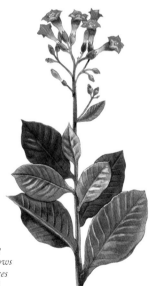

RIGHT *The tobacco plant is a half-hardy annual, native to South America. It grows to a height of 4-6ft. (1-2m.) and produces leaves 3ft. (1m.) long. Its heady-scented, rose pink flowers bloom in late summer.*

Basil Ocimim basilicum

 AROMATHERAPY

Basil is a good nerve tonic and acts as a natural tranquilizer, aids concentration, and is helpful for headaches, migraines, and head colds. It combines well with other oils, such as thyme.

Used as an inhalation or in a bath, it helps fight fatigue, anxiety, and depression. When used in massage it aids muscular spasms in the intestine and bowel; it also aids urinary infections and prostatitis. When massaged over the stomach area, it regulates the menstrual cycle and is helpful in a compress for engorged breasts. It acts in an anti-inflammatory way and as a decongestant of varicose veins. Basil also acts as an insect repellent, helps to shrink warts, and relieves snake bites. Can be used as a mouthwash when treating mouth ulcers and gum infections. For babies, tea tree is an excellent treatment for diaper rash and cradle cap.

 PROPERTIES

- Anti-infectious
- Anti-inflammatory
- Antibacterial
- Antispasmodic
- Regulator of nervous system
- Vein decongestant

Contraindications
- Basil is best used in moderation since there are concerns about its toxicity.
- It can act as a powerful depressant if overused.

 RIGHT *Basil essential oil is extracted by steam distillation from the leaves and white flowering tops of the pungent-smelling basil bush. The bush is native to Greece; the Greek name for basil is basileus, meaning king," and it was indeed favored by the nobility. It has long been cultivated in France and India. The oil is yellowish in color. It is especially helpful for clarity of thought and restoring harmony and acts as a regulator and tonic of the nervous system.*

! CAUTION

Best avoided during pregnancy and on babies and children.

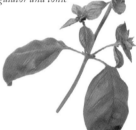

Olive Olea europaea

 FLOWER ESSENCE

Olive is one of the remedies for those who are not sufficiently interested in present circumstances. It is used for extreme fatigue of the mind, body, or spirit. People in need of Olive feel totally exhausted in every way. Life is hard and without pleasure. They feel that they have no more strength and at times hardly know how they manage to keep going. They depend very much on others for help. The leaves of the olive tree are used therapeutically as well as the oil from the fruit.

 FOOD USES

Eating olive oil may reduce the risk of circulatory diseases. It is beneficial to those suffering from hyperacidity since it reduces the level of gastric secretions. The oil can help in the treatment of constipation and peptic ulcers.

It is also useful for dry skin and hair, particularly for the treatment of dry, flaky scalp. The leaves of the olive are used to treat high blood pressure, stress, and abrasions to the skin.

 METHOD

The Sun Method *(see page 42)*
- Flowers blossom in the spring. They are small and inconspicuous, growing in clusters from the leaf axil. Pick the entire flower cluster from as many trees as possible.

Lesson
Renewal and regeneration
Hornbeam is the other remedy used for exhaustion. The exhaustion in Hornbeam comes from living on will-power. Olive deals with total exhaustion for people who feel drained to the core. Olive helps people relax and switch off so that the simple things of life—a warm bath, a walk in the sunshine, watching children, or sharing with friends -can refresh the spirit. With the spirit refreshed renewal is possible.

 PROPERTIES

Olive oil is an excellent source of vitamin E; it is high in monounsaturated fats and has a high energy value (899Kcal. per 100g.). It does not contain any minerals. Olive oil has a beneficial effect on the circulatory and nervous systems. It also benefits the digestive system.

Special Notes
People on low-fat diets may have to avoid eating olive oil.

RIGHT *The evergreen olive tree grows to 30ft. (10m.) with many thin branches. The smooth, narrow leaves are 2in. (5cm.) long, gray-green on top and silvery underneath. The fruits of the olive are eaten as an aperitif and compressed to exude the soothing olive oil.*

Marjoram *Origanum majorana*

 AROMATHERAPY

Used in steam inhalation, marjoram oil will often clear the chest and ease respiratory difficulties quickly. Asthma, bronchitis, colds, sinusitis, and whooping cough are all treated with marjoram. As a massage oil or in the bath, marjoram helps treat anxiety, insomnia, and high blood pressure, and it also assists narrowing of the arteries. As an analgesic it is good for muscle pains, strains, arthritis, and rheumatism—it works particularly well as a compress on specific areas of the body. If massaged over the abdomen it helps painful periods and is good for PMS. It is safe to use externally during pregnancy. It combines well with other oils, such as bergamot, lavender, and rosemary. Burned in a room, specific is a warm, relaxing sedative oil.

 FOOD USES

Marjoram leaves add a distinctive flavor to Greek and Italian dishes and when used in cooking may aid digestion.

 PROPERTIES

- Analgesic
- Antibacterial
- Antiseptic
- Diuretic
- Neurotonic
- Vasodilator
- Acts upon nervous system
- Treats PMS

Contraindications
Marjoram has sedative properties, so avoid overuse.

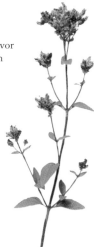

LEFT *Marjoram essential oil is extracted by steam distillation from the dried flowering herb. Marjoram, long known as a herb in cooking and in herbal medicine, can be found in the Mediterranean, Europe, Iran, and North Africa. The oil is a pale yellow or pale amber color and has a warm, peppery aroma.*

! CAUTION

- Do not use on babies
- Avoid internal use while pregnant

Star of Bethlehem *Ornithogalum umbellatum*

 FLOWER ESSENCE

Star of Bethlehem is one of the remedies for those who suffer despondency and despair. Star of Bethlehem is included in the Rescue Remedy to ameliorate the effects of shock—for example, the shock of bad news, loss, an accident, birth (for mother and baby). Shock makes the body jump as shock waves ripple outwards and affect every cell of the body. Time is needed for everything to settle back down, but sometimes the trauma of shock may be so extreme that the effects are still resonating years later. Star of Bethlehem can be given after the shock of an operation or after childbirth. It can be given to the mother and/or the child. Put four drops of the remedy into a pint of water. Use to sip or moisten the mother's mouth, as a compress or as a skin wash or bath. For those who refuse to be consoled this remedy also brings comfort.

 METHOD

The Boiling Method *(see page 43)*
The flowers bloom from April to May. Gather when the flowers are fully open, pick the whole cluster together with a few inches of the main stem. The flowers open only in the sunshine so it is important to gather on a clear, sunny day.

Lesson
Peace and comfort
The effects of shock must be fully acknowledged and not trivialized. Star of Bethlehem helps acknowledge and release any residual blockages so that the body and mind can find equilibrium and comfort.

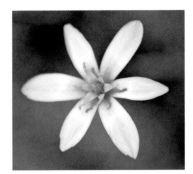

ABOVE *The star of Bethlehem is closely related to the onion. The slender flower stems and long thin leaves grow from the center of a small bulb. They reach 9–12in. (23–30cm.) high.*

Ginseng Panax ginseng, Chinese ginseng

 HERBALISM

Use a decoction, tincture, or tablets for convalescence, exhaustion, weakness in old age, and with other strengthening herbs for persistent infections, especially of the lungs and the digestive system. Ginseng is an aphrodisiac for men and is especially good for loss of sex drive due to stress or prolonged illness. It may be combined with damiana for sexual anxiety. Use for agitation, forgetfulness, and lack of concentration. It helps the body to cope with stress and with the side effects of chemotherapy for cancer. Ginseng is useful when studying for exams and during training for athletic events. Chew a few small pieces of root to hasten labor. It is useful for jet lag.

 PROPERTIES

• Replenishes vital energy
• Strengthens the immune system, an adaptogen
• Soothes the spirit and increases concentration

Notes and Dosages
• Ginseng is best suited to old and weakened people.

• Young and strong people may find it overstimulating, in which case they should avoid it or take much smaller doses or try Siberian Ginseng.

• In general take 1g. of powdered root, 3g. of cut root in decoction or 20 to 30 drops of the tincture twice daily.

• There are many different forms of ginseng, including capsules, pills, instant tea, and even creams for damaged skin—follow the instructions on the package.

• Women can take ginseng but Chinese angelica is often more suitable, especially in weakness and debility.

 CAUTION

• Do not use during pregnancy
• Not to be used for children except under professional guidance
• Avoid in high blood pressure

Contraindications
Ginseng can have adverse effects, especially when taken in excessive quantities or over long periods. It is best not taken continuously. A two-week break every two months is recommended. Ginseng is stimulating and should not be taken with other stimulants such as strong tea and coffee.

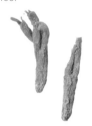

ABOVE *Ginseng is a yellowish, radishlike herb that is used as a culinary root vegetable in China, particularly in making soup. It is expensive and not widely available in this form in the West. Ginseng root is the most famous of the Far-Eastern tonics.*

Geranium Pelargonium odoratissimum

 AROMATHERAPY

Used as a massage oil, geranium acts as a tonic to the nervous system and helps menopausal problems including hot flushes. Massaged over the stomach area it is excellent for relieving symptoms of constipation, diarrhea, and enteritis. Massaged over breasts it helps to relieve mastitis. Soaked on a Q-tip, geranium is good for healing wounds and burns. If used in the bath, it will help skin conditions such as eczema, shingles, and chilblains. Geranium combines well with other essential oils, such as bay, orange, rose, bergamot, and lemon, and used in a burner or a vaporizer in a room it has a fresh, balancing effect on the atmosphere. It is an excellent insect repellent.

 PROPERTIES

• Antibacterial
• Antidepressant
• Antifungal
• Anti-inflammatory
• Anti-infectious
• Antiseptic
• Antispasmodic
• Diuretic
• Deodorant
• Useful for treating PMS

Contraindications
• Use half the measure while pregnant.

• Use with care, and in half measures for babies, infants, and children.

 CAUTION

Should not be used if there are tumorous growths

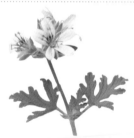

ABOVE *Geranium essential oil is extracted by steam distillation from the leaves and stems of the geranium plant. First distilled in France, it is now produced in Reunion, an island in the Indian Ocean, and in Algeria, China, and Egypt. It has a wonderful, strong, heady aroma, and its oil is a yellowish-green or brown color. Geranium is much used in the perfume industry.*

Bay Pimenta racemosa, Pimenta acris

 AROMATHERAPY

Used as a massage oil, bay is an excellent general tonic; it is uplifting, replenishing the body's vital force, and aids depression. When massaged into the hair, it assists growth and helps develop strength. When used as an inhalation or in a vaporizer, bay acts as a strong pulmonary antiseptic and is good for the common cold, sinusitis, bronchitis, and pneumonia. A few drops of bay in a bath acts as an excellent tonic. It combines well with other oils, such as geranium and orange. Marjoram leaves add a distinctive flavor to Greek and Italian dishes and when used in cooking may aid digestion.

 PROPERTIES

- Antidepressant
- Regulates the rheumatic system
- Antiseptic
- Aids digestion

! CAUTION

- Do not use on babies, infants, and children
- Avoid during pregnancy, but good burned in a room

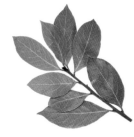

ABOVE *The bay is an evergreen shrub whose shiny leathery leaves produce clusters of yellowish-green fowers in the spring. It grows wild in the West Indies. Bay essential oil is extracted by steam distillation and varies in color from yellow to dark brown. It gives off a lovely spicy, warm, mellow aroma. It acts as an antidepressant, aids the digestive and rheumatic systems, and is an antiseptic.*

Anise or Aniseed Pimpinella anisum

 AROMATHERAPY

Aniseed helps the digestive and respiratory systems. As a massage, aniseed oil can help muscular aches and pains, bronchitis, indigestion, and flatulence. It is used in orthodox medicine to disguise unpleasant tastes.

 FOOD USES

A tea made from aniseed can be helpful in reducing gas in the stomach and bowel. Aniseed is useful in the treatment of bronchitis and mucous coughs; it thins mucus secretions and aids their expulsion from the lungs and bronchial tubes. Aniseed is reputed to be helpful in cases of asthma and loss of libido. External applications of aniseed oil may deter body lice.

 CHILDREN

Aniseed tea can help infant colic and catarrh.

 PROPERTIES

- Anise benefits the digestive and respiratory systems.

Special Notes
- No safe dosage has been established for aniseed.
- When taking commercially prepared health products, follow the manufacturer's directions for use. If ill-effects occur, stop taking immediately and seek medical advice.
- Aniseed usually has no harmful effects when eaten in small quantities as part of the normal diet, or when taken medicinally for a short time, but some people may be at risk.

RIGHT *Anise is an umbelliferous plant belonging to the parsley family. The aromatic seeds, which have a taste similar to that of licorice, are used for culinary and cosmetic purposes, to make the alcoholic drink anisette, and for therapeutic purposes. An essential oil is extracted from the seeds.*

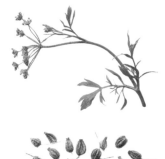

 CAUTION

Aniseed oil can be used for very similar conditions, but because of its high concentration and possible toxicity, only one drop should be used externally.

Pine Pinus sylvestris

 HERBALISM

Pine buds are still used in European herbal medicine for treating lung infections. The resin from pine trees can be crushed and added to teas for the same purpose. A useful ointment for stubborn skin diseases and for healing old wounds can be made by grinding the resin into an equal amount of honey.

 FLOWER ESSENCE

Pine is one of the remedies for those who suffer despondency or despair. It is a very specific remedy for those who blame themselves and are suffering from feelings of self-reproach. Even when successful they are never content with the results and always feel that they could have done better.

 AROMATHERAPY

Pine essential oil used in massage, in the bath, or as an inhalation is a powerful respiratory antiseptic, good for pneumonia, bronchitis, asthma, flu, coughs, and colds. It clears mucus from the chest. It is helpful for hay fever. Massaged over the abdomen, pine can be used to treat urethritis, uterine congestion, pyelitis, and complaints of the prostate gland. As a douche, pine is used for NSU (nonspecific urethritis) and venereal infections. Burned in a room, it clears the mind and is uplifting, and particularly good for general aches and pains. Used as a footbath, it eases aching feet and acts as a deodorant. Pine is a natural parasiticide against scabies and lice. Burn in a room for respiratory ailments in babies.

> CAUTION
> • Do not overuse
> • Use at half measure while pregnant

 HOMEOPATHIC

Nettle rash, itching all over. Coughs—dry and tight. Ribs feel weak and thin as if they will collapse if touched. Weak ankles, especially in children. Rheumatism and gouty pains. Joints are stiff, hot, swollen, and tender.

 METHOD

The Boiling Method (see page 43)
Flowers bloom in the early summer. Male and female flowers grow on the same tree. Male flowers are more abundant, forming small yellow clusters. Female flowers become cones and are found singly or in small groups at the tip of year-old growth. Pick twigs about 6in. (15cm.) long with male and female flowers. Pick when the male flowers are thick with pollen.

Lesson
Appropriate response, responsibility
Pine people feel the need to control all aspects of their lives and have a script of what should happen. They burden themselves with duty and a personal responsibility for the world. Pine helps us see beyond the script and understand that "responsibility" is the ability to respond. If we respond honestly and freely there can be no blame.

 PROPERTIES

• Antiseptic
• Anti-infectious
• Antifungal
• Antidiabetic
• Neurotonic
• Decongestant of the lymphatic system
• Parasiticide

 DOSAGE

5-10 drops mother tincture, three times a day, or 6c potency three times a day.

Contraindications
Use with care if skin is sensitive.

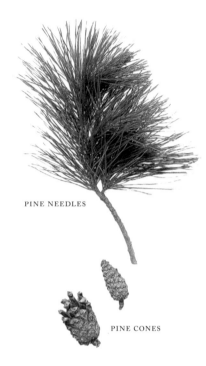

PINE NEEDLES

PINE CONES

ABOVE *The Scots pine is a tall, straight evergreen growing to a height of 100ft. (30m.), in pine woods and heathlands. The leaves, which grow in pairs in dense tufts, are 2in. (5cm.) long and very slender. They fall every two or three years. Pine essential oil is extracted by steam distillation from the needles and fresh young cones of the pine tree, which is grown widely throughout Europe, North America, and Russia. The oil is colorless or a pale amber color and has an uplifting, fresh, balsamic aroma. Pine is one of the most extensively used essential oils—particularly in perfumery, disinfectants, insecticides, and detergents.*

Plantain Leaf Plantago major, Plantago lanceolata

 HERBALISM

A compress or lotion is helpful for soothing and healing insect bites, allergic rashes of any kind, and infected eczema. Use for cleaning bites and wounds, and for drawing stings and splinters. Plantain promotes quick healing of spots, pimples, acne, and bruises. It soothes neuralgic pains and shingles rash. Use the cream or ointment for slow-to-heal cuts and bleeding hemorrhoids; use the tea or the tincture for running nose from allergies, dust, smoke irritation, colds; dizziness and tinnitus associated with catarrh; irritable bowel; irritable bladder; and chronic cystitis. Use with meadowsweet and yarrow for bleeding stomach ulcers; use with yarrow for heavy menstrual bleeding.
The tea is a cooling drink for persistent fevers and is a useful addition to any medicine given to "hot" people. Use infusion as a mouthwash for sore and bleeding gums.

 CHILDREN

Plantain is totally safe at any age. For infants with allergies, runny noses, and rashes, a simple treatment is to add two cups of strong plantain tea to their bath.

 PROPERTIES

• Soothing
• Astringent
• Healing—an excellent wound herb

Notes and Dosages
• The tea is the best method of administration. Use at double strength (two teaspoons per cup) for most purposes.
• A quick way of making a compress for first-aid when away from home is to chew two or three plantain leaves and bind them on to the cut or sting with a clean cloth. (Chew your own leaves.)
• Plantain seeds are a gentle bulk laxative. Collect them when fully ripe by picking the whole stem and hanging it over a sheet of paper. Take 1 teaspoon with a glass of water two or three times daily, before meals.
• Psyllium seeds are a type of plantain seed and are easily available.
• Green plantains are a type of banana—not to be confused with the herb.

Contraindications
Always have internal bleeding medically assessed before treating yourself.

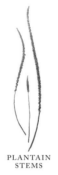
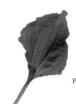

PLANTAIN
LEAF

PLANTAIN
STEMS

ABOVE *Plantain is a common weed of pathways and lawns. The leaves of the broad-leaved plantain or the ribwort plantain are used in herbalism.*

Patchouli Pogostemon cablin

 AROMATHERAPY

Used in massage or in a bath, patchouli has a soothing influence on the nervous system. It is excellent for depression, stress, anxiety, and nervous exhaustion. Its mellow, warming aroma assists frigidity and is a known aphrodisiac. Massaged over the stomach it aids both constipation and diarrhea. Used in a vaporizer, patchouli breaks down mucus produced by infections and helps to bring down a temperature. It is good for conditions such as acne, eczema, allergies, hemorrhoids, sores, and minor burns. As a footbath, it helps to clear fungal problems and athlete's foot. Burned in a room, patchouli mellows the atmosphere. It combines well with other oils, such as rose, geranium, orange, cedarwood, and sandalwood. It is good for stretch marks.

 PROPERTIES

• Antidepressant
• Anti-inflammatory
• Antiseptic
• Aphrodisiac
• Fungicidal
• Febrifuge—reduces fever

 CAUTION

• Not for babies or infants
• Avoid anything but vaporization while pregnant

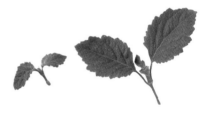

ABOVE *Patchouli essential oil is extracted by steam distillation using the leaves of the tall, bushy patchouli plant found in Asia, Europe, and the United States. The leaves are fermented before distillation. Patchouli was a well-known "flower power" aroma in the 1960s, when it was used as a warm, relaxing incense. The oil is thick and varies from a dark burgundy red to a browny amber; it has a distinctive musky, warm, spicy aroma. Widely used in the perfume industry.*

Aspen Populus tremula

 FLOWER ESSENCE

Aspen is one of the remedies for those who have fear. Dr. Bach says that Aspen is for "vague unknown fear, for which there can be given no explanation, no reason." These are generalized, deep, and unknown fears, accompanied by an inexplicable sense, sometimes physical, of foreboding and doom. This fear can be so deep that the person may be too frightened to express it, or they may not acknowledge the sensation as fear but feel doom frozen somewhere inside. This shapeless fear is not open to argument or intellectual reassurance; it is met with faith and trust.

 METHOD

The Boiling Method *(see page 43)*
Gather male and female catkins. They appear on the same tree, just before the leaves appear, in the early spring. Pick twigs, about 6in. (15cm.) long, which have male and female catkins and leaf buds. Pick enough twigs to fill a saucepan ¾ a full. Pick from several different trees.

Lesson
Courage to face the unknown
• Aspen helps face fear openly and proceed even when afraid
• Rock Rose, one of the twelve healers, also deals with unknown fear and can be very supportive if taken with Aspen

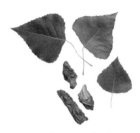

ABOVE *Aspen is a slender, medium—sized, deciduous tree with smooth, grayish bark and dark green leaves. The leaves tremble with the slightest breeze.*

Cherry Plum Prunus cerasifera

 FLOWER ESSENCE

Cherry plum, one of the remedies for fear, is included in Rescue Remedy. Dr. Bach says this remedy is for "fear of the mind being overstrained, of reason giving way, of doing fearful and dreaded things, not wishes and known wrong, yet there comes the thought and impulse to do them." Cherry Plum is for desperation, the fear of losing control over the mind. Thoughts may be suicidal, compulsive, or destructive. This turmoil may happen during a period of great emotional or physical change.

 FOOD USES

Stew the fruit gently and serve with yogurt for a healthy dessert. Cherry plums contribute some vitamin A and C to the diet and are a good source of potassium, which is needed for a healthy fluid balance and the maintenance of cells and nervous tissue.

 METHOD

The Boiling Method *(see page 43)*
The pure white flowers appear in the early spring before the leaves. Pick the flowering twigs, which are about 6in.(15cm) long. Pick from as many bushes as possible and from all parts of the tree.

Lesson
Release, letting go
Cherry Plum makes it possible to release—to let go of the bottled energy of fear that is producing the turmoil. It teaches us to lose the fear of the fear so that there is space for the mind to move on—as in the case of a rock climber, frozen by fear to the rock face. However frightening it may be, he must let go of the handhold to find another and continue the climb.

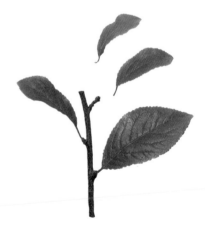

ABOVE *The cherry plum is the small, edible fruit of a small, thorny, deciduous tree, 12-15ft. (3–4m.) high. The tree is usually grown for its spring blossom rather than as a food source.*

Ipecacuanha (Ip.) Psychotria ipecacuanha

 HOMEOPATHIC

Ipecacuanha is useful for ailments that occur after bouts of irritability and anger. It is also useful for nausea and vomiting, especially in cases where vomiting does not quell nauseous sensations. Ipecacuanha root is also used in conventional expectorant cough remedies.

 CHILDREN

Ipecacuanha can be very useful, if the remedy picture fits, for children suffering from bronchitis characterized by coarse rattling cough and mucus in the chest which cannot be shifted by coughing.

 SYMPTOM PICTURE

Mental and Emotional Symptoms
The person is haughty, finds things contemptible, irritable, angry, and morose.

Physical Symptoms
• The person has a clean tongue, lots of saliva and is thirstless. Gastrointestinal tract: Stomach upset—constant nausea, not relieved by vomiting. Diarrhea, with green stools, severe griping pains cause nausea. *Lungs:* Excessive mucus in airways with spasm, difficult to cough up phlegm. May have fits of retching and coughing at the same time—feels he is suffocating. Coughs until red or blue in the face—choking and gagging. Asthma, whooping cough, bronchitis.

Women's complaints: Morning sickness in pregnancy, with constant nausea unrelieved by vomiting, clean tongue, lots of saliva, thirstless, worse for thought of food.
Hemorrhages: From anywhere—lungs, kidneys, stomach, bowel, uterus, nose. Hemorrhage of bright red blood that flows out steadily and also gushes. Blood loss causes constant nausea with above symptoms.

Dosage:
Generally use a 6c or 30c potency but for sudden hemorrhage use a 200c potency in water, take a teaspoonful every hour until blood-flow is stemmed.

Antidotes: Arnica, Ars. alb., Nux vom., Tabacum
Complementary Remedies: Ant. tart., Arnica.

Pulsatilla (Puls.) Pulsatilla pratesis var. nigricans, wind flower, field anemone, pasque flower

 HERBALISM

In herbal medicine Pulsatilla, or anemone, is considered to be a relaxing nervine and analgesic. It may be added to mixtures for any pain of the sexual organs. It is helpful for tranquilizer withdrawals. Use 10-30 drops of the tincture three times daily or add a little to your herbal teas.

 HOMEOPATHIC

Pulsatilla is a remedy often indicated for catarrhal children if the symptoms fit. Constitutional type: Fair complexion, light hair, slight build, easily flushed, shy, and sensitive, or more solid, deeper complexion, sluggish reaction.

 CHILDREN

Pulsatilla best fits symptom pictures displayed by children and babies, but can also be used by adults.

 SYMPTOM PICTURE

Mental and Emotional Symptoms
• Mild and yielding disposition, wants to please, to be liked.

• Fear of the dark.

• Changeable; can be stubborn.

• Children can be whiney and clinging. Need affection and compassion, like to be cosseted.

Physical Symptoms
• Rheumatism with wandering, fleeting, shooting pains.

• For childhood diseases—measles, mumps, chickenpox where the child is tearful, clingy. *Gastrointestinal tract:* Slow digestion/indigestion worse for fatty foods. Stomachache or nausea from overeating. *Headache:* Headache from rich food or excitement, one-sided throbbing pains in head. Eye on affected side has scalding tears. Better for firm pressure, worse for evening.
Eyes: Conjunctivitis with thick yellow discharge, eyes itch, burn. Especially in babies.
Fever: High fever, chilly better uncovering, thirstless, worse in the evening. Heat and sweating may be one-sided.

Coughs, colds, and catarrh: Catarrh thick and yellow-green, worse in a stuffy room, child may be snuffly, prone to glue ear. Sore throat dry, scratchy, better for cold liquids but thirstless. Cough dry at night, better sitting up.

Remedy Picture
• Thirstless with a dry mouth.

• Chilly but better for cold fresh air, cold drinks.

• Dislikes and is worse for fatty, greasy foods, butter, pastries.

• Better for slow movement, gentle walking in fresh air.

• Worse for getting wet.

• One-sided symptoms; onesided sweat, one hand or foot hot, the other cold.

• Bland yellow-green discharges.

Dosages: 6c or 30c
Generally use a 6c or 30c potency but for sudden hemorrhage use a 200c potency in water, take a teaspoonful every hour until blood-flow is stemmed.

Antidotes: Coffea
Complementary Remedies: Belladonna, Silica

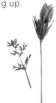

ABOVE *The field anemone is a wild flower that grows on the chalklands of Europe. The whole plant is used to make remedies, but the fresh leaves irritate the skin, so dry them before use.*

Oak Quercus robur

HERBALISM

In herbalism oak bark, or galls, are considered to be a strong astringent. The decoction is used as a mouthwash for loose teeth and bleeding gums. Finely powdered bark is used as a snuff for nasal polyps. Oak leaf tea is used for low blood pressure and general weakness.

FLOWER ESSENCE

Oak is one of the remedies for those who suffer despondency or despair. Oak people are strong and brave fighters. They struggle through events and physical illnesses even when there is no hope, and blame themselves when there is no change. Their strength is inappropriate and they exhaust themselves by pushing on in one narrow direction.

METHOD

The Sun Method *(see page 42)*

The Sun Method *(see page 42)*
The oak flowers in the spring with the young leaves. Pick the female catkins only from as many trees as possible. The male catkins are the most obvious. They usually grow on the previous year's growth, forming loose drooping clusters about 1.5in. (4cm.) long. Female flowers are found on the same tree. They are small and inconspicuous and grow from the upper leaf axil of the new shoots.

Lesson
Flexibility

Strength is a virtue, but it is pointless pushing against an immovable object. More and more strength will not help and fighting becomes frustratingly exhausting. Oak helps us surrender and accept there are many different ways of being. It helps us to have the true inner strength to go with the flow, or to pull back and face the unknown in other directions, to share responsibility and accept different/difficult answers. See also Gentian and Larch.

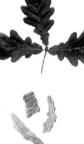

RIGHT *Oak is the archetypal deciduous tree, growing slowly into a tall, strong, and majestic being. It has a thick, straight, gray-brown trunk and many spreading branches. The wood is strong and was used for ship-building, poles, and masts. It grows in woods, groves, hedgerows, and meadows.*

Rehmannia Rehmannia glutinosa

HERBALISM

A decoction or tincture is useful for weakness and lack of energy with pallor, anemia, persistent low fever, constipation, palpitations, and dizziness. The dried, cooked root is combined with Chinese angelica for weakness in women from overwork and after childbirth, especially with low back pain and scanty or irregular menstruation. Used as a decoction.

PROPERTIES

• Tonic and upbuilding

Notes and Dosages
• Rehmannia is also called Di huang. It is available from specialist herb shops and Chinese herbalists.

• Cooked rehmannia is called Shu di huang.

• *Dose*—1 teaspoon tincture three times daily or 5-.7oz. (15-20g.) of the root daily, by decoction.

Contraindications
Prolonged use may upset delicate digestive systems, in which case it is often combined with a little bitter orange peel.

CAUTION

• Do not exceed the stated dose, except under the guidance of a professional herbalist
• Avoid within diarrhea

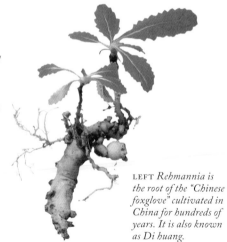

LEFT *Rehmannia is the root of the "Chinese foxglove" cultivated in China for hundreds of years. It is also known as Di huang.*

Wild Rose Rosa canina

HERBALISM

The flower buds from Rosa canina, or dog rose, were used as a gentle astringent for children's diarrhea. The hips are an excellent source of vitamin C and their syrup is used in many cough medicines.

FLOWER ESSENCE

Wild rose is one of the remedies for those who are not sufficiently interested in present circumstances. Dr. Bach recommends Wild Rose for those who without apparently sufficient reason become resigned to all that happens. They glide through life passively, taking it as it is, without motivation or expectation. They are only half alive. Apathy is not the cause but the response to a disinterest in life. "What is the use?" They have given away their power and interest in life.

METHOD

The Boiling Method *(see page 43)*
The wild or dog rose flowers throughout the summer. Pick about 6in. (15cm.) of stem, including the open pink flower and leaves. Pick from as many plants as possible. Pick from all parts of the plant, the center and rambling edges.

Lesson
Interest and action
Life is full or color and joy. Wild Rose helps us to interact with all aspects of life and make an impact by creating our own unique and dynamic reality.
See also Gorse.

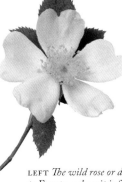

LEFT *The wild rose or dog rose is native to Europe, where it is found in hedges and country lanes. It has simple, open, pink flowers. It grows as a bush or shrub with prickly leaves and thorny stem. The wild rose is used as a symbol for innocence and romance the world over.*

Cabbage Rose Rosa centifolia, French rose, Maroc rose

AROMATHERAPY

Known as the Queen of Flowers, the rose undoubtedly produces the most feminine essential oil. It is excellent in treating PMS and menopausal problems; when massaged over the stomach area it assists heavy periods, miscarriage, infertility, and frigidity. Used by men, it can also increase the sperm count. It can also help in anorexia and ME, works on the digestive system and is good for gastric ulcers.Dabbed on absorbent cotton, it can help earache. Burned in the room, it has an uplifting, relaxing effect, and used in a vaporizer its rejuvenating qualities assist various skin conditions. Rose combines well with other oils such as bergamot, geranium, jasmine, patchouli, and sandalwood.

CHILDREN

Rose is safe to use on babies, infants, and children; used in a massage or the bath, it is a natural relaxant for strong emotions and promotes inner well-being. It helps with hyperactivity, insomnia, skin problems, constipation, and also with stomach upsets.

PROPERTIES

- Antibacterial
- Antidepressant
- Anti-inflammatory
- Aphrodisiac
- Reinforces immune system
- Relieves varicose veins
- Relieves menstrual symptoms
- Supports reproductive system

Contraindications
None

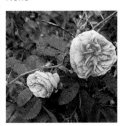

ABOVE *Rose essential oil is extracted from the flowers of the rose bush by means of volatile solvents. Originally found in China and Russia, the rose is now extensively cultivated in Morocco and France. The color of the oil ranges from pale yellow to brownish red and has a pungent, warm, rich floral odor.*

Bulgarian Rose *Rosa damascena, Damask rose*

 AROMATHERAPY

The bulgarian rose has the same properties as the Cabbage Rose (see page 193). The oil is distilled from the fresh petals. It is good for dry and mature complexions, wrinkles, broken capillaries, and herpes; poor circulation; asthma and hay fever; nausea; menstrual problems; depression, insomnia, nerviness, and stress.

 CHILDREN

It is safe to use for babies, infants, and children.

 FOOD USES

Rose water is used in cooking; rose petals make a delicate preserve.

 PROPERTIES

- Antidepressant
- Antispasmodic
- Laxative
- Regulates appetite
- Sedative
- Tonic

Contraindications
None

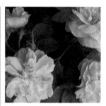

ABOVE *The Bulgarian rose grows on a small shrub between 3-6ft. (1-2m.) high. The fragrant flowers are pink.*

Rosemary *Rosmarinus officinalis*

 HERBALISM

Use as a tea or tincture for depression and headaches associated with gastric upsets. Use with chamomile for stress and tension headaches. It is helpful for circulation, taken on a regular basis. Rosemary is a useful addition to any herbal medicine for conditions associated with cold and poor circulation. Use it with devil's claw or willow bark for rheumatism and arthritis that is worse in the cold weather or when the pains move around from joint to joint; with sage for exhaustion with feelings of cold; with horsetail and skullcap for hair loss due to stress and worry. Rosemary is good for poor digestion, gallbladder inflammation, gallstones, and feelings of liverishness. As a gargle, it relieves sore throats; it is a useful substitute for sage during pregnancy. Use the infused oil for massage for cold limbs and aches and pains. Rosemary vinegar keeps hair in good condition and reduces dandruff. Use 4 teaspoons in the final rinsing water when you wash your hair.

 CHILDREN

Add a pint or two of rosemary tea to the bath for children who always "feel the cold."

 FOOD USES

Use rosemary as a flavoring for meat and vegetables, especially lamb and/or roasted potatoes. Add sprigs of rosemary to vinegars and olive oil and use in dressings and marinades. It may help in the treatment of digestive problems, but in the forms noted above, and in such small quantities, it is of relatively minor use as a medicine.

 PROPERTIES

- Lifts the spirits
- Improves circulation
- Carminative
- Gentle bitter tonic

Notes and Dosages
- Can be used freely.
- Rosemary is used in many cosmetic preparations.

- Rosemary works best on "cold" headaches. If your head feels hot during a headache then lavender will work better.

Contraindications
Generally safe but should not be used in internal medicinal doses by pregnant women. Do not swallow when gargling.

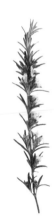

 CAUTION

Avoid in migraines when there is a feeling of heat in the head.

LEFT *Rosemary, the popular cooking herb, is an attractive bush with pretty blue or pink flowers in the spring.*

Raspberry *Rubus idaeus*

 HERBALISM

Take tea, tablets, or tincture of raspberry leaves three times daily for the last three months of pregnancy to strengthen and relax the womb and promote an easy birth. Add an equal amount of motherwort for the last three weeks. Drink chamomile and raspberry leaf tea during labor and continue for three or four weeks afterward to retone the womb quickly and to help milk flow. Use a strong tea as a mouthwash for sore mouths, sore throats, weak gums, and mouth ulcers. Drink the tea with motherwort for period pains with heavy bleeding. Use it with marshmallow and agrimony for diverticulitis.

 CHILDREN

Tea for diarrhea and as a mouthwash for oral thrush. For infants put raspberry leaf tea in a sterilized spray bottle and spray directly into the mouth three or four times daily.

 FOOD USES

Raspberries are one of the summer fruits that are best eaten raw in order to benefit from the vitamins and other nutrients they contain.

 PROPERTIES

- Astringent
- Anti-inflammatory
- Antispasmodic, especially applicable to the womb

Notes and Dosages
- 1 teaspoon of cut leaves to a cup of water for tea or one teaspoon of tincture.
- For tablets follow the dose on the box.
- If you pick your own leaves be sure that they have not been sprayed.
- To prepare for birth the herb needs to be taken for at least two months. This is an old gypsy remedy that has been validated by modern research. Some women drink raspberry leaf tea throughout their pregnancies but, since the last two or three months are the most important, it is best to wait.
- Raspberry vinegar is made by steeping the fruit in cider vinegar for two weeks and then straining off. It makes an excellent mouthwash or gargle for weak gums and sore throats. Dilute with four parts of water to use.

RASPBERRY

 CAUTION

Avoid large doses of raspberry leaves in the first four months of pregnancy.

ABOVE *The leaves from the raspberry bush gathered from the wild or from gardens are used in herbalism.*

Yellow Dock *Rumex crispus*

 HERBALISM

A decoction or tincture is an effective but gentle laxative; it is especially useful for chronic constipation since it does not induce dependency. Use yellow dock as a bitter tonic for liver congestion with poor fat digestion, feelings of heaviness after eating, and mild jaundice; for stomach acidity; with chamomile and marshmallow for irritable bowel with constipation. It can also help in cases of food poisoning and intestinal infections, to clear the source of irritation from the digestive system. Yellow dock is also useful for chronic skin diseases, especially with hot, dry skin, and nonspecific itchiness. Try it with marigold or echinacea for boils; with burdock for psoriasis and intractable eczema; and with nettles for urticaria (nettle rash). Use as a mouthwash for infections and sore throats.

 CHILDREN OVER EIGHTEEN MONTHS

Safe laxative. Add to teas for eczema if the child is hot.

 HOMEOPATHIC

For dry, spasmodic, hacking coughs with rawness and dull aching in chest. Coughs are worse at night. For pustular skin eruptions, impetigo, and acne that burns and itches, and for nettle rash.

 PROPERTIES

- Astringent
- Laxative
- Bitter tonic
- Alterative

 CAUTION

Avoid in chronic diarrhea

Notes and Dosages
Make the decoction using 5oz. (12g.)to 1pt. (500ml.) water.

- For constipation take 1 cup of decoction or 2 teaspoons of tincture daily. More might be needed for short periods. Half this dose for chronic conditions, for children, and for constipation in pregnancy. The best laxative for infants is syrup made from dry figs.
- Traditionally used in bowel cancer.

Dosage
6c potency three times a day.

Contraindications
Always consider your diet in stubborn constipation.

RIGHT *Yellow dock is a common wild plant, with narrow, wavy leaves. The root is used in herbalism.*

Ruta Graveolens (Ruta Grav.) Ruta graveolens, rue

 HERBALISM

A weak rue tea (quarter of a teaspoon to one cup of boiling water) is used as a wash for tired eyes and as a compress for sprains. It also helps to regulate periods.

 HOMEOPATHIC

Ruta is used for sprains and injuries to the tendons and periosteum (bone covering) from overexertion.

 SYMPTOM PICTURE

Mental and Emotional Symptoms
Quarrelsome, restless, dissatisfied; prone to despair and languor.

Physical symptoms
Eye-strain: Eyes are hot, sore, and aching, worse for reading, sewing, close eye-work, or working in a dim light. Backache: In the nape of neck, lumbar region. Worse in the morning before rising. Better for lying on back and for pressure. Joint and bone pains: From sprains and overuse. Extremely sore, tender, bruised. Legs may give way when trying to stand. Lameness of affected part. Ruta has an affinity to the wrists and ankles.

Remedy Picture
• Worse for lying, sitting, cold air, wind, damp, pressure on the affected part.
• Better for warmth, rubbing, lying on back.

Dosage: 6c
Antidote: Camphor
Complementary Remedies: Calc. Phos.
Follows well after Arnica and Rhus tox.

Contraindications
Rue is a strong herb and should not be used internally except with professional guidance.

 CAUTION

• Avoid handling the fresh herb in sunshine since this often causes a rash
• Do not take when pregnant

LEFT *Rue is a hardy evergreen shrub native to Europe.*

White Willow Bark Salix alba

 HERBALISM

A decoction or tincture is useful for gout and all types of arthritis, especially with inflamed joints and when associated with autoimmune diseases. Use with fennel seed for multiple painful joints; with cramp bark for inflammatory back pains, lumbago. It can also be helpful for chronic diarrhea. Use it with rosemary for headaches. Use for sexual overstimulation, wet dreams, premature ejaculation. White willow is also good in convalescence, low grade recurrent fevers, and feeling of being overheated in the evenings.

 PROPERTIES

• Reduces inflammation and fever
• Mild painkiller
• Antiaphrodisiac
• Tonic

Notes and Dosages
• There is no benefit in taking larger doses. It is best to take standard doses *(see pages 21-25)* and persist.
• Willow bark contains aspirinlike compounds but it does not upset the stomach.
• It can be used to reduce dependency on aspirin and other anti-inflammatory drugs.
• The American black willow bark

is considered to be more specifically antiaphrodisiac.

Contraindications
Willows are quite variable and difficult to tell apart. None are poisonous but for the best effect buy the bark from a reputable dealer.

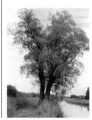

LEFT *The white willow is an imposing tree with rough, light-brown bark on the trunk and gray-white bark on the branches.*

Willow Salix alba "Vitellina," golden willow, yellow willow

 FLOWER ESSENCE

Willow is one of the remedies for those who suffer despondency and despair. It is useful for people who find the injustices of life hard to accept; those who have become embittered and complain with resentment. Life has become a personal trial to endure, without hope or happiness. They blame the world when things go wrong. "It's not fair," they say, like the tantrum of a two-year-old child. With this rigid outlook they do not see that they are creating their own oppression.

 METHOD

The Boiling Method (see page 43)
There are many different varieties of willow. Vitellina is a variety of Salix alba, the common white willow, grown for its particularly brilliant yellow twigs in winter. Male and female flowers grow on different trees and appear in the spring with the new leaf growth. Pick about 6in. (15cm.) of twig, together with catkins, of either sex, and the new leaves. Gather from many different trees.

Lesson
Mature and natural balance
Willow helps us see that we create our own reality by focusing on different elements of our life. Willow may also be taken for a brief temporary embitterment. Pine also deals with aspects of blame. See also Oak and Vervain.

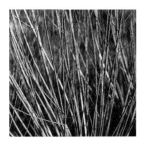

ABOVE *The willow is a delicate deciduous tree with rough, deeply fissured bark. The shoots are thin and flexible. The thin, lance-shaped leaves grow alternately. They are silvery underneath and shimmer with the wind.*

Sage Salvia officinalis

 HERBALISM

Use a strong tea or tincture as a gargle and mouthwash for sore throats, laryngitis, tonsillitis, mouth ulcers, and inflamed and tender gums. Sage is often included in herbal toothpastes. Add a few drops of myrrh essential oil for a stronger action. The tea or tincture is useful for indigestion, wind, loss of appetite, and mucus on the stomach. Use for depression and nervous exhaustion, postviral fatigue, general debility. Sage strengthens lungs made weak by infection and allergy. Take a cold tincture or the tea for excessive sweating and night sweats. Sage is valuable in containing night sweats in serious infections including HIV. Use with motherwort for menopausal hot flushes and to prevent period pains; use with fennel and marshmallow for premenstrual painful breasts. Cold sage tea taken every few hours will usually dry up breast milk. Use it with gingko for weakness, confusion, and poor memory in the elderly. Use the tea as a rinse to delay graying of hair.

 FOOD USES

Use sage to flavor pork, liver, and stuffings for poultry. It may help in the treatment of indigestion.

 PROPERTIES

• Astringent
• Stimulant
• Antiseptic
• Carminative
• A bitter tonic, especially strengthening for women

Notes and Dosages
• Standard tea, three cups a day for acute conditions, one or two cups a day for chronic conditions. Traditional wisdom has it that one cup daily would maintains health in old age.
• For mouthwashes and hair rinses allow a fifteen-minute infusion.
• Do not take fennel or sage combination remedies in pregnancy.

 CONTRAINDICATIONS

The small amounts used in cooking are safe.

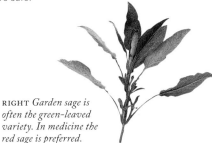

RIGHT *Garden sage is often the green-leaved variety. In medicine the red sage is preferred.*

 CAUTION

• Do not take as a medicine in pregnancy or when breast-feeding
• Avoid in epilepsy

Clary Sage Salvia sclarea

 AROMATHERAPY

When used as a massage oil, clary sage acts very quickly on the nervous system. It is a renowned antidepressant and is excellent for postnatal depression, menopause, and period pains. When massaged over the legs it helps varicose veins. If massaged over the lower back while in childbirth, it eases labor pains. Clary sage is also a known aphrodisiac and is useful in the treatment of impotence and frigidity. Burned in a room, it provides a calm atmosphere; used in a bath, it calms the nervous system. Clary sage combines well with other oils, such as jasmine, geranium, and lavender.

 FOOD USES

Add the flowers to salads and use the leaves in fritters to stimulate the appetite.

 PROPERTIES

• Antidepressant
• Relieves stress and nervous tension
• Soothes painful periods
• Antibacterial
• Relieves muscular spasm

Contraindications
• When used therapeutically, clary sage can have adverse effects, particularly for women taking oral contraceptives or HRT, and those with high blood pressure.
• Medicinal doses should not be taken before driving.
• Clary sage is a powerful oil and should not be used on a continuous basis.
• Generally safe, but as a precautionary measure do not eat clary sage during pregnancy.

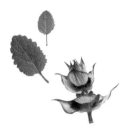

ABOVE *Clary sage essential oil is extracted by steam distillation from the flowering tops and green leaves of the tall, noble herb plant. It can be found and is grown extensively in Russia and is also produced in Morocco and the south of France. In Germany it is known as muscatel sage and is combined with elderflowers to make muscatel wine. The extracted essential oil is colorless, pale yellow, or pale green and has a strong, gentle herby smell.*

 CAUTION

• Do not use on babies, infants, or children
• Do not use on young menstruating adolescents
• Do not use with breast problems, ie. mastitis
• Avoid during pregnancy

Elderflowers Sambucus nigra

 HERBALISM

The tea or tincture is helpful for sinusitis, colds, running nose, hay fever, and flu. An excellent traditional remedy for colds and flu is a tea made of equal parts of elderflowers, yarrow, and peppermint, taken hot, 1 cup every two hours. Inhale the steam deeply as you drink it. To prevent hay fever take three cups a day, starting two months before your regular season begins. Use a lotion or compress for sore and runny eyes and sunburn. Use a lotion or cream for skin blemishes and greasy skins.

 CHILDREN

Give elderflower tea freely to break fevers. Sweeten with honey if your child likes sweet things. Use it as a lotion to soothe the rashes that come with fevers. For colds and runny noses in infants, add 3 or 4 cups to their baths.

 PROPERTIES

• Drying and restorative for nose lining, eyes, and sinuses
• Induces sweating
• Diuretic
• Soothes and tones greasy and hot skin

Notes and Dosages
• Take freely for colds and fevers.
• Elderflowers are found in many cosmetic preparations. Elderflower water was a favorite astringent skin soother of our grandmothers' days. It is still available.
• The fresh flowers may be eaten to relieve hay fever. They also make delicious fritters and pancakes and may be used to flavor salads, water ices, and jam. Elderflowers and gooseberries make an especially tasty combination.
• Elderflower cordial is a popular hot weather drink with children. It is made in the same way as the syrup *(see page 21)* and then diluted with cold, fizzy water to taste.

• Elderleaf ointment works well on painful hemorrhoids.
• Elderberry wine is a traditional drink for neuralgia and sciatica.

Contraindications
Elderflower products may be too drying for some people.

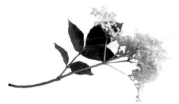

ABOVE *The small elder tree grows abundantly on wasteland and is easy to identify. Its froth of creamy white flowers in the summer and clusters of small, deep purple berries in the fall are both used in herbal remedies.*

Sandalwood Santalum album

 AROMATHERAPY

When burned in a room, sandalwood is a natural mind, body, spirit balancer; use in meditation. It aids emotional and physical problems. In massage or in a bath, it calms the nervous system. A good oil for men—it helps treat impotence and works as a relaxant and aphrodisiac. Massaged over the stomach area, it has an antiseptic effect on the gallbladder, helps diarrhea and dysentery, and acts on the urinary tract treating general venereal problems, NSU (non-specific urethritis) leucorrhea, and gonorrhea. As a douche, sandalwood is used to treat cystitis. It helps fluid retention and varicose veins. Used in a vaporizer or in massage, sandalwood helps bronchitis, mucus congestion, bronchitis, laryngitis, and respiratory problems. It acts as an astringent for eczema, sores, and dry skin. Sandalwood combines well with other oils, such as benzoin, cypress, jasmine, ylang ylang, vetivert, and palmarosa.

 CHILDREN

Used at a very weak strength, Sandalwood soothes diaper rash.

 PROPERTIES

- Antiseptic
- Decongestant
- Anti-inflammatory
- Calming and soothing
- Meditative
- Assists lymphatic system

Contraindications
- If your kidneys become irritated, or if you have suffered from kidney complaints in the past, use at half dosage.

- Avoid using sandalwood in massage while pregnant (although it is perfectly safe in a vaporizer or burned in the room).

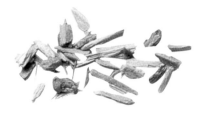

BARK

ABOVE *Sandalwood essential oil is extracted by steam distillation from the roots and innermost heartwood of the tree. Sandalwood, a small tree, originated in India and has been used since ancient times in temples and funerary ritual and for furniture. The Chinese also used sandalwood for its medicinal qualities. The oil is a yellow or dark yellowy-brown color and exudes a thick, subtle, mellow woody aroma.*

Schisandra Schisandra chinensis

 HERBALISM

A decoction or tincture is helpful for weakness with nervous exhaustion and sleeplessness exhaustion from prolonged hard work. It is also helpful in restoring lost sex-drive in men and women. It restores softness to the skin and can be used for dry and chronic coughs.

 PROPERTIES

- Astringent
- Nourishing
- Soothing
- Expectorant

Notes and Dosages
- Schisandra is called *wu wei zi* by Chinese herbalists and is available from specialist herb shops.
- *Dosage:* tincture—1 teaspoon three times daily; dried berries—3oz. (10g.) daily by decoction.

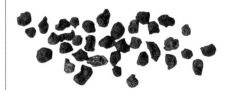

DRIED SCHISANDRA BERRIES

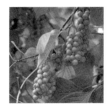

ABOVE *The red berries of this ornamental vine from China are used in herbalism.*

Sabadilla (Sabad.) Schoenacaulon officinale, Cevadilla

 HERBALISM

Sabadilla is usually recommended for hay fever and colds with a lot of spasmodic sneezing and mucus production. The person is usually chilly, with chills starting from below and moving upward, and very cold hands and feet. Thinking brings on a headache.

 CHILDREN

Sabadilla may be indicated for worm infestation, tonsillitis, and diarrhea with constant cutting pains.

 SYMPTOM PICTURE

Mental and Emotional Symptoms
Nervous, timid, hypochondriac; women may believe they are pregnant.

Physical Symptoms
• Frequent bouts of sneezing with irritation in the nose; it itches and tickles.
• Runny nose, worse for smelling flowers.
• Eyes watery and red, worse for sneezing, coughing, walking outdoors.
• Sneezing may cause a frontal headache.

Remedy Picture
• Acute sense of smell.
• Face may be hot and red, lips burn, mouth itches. Left-sided sore throat.
• Worse for cold air, cold drinks, full moon.
• Better for heat, warm food and drink, swallowing.

Dosage: 6c
Antidote: Pulsatilla
Complementary Remedy: Sepia.

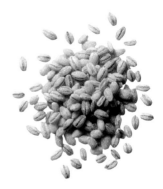

ABOVE *Sabadilla is a member of the lily family and is native to Mexico, Guatemala, and Venezuela. The seeds are used to make the remedy. They have long been known as an efficient vermifuge.*

Scleranthus Scleranthus annuus

 FLOWER ESSENCE

Scleranthus, one of the twelve healers, relates to indecision and steadfastness. It is one of the remedies for those who suffer uncertainty, are unable to decide, and suffer much from hesitation and procrastination. First they think one thing and then another. They may want several things at once, swinging between emotional and intellectual argument. They become easily confused and cannot make up their minds or apply themselves steadfastly. Scleranthus people are usually quiet and are not inclined to discuss their options with others.

 METHOD

The Sun Method (*see page 42*)
Gather the flowering stems from as many plants as possible. Cover the water surface thickly.

Lesson
Stability and balance
Before we can act decisively, an argument must feel right on all levels. It must feel correct "inside," to the guts, heart, and mind. Scleranthus helps us find the stability to listen to our inner selves and integrate the emotional and intellectual extremes into a balanced and sustained action.

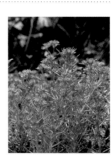

ABOVE *Scleranthus is a small, bushy, spreading plant growing 4in. (10cm.) high on sandy soils and in fields. It has short, thin stems that divide and divide, branching into a tangled mass. Scleranthus flowers are green, have no petals, and grow at the forks and end of the stem.*

Skullcap Scutellaria galericulata

HERBALISM

A tea or tincture is useful for anxiety, tension headaches, premenstrual tension, examination nerves, and postexamination depression. Use skullcap with valerian or chamomile and linden flowers for insomnia and disturbed sleep and for tranquilizer withdrawal; use it with vervain for workaholics. The mixture is relaxing without sedation; use it with wild oats, valerian, and sage to support anxious people with stressful jobs. Skullcap is a supportive treatment in epilepsy and for people on major tranquilizers. It reduces anxiety without interfering with their medication.Used at a very weak strength, Sandalwood soothes diaper rash.

HERBALISM

• Strengthens and calms the nervous system
• Antispasmodic

Notes and Dosages
• Standard doses (*see pages 21-25*).
• There are many relaxing tablets available containing skullcap and other herbs; follow the dosage on the box.

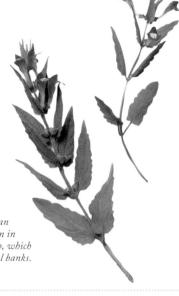

RIGHT *Herbalists use American skullcap, which is easily grown in gardens, or European skullcap, which grows wild on river and canal banks.*

Saw Palmetto Berries Serenoa repens

HERBALISM

A decoction, tincture, or tablets are helpful for prostate enlargement, cystitis, and inflammation of the urinary tract. Use with horsetail for urinary incontinence and cystitis due to prostate problems. Use with damiana for weakness and impotence. It helps restore weight after severe illness.

CHILDREN

Use with marshmallow for failure to thrive, 10 to 15 drops of the combined tincture three times daily in pure fruit juice

PROPERTIES

• Strengthening tonic
• Urinary antiseptic
• Alterative
• Stimulates sex hormones

Notes and Dosages
Decoction: ½ teaspoon of the crushed berries to one cup of water. Adult dose one or two cups daily.

Tincture: 20 to 40 drops, in water, three times daily.

• Modern research in Germany has demonstrated that the tablets are useful in prostate enlargement.
• Traditionally used for fattening animals.

Contraindications
Always have suspected prostate enlargement medically assessed.

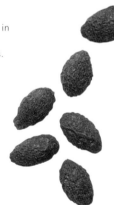

LEFT *The fruit of this small, palmlike plant grown in the West Indies and southern United States is used in herbalism.*

Sepia (Sep.) Sepia officinalis, cuttlefish

HOMEOPATHIC

Sepia is often perceived as being a remedy needed predominantly by women but can also be required by men and children. It has a positive effect on the liver and blood flow and female hormones.

Constitutional type: Tall, slender women. Chilly, cannot get warm yet sweat easily at the slightest exertion. Dark-haired, pale or sallow complexion with yellow or brown saddle across the nose and moth marks on the forehead, dark shadows under the eyes. They are soft featured rather than hard and angular with a doughy face and dull expression. Weak, lax muscles, pot-bellied, droopy, prone to prolapse of the uterus. Catch cold easily.

SYMPTOM PICTURE

Mental and Emotional Symptoms
• Worn out from life's hard grind.

• Joyless. Life is a drudge. Indifferent to loved ones.

• Very sensitive to noise, music, odors. Longs to be carefree.

Physical Symptoms
Headache: Surging, darting, tearing, throbbing pains. Feet icy-cold with headache. Very hungry yet averse to food; better for eating.

Cough: Short, dry, hacking cough. Chest feels hollow or tight and sore. Tastes rotten eggs in mouth. Profuse yellow phlegm. Worse for lying down.

Backache: Backache in small of back. Icy coldness between shoulder blades. Back is weak and stiff, aching with dragging pains. Better for firm pressure, walking. Worse for sitting, bending, around menstruation.

Skin: Itches generally, weepy and crusty in bends of joints—elbows, behind knees. Herpes—especially around the mouth. Brown warts. Hair loss from depression.

Gastrointestinal tract: Nausea from sight or smell of food, worse in the morning, better for eating. Morning sickness. Gnawing hunger with nausea. Constipated.

Urinary tract: Incontinence of urine. Worse for running, laughing, coughing, sneezing. Bedwetting in children within the first hour or two of being asleep.

Women's complaints: Heavy, weak, congested uterus with bearing-down pains, tendency to prolapse. Painful periods—may be late with light flow or early and heavy.

Menopausal hot flushes as if drenched with hot water, red face, thirstless. Dryness of vagina and vulva with pain on waking.

Remedy Picture
• Cold with cold hands and hot feet or vice versa.

• Left-sided complaints.

• Yellow discharges—sour, smelly, irritating.

• Sensations of lumps or balls either stuck or moving in the abdomen and pelvis.

• Dragging sensations.

• Sweat—sour, cold, or hot, profuse, from pain or exertion.

• Worse in the early morning and evening, damp, cold, cold air, after sweating, exhausting mundane chores in a damp atmosphere.

• Better for sleep, eating, brisk walking, rapid movement. Dry weather, warmth, pressure.

• Desires vinegar, wine, sweets.

• Dislikes and is worse for bread, milk, fatty foods, acid, and meat.

Dosages: 6c or 30c
Antidotes: Sulfur
Complementary Remedies: Nux vom., Natrum mur., Sabadilla

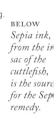

BELOW *Sepia ink, from the ir sac of the cuttlefish, is the sourc for the Sep remedy.*

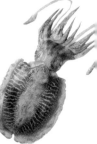

Milk Thistle Seed Silybum marianum

HERBALISM

Use a decoction or powdered seeds for liverishness and liver disease, poor fat tolerance, pale stools, and to protect the liver when taking strong drugs and medicines. It can treat high blood pressure with liverish symptoms. It is useful for depression following hepatitis, gallbladder stones, inflammation, Candida infection, and food allergies. As the name implies, it promotes the flow of milk in breast-feeding mothers and can be safely drunk as a tea throughout the nursing period.

PROPERTIES

• Strengthens and clears the liver and gallbladder

• Promotes milk flow in nursing mothers

Notes and Dosages
• Standard decoction, ½ a cup three times daily for at least six months.

• Tablets are also available—follow the instructions on the package.

• Recent research indicates it may be useful in hepatitis C.

Contraindications
• Liver disease should be treated by a professional.

• Milk thistle can be used as a supportive medicine—it will only help, but do tell your practitioner.

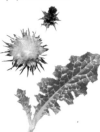

LEFT *Milk thistle is a tall, beautiful thistle that can easily be grown in gardens. The seeds resemble sunflower seeds.*

Mustard Sinapsis arvensis, Sinapsis alba and Brassica nigra

 FLOWER ESSENCE

Mustard is one of the remedies for those not sufficiently interested in present circumstances. A dark cloud of gloom or deep depression comes from nowhere and blocks out the sun with heavy feelings of melancholy and sadness. There may be no reason for the feeling, and it may lift just as suddenly as it arrived. Under the "dark cloud," it is hard for the sufferer to muster any feeling of happiness or hope.

 FOOD USES

Mustard plasters and poultices are very effective treatments for chest infections. Mustard oil is beneficial in relieving pain in arthritic joints, and chilblains, and can help in the treatment of skin eruptions. A mustard footbath (one teaspoon of mustard powder added to a bowl of hot water) is a traditional remedy for colds and headaches.
Mustard powder mixed with water makes a powerful emetic when taken in large doses. Mustard can be used as an expectorant.

 METHOD

The Boiling Method (*see page 43*)
(*Synapse arvensis*)
Mustard flowers throughout the late spring and early summer. Pick bright open flowers and the whole flowerhead above any faded flowers and seed pods. Pick from a wide area and from as many plants as possible.

Lesson
Hope
All clouds pass. Mustard lightens our mood and gives us faith to keep on going. Although these attacks seem to come from nowhere, they are not independent. The mood comes to fill a vacant space, a vacuum of the spirit. This may be very deep and subconscious and other remedies may be needed to support the core of the person.

 PROPERTIES

Black mustard and white mustard are warming herbs that stimulate the circulatory and digestive systems. White mustard relieves pain and is a diuretic and an antibiotic.

Special Notes
• The seeds of white mustard should not be handled or used by anyone but a qualified practitioner.
• The seeds and oil of black mustard may cause blistering of the skin in sensitive people after prolonged contact.

Contraindications
White mustard seed is a potent irritant when in contact with the skin and mucous membrane.

BELOW *Mustard is a common annual of fields and waysides, growing 1–2ft. (30–60cm.) high. Wild mustard greens are eaten like spinach or put in salads for their slightly peppery taste. Both black (*Brassica nigra*) and white mustard (*Sinapsis alba*) are used in cooking and medicines. The leaves, flowers, seeds, and oils of black mustard are used, but only the seeds of white mustard. A third type, brown mustard (*B. juncea*) also known as Indian or Chinese mustard, has only culinary applications.*

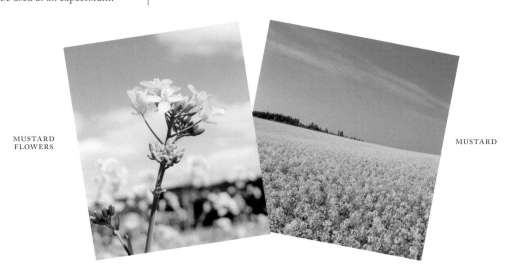

MUSTARD
FLOWERS

MUSTARD

Ignatia (Ign.) Strychnos ignatii, Ignatia amari, St. Ignatius bean

 HOMEOPATHIC

Signatia is useful for acute ailments from grief, and emotional shock. It is also useful in eating disorders, especially where the sufferer craves cold, raw, unappetizing foods.

 SYMPTOM PICTURE

Mental and Emotional Symptoms

• Silently grieving. Grief from death of a loved one or a broken friendship.

• Sudden bursts of weeping.

• Feel stressed.

• Insomnia from emotional upset. Light sleeper with repetitive dreams. Trembles with grief. Mood swings—one moment happy and laughing, then sad and crying.

Physical Symptoms

Headache: From grief. Head feels empty yet heavy. Pain as if a nail were boring out through the side. Congestive, throbbing. Worse for stooping, tobacco smoke. Better for firm pressure.

Roaring in ears: Relieved by music.

Gastrointestinal tract: Hunger not relieved by eating. Hiccups and belches after eating and drinking. Craves acid foods.

Sore throat: With stitching pains that shoot into ears, better for swallowing. Sensation of lump in throat not relieved by swallowing.

Cough: Worse at night, dry, spasmodic cough in quick bursts, the more they cough, the more they have to cough.

Fever: Thirst only during chill. Red face with chill, wants to be covered.

Convulsions or fits: After a fright—especially in children who have been severely told off, then become extremely hot and upset and have a febrile convulsion.

Remedy Picture

• Frequent yawning, sighing and sobbing. Worse at night, coffee, tobacco and alcohol.

• Swollen, inflamed tissues that are painful when not being touched and are better for firm pressure, lying on the painful side.

Dosages: 6c or 30c

Take Ignatia in the morning if possible—it may cause insomnia if taken at night.

Antidotes: Arnica, Cocculus, Chamomilla, *Pulsatilla*

Complementary Remedy: Natrum Mur.

> **ORIGINS OF IGNATIA**
> Ignatia is made from seeds found in the bitter fruits of the St. Ignatius bean.

Nux Vomica (Nuxvom.) Strychnos nux-vomica, poison nut tree

 HOMEOPATHIC

Nux vomica is often needed by business men and women who work hard and desire stimulating foods, e. g. spices, coffee, and alcohol. It is also sometimes required by children when the symptoms fit. It is a good "hangover" remedy if the symptoms fit.

 SYMPTOM PICTURE

Mental and Emotional Symptoms

For overstimulated people. Oversensitive and irritable, faultfinding, feel uneasy, and violent.

Physical symptoms

Headache: Dull, aching, squeezing, throbbing. Worse in the morning, light, moving eyes, stooping. Drunken headache.

Coughs and colds: Nose blocked at night, runs by day. Worse in a warm room, better for cold air. Tight, dry, cough and headache.

Fever: Burning hot all over but cannot uncover without chill.

Women's complaints: Irregular periods, too early, too long, black blood. Period pain felt in sacrum.

Gastrointestinal tract: Likes fat, spices, coffee, alcohol, tobacco but is worse for them. Indigestion an hour or two after eating. Retches and strains to vomit.

Constipated: Has the urge but cannot pass anything.

Remedy Picture

Very chilly. Worse for cold things, drafts, dry and windy weather, winter. Better for warmth, being well-wrapped up. Worse at 3 to 4 a.m. and on getting up in the morning. Better in the evening.

Dosages: 6c or 30c

Antidotes: Ars. alb., Chamomilla, Cocculus, Pulsatilla, Thuja

Complementary Remedies: Sulfur, Sepia

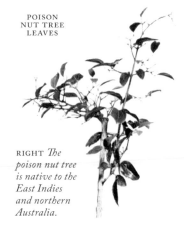

POISON NUT TREE LEAVES

RIGHT *The poison nut tree is native to the East Indies and northern Australia.*

Comfrey or Symphytum (Symph.) Symphytum officinale, knit-bone

 HERBALISM

Comfrey is the pre-eminent herb for rapid healing of cuts, wounds, sprains, bruises, and broken bones. It can be taken as a tea or tincture and used as a poultice, cream, ointment, or lotion. Make sure deep wounds are well cleaned, using marigold tea for example, before applying the comfrey. It works best on new and old bruises. Comfrey is also a good cream for cracked, dry skin. Use with chamomile and meadowsweet for gastritis and stomach ulcers. Add a few drops of a warming essential oil, such as black pepper, to the infused oil to make a good liniment for arthritis, bunions, and aches and pains arising from old injuries. Add a few drops of a soothing, antiseptic essential oil, such as lavender, to comfrey cream for use on slow-to-heal wounds and bed sores. Use as a syrup for long-standing dry coughs. Comfrey is such a powerful, rapid healer that care must be taken when using it on deep cuts. It may promote the formation of tissue over an unhealed wound sealing in infection and causing abscesses.

As a homeopathic remedy, Symphytum is used for injuries to the bones and eyeballs.

 PROPERTIES

• Promotes rapid healing

• Mucilaginous

Notes and Dosages
• Comfrey root is often used in creams and ointments but it should not be used internally except with professional guidance.

• Comfrey has been shown to cause liver disease in laboratory rats. There is a lot of dispute about the relevance of these findings to human use. In Britain, the Ministry of Agriculture, Fisheries and Food has determined that Comfrey leaf tea is quite safe for everyday use by adults.

 SYMPTOM PICTURE

Symphytum is primarily a first-aid remedy in homeopathic terms and so there is no extensive remedy picture.

Physical Symptoms
Fractures: It eases the pain (severe aching or pricking pain) and encourages the bones to heal; can be given for old injuries (broken bones and sprains) when they remain painful and weak.
Eyeball: Sore and bruised after a direct blow to the eyeball. Give Arnica first to deal with the shock and bruising, follow with Symphytum to allay pain and encourage healing.

Dosages: 6c
Antidotes: None
Complementary Remedies: Arnica, Calc. phos., Calc. fluor., Ruta

 CAUTION

Do not use internally in pregnancy or for infants.

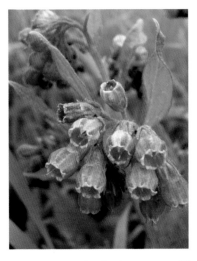

BELOW & ABOVE *Comfrey is a common wild plant with large, bristly leaves, and clusters of purple, bell-shaped flowers. The flowers and top leaves are used in herbalism.*

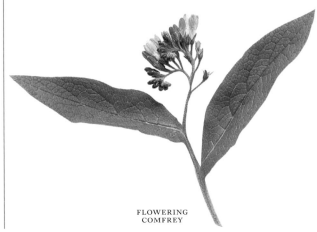

FLOWERING COMFREY

Clove Syzygium aromaticum

 AROMATHERAPY

Clove, when used as a massage oil, is excellent for rheumatism, arthritis, sprains, and stains. Massaged over the stomach, it aids dyspepsia, flatulence, and stomach problems. Massaged over lower back during childbirth, it eases labor pains. Dotted on absorbent cotton, it acts very effectively on abscesses and toothache. As an antiseptic oil, it will help heal and prevent infection in wounds and ulcers. Clove is often used in the treatment of scabies and has been known to be used in treating cancer. Used in a vaporizer or burned in a room, it enhances concentration and acts as an aphrodisiac. Clove also acts as an effective insect repellent and has action against intestinal parasitic conditions. It combines well with other antiseptic oils, such as lavender, thyme, and bergamot.

 FOOD USES

Clove is a warming, aromatic herb much used to flavor savory and sweet dishes. Clove tea is a warming, stimulating drink that causes sweating. It is useful for fevers, vomiting, and nausea.

 PROPERTIES

- Stimulant
- Antispasmodic
- Antineuralgic
- Antiseptic
- Anticancer
- Vermifuge (infestations)

Contraindications
Dilute clove oil well because it can irritate the skin.

 CAUTION

- Do not use the oil on babies, infants, and small children
- Avoid cloves and clove oil during pregnancy; cloves can cause uterine contractions

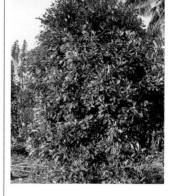

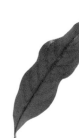

ABOVE *The clove tree is a small evergreen related to the myrtle, with pale gray leaves and a smooth bark. It is found in Sri Lanka, Madagascar, Reunion, and Malaysia. Cloves, the unexpanded dried flower buds, and their oil are used therapeutically. Clove essential oil is water-distilled from the clove buds and is a pale yellowy color. It has a strong, pungent, spicy aroma.*

Tamus Tamus communis, black bryony root and berries

 HOMEOPATHIC

Tamus is a poisonous plant that is no longer used as a medicinal herb internally. It is very effective when used as an ointment externally to soothe unbroken chilblains.

 DOSAGE

Apply the ointment twice a day to clean, washed and dried feet—or as directed on the label.

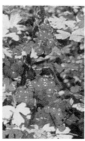

BLACK BRYONY
BERRIES

LEFT *Black bryony, a half-hardy shrub, is very poisonous and should not be touched.*

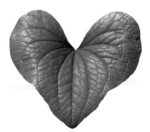

Feverfew Tanacetum parthenium

HERBALISM

The fresh plant tincture or fresh leaves are eaten for migraine and severe headaches. Combine with skullcap for persistent headaches and with valerian for migraine linked with anxiety and tension. Feverfew is also useful for period pains, vertigo, and arthritis. The compress relieves painful, swollen, and hot joints.

PROPERTIES

- Anti-inflammatory
- Antispasmodic
- Bitter
- Antithrombotic
- Emmenagogue

Notes and Dosages

- The various tablets and pills available are often useless. The best preparation is the tincture made from the fresh plant.
Dose: 1 teaspoon in a little water at the first signs of a migraine, repeat in two hours if necessary.

- For repeated attacks and as a treatment for arthritis and other chronic complaints, take one teaspoon every morning.

In combination: Add an equal part of a tincture of the other herb and take three teaspoons of the combination daily.

- If you have a plant, take two or three medium-sized leaves. To keep the plant growing cut the flowers off as they form.

Contraindications

The fresh leaves are acrid and can cause mouth ulcers. To prevent this wrap them in a small piece of bread.

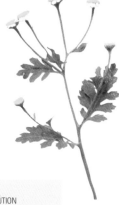

RIGHT *Feverfew is easily grown in gardens and often found self-sown. Both the small flowered daisy and the leaves are used in herbalism.*

 CAUTION

- Do not take during pregnancy
- Do not take if you are using drugs to thin the blood, such as warfarin

---

Dandelion Taraxacum officinale

HERBALISM

Use dandelion leaves with uva ursi or thyme for cystitis and urethritis. The fresh white sap in the flower stalks will banish warts if dabbed on regularly. Take a decoction of dandelion roots for all types of liver problems, gallstones, and gallbladder inflammation. Use the roots for mild jaundice with a yellowish cast to the skin, a bitter taste in the mouth, and dull eyes; for indigestion, loss of appetite, and constipation in pregnancy. Use in combination with burdock or other alterative herbs for arthritis and stubborn skin disease; with horsetail for degenerative arthritis and chronic bladder weakness. Research shows that regular use of dandelion roots helps reduce blood cholesterol. The liver plays a crucial role in detoxification and nutrition, so dandelion root is helpful in most chronic and wasting diseases and helps the body to cope with strong chemical drugs.

FOOD USES

Make a salad of blanched dandelion leaves and fresh herbs. The leaves can also be cooked and eaten like spinach and the flower petals made into wine. Eat the leaves as a spring tonic to cleanse the system after winter. Use dandelion leaf tea for all types of water retention and edema; especially useful for swollen ankles associated with heart and circulatory problems. Dandelion may help in the treatment of urinary disorders, eczema, and asthma. It is safe when eaten as part of the normal diet.

PROPERTIES—LEAVES

- A powerful diuretic
- Nourishing

PROPERTIES—ROOT

- Restorative liver tonic
- Promotes good digestion
- Alterative

Notes and Dosages—Leaves

- Use 2 or 3 teaspoons of the dried herb to a cup of boiling water. Drink freely. Take sufficient to produce a good flow of urine.
- Contains vitamins A, B, and C and many trace minerals; it is especially high in potassium.
- The fresh leaves are a tasty salad ingredient.

Notes and Dosages—Root

- Take at least 3 cups of decoction a day for six months.
- *Tincture:* Take 4 to 6 teaspoons daily, but the decoction is best for liver problems.
- Dandelion "coffee," made by roasting the root, has a pleasant, slightly bitter taste and keeps much of the strength of the unroasted root.

LEFT *Both the leaves and roots of this familiar, yellow-flowered weed are used in herbalism. Dandelion is the best example of the maxim, "there are no weeds in a herbalist's garden."*

Thuja (Thuj.) Thuja occidentalis, tree of life, arbor-vitae, swamp cedar

 HERBALISM

Thuja is used in herbalism for bronchitis, acute fevers, pain on ovulation, cystitis with pus in the urine, and itchy skin diseases. Use the tincture. The adult dose is 15-20 drops three times daily. The children's dose is 5 drops three times daily.

 HOMEOPATHIC

Thuja is often taken as a general remedy for warts; however, the other symptoms should be there to base the prescription on. If in doubt consult a qualified homeopath. Constitutional type: Often short with a slight build, greasy, waxy, pale complexion, prone to chronic thick green catarrh, pustular acne, and warts.

 SYMPTOM PICTURE

Mental and Emotional Symptoms
• Sensitive to other people's moods and to music.
• Paranoid, has fixed ideas; feels brittle, feels as if something is alive in stomach.
• Children can be slow to develop mentally.

Physical Symptoms
• Headache where there is left-sided pain as if pierced by a nail, can be brought on by tea-drinking.
• Chronic thick green mucus causes a permanent runny nose, blocked ears with creaking noise on swallowing, chronic ear infections, chronic sore throat, laryngitis.
Skin: Sweet-smelling sweat, dirty-looking skin; pustular spots, boils, carbuncles; warts, large, bleed easily.

Remedy Picture
Left-sided complaints.
• Worse at night and early morning, at 3 a.m. and 3 p.m., waxing moon, from bad effects of vaccination, sunshine and bright lights, warmth of bed, fatty food, coffee, damp, warm weather, rest.
• Better for lying on left side, while drawing up a limb.
• Chilly—likes cold food and drinks.
• Exhausted.
• Dislike meat and potatoes.
Dosage: Thuja is a remedy that should be treated with respect. It is not a first-aid remedy in the way that Arnica is for bruising or Aconite is for shock. It should only be given if truly indicated as the similar remedy (similimum), in which case take a single dose of a 6c potency and wait; it is best not to repeat the dose too frequently.
• Thuja tincture (Q)—may be applied externally 3 times a day to warts.
Antidotes: Camphor, Merc., Sulfur
Complementary Remedies: Ars. alb., Silica

 CAUTION

Do not use in pregnancy.

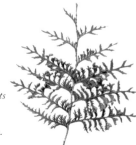

RIGHT *Thuja is a coniferous tree, a member of the cypress family. It grows up to 65ft. (20m.) high, and its leaves, stems, and bark are used for medicinal purposes.*

Linden Tilia europaea, Tilia x vulgaris, lime

 HERBALISM

The tea or tincture is helpful for anxiety and insomnia. Linden flower makes a pleasant combination with chamomile. Long-term use strengthens the nervous system and improves stress tolerance. It improves digestion. Use with hawthorn tops as a tea for mild high blood pressure.

 CHILDREN

Induces sweating and reduces temperature in fevers. Normal tea strength can be taken freely.

 PROPERTIES

• Calming and soothing
• Strengthens nerves
• Diaphoretic

Notes and Dosages
May be taken freely.

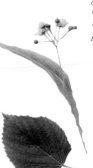
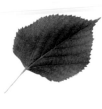

BELOW *The flowers of a linden or lime tree, often grown in parks and along streets, are used in herbalism. It makes a pleasant drinking tea that mixes well with other herb teas. Linden tea is a popular everyday drink in France.*

Thyme Thymus vulgaris

 HERBALISM

The tea, tincture, or syrup is useful for any cough with infected or tough phlegm. Thyme tea is helpful in asthma, taken regularly. Use it as a gargle for sore throats and drink it for indigestion and wind. Use it with marshmallow for cystitis and intestinal infections. It can also be used as a diluted tincture or vinegar wash for fungal infections.

 CHILDREN

Syrup for coughs, whooping cough. Infused oil as a gentle chest rub for infants. Strong tea for worms. Weak tea for nightmares.

 AROMATHERAPY

The essential oil is good for rheumatism, venereal diseases, cystitis: use in the bath. It can also be used for gastroenteritis (massage over stomach) and chest complaints (massage over chest).

 FOOD USES

Common thyme has many uses in cooking, particularly as a flavoring for savory dishes. Used as a culinary herb it may be of some benefit in the treatment of indigestion and diarrhea in children.

 PROPERTIES

- Antiseptic
- Antibacterial
- Antifungal
- Expectorant
- Digestive tonic

Notes and Dosages
- Take freely. Large doses may be needed for coughs.
- For infant's coughs, two or three teaspoons of syrup up to four times daily or two cups of tea in their bath.
- For children's worms, ¼-½ cup strong tea before breakfast, for two weeks.
- For nightmares 2-6 teaspoons tea before bed.
- Wild thyme is stronger.

Contraindications
Pregnant women and those suffering from epilepsy should avoid taking in medicinal doses, although the small amounts used in cooking are safe.

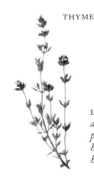

THYME

LEFT *The leaves and flowers of this popular cooking herb are used in herbalism.*

Rhus Toxicodendron (Rhus. Tox.) Toxicodendron radicans, poison ivy

 HOMEOPATHIC

Rhus toxicodendron is a remedy with an affinity for the joints and skin. Choose it for symptoms that appear after getting wet or overworking. It is also useful for recovery after surgery.

 SYMPTOM PICTURE

Mental and Emotional Symptoms
Restless and irritable, depressed. Bursts into tears without knowing why.

Physical Symptoms
- Fever, very hot and restless, cannot lie still, feels chilly and wants to be covered.
Rheumatism: Hot, painful, swollen joints with tearing pains and stiffness. Very restless, constantly changes positions. Worse when getting up and starting to move. Better for continued movement, until he or she tires and has to rest, but is soon driven by restlessness to get up again.
- Also for strained, overused muscles with above symptoms.
Skin: Nettle rash, raw, oozing eczema, blisters, and cold sores (herpes) with itching, burning, tingling. The more they scratch, the more they need to scratch. Chickenpox and cold sores that are intensely itchy and painful benefit from Rhus tox.
Mumps: Left-sided swollen parotid gland, highly inflamed and enlarged, with cold sores on lips. Worse for cold air, cold water.

Remedy Pictures
- Worse at rest, beginning to move, prolonged exercise, in the damp, cold wet weather.
- Can often feel approach of wet weather in joints.
- Better for gentle motion, heat, hot baths, massage and rubbing, changing position.

Dosage: 6c
Antidote: Coffea
Complementary Remedy: Bryonia

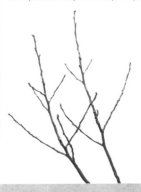

LEFT *Poison ivy is a sumac, a native of North America. Skin contact with its leaves brings up an extremely itchy, irritating rash.*

Damiana Turnera diffusa

 HERBALISM

The tea and tincture is used for impotence and sterility associated with anxiety, especially in men. Use it for physical weakness, depression, mental stupor, and nervous exhaustion in both sexes; for prostatitis and chronic cystitis; for poor digestion with constipation and lack of appetite.

 PROPERTIES

• Stimulant tonic for the nerves and reproductive system
• Aphrodisiac

Notes and Dosages
• ½ cup of the tea or 1 teaspoon of the tincture twice daily.

• Alternatively combine damiana with other herbs and use 1 cup of the combination tea, or 1 teaspoon of tincture, twice daily.

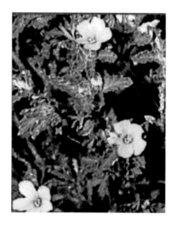

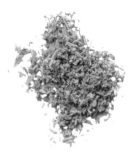

LEFT *Damiana is a small, strongly aromatic shrub grown in Mexico and South America. The damiana leaf is used in herbalism.*

Gorse Tulex europaeus

 FLOWER ESSENCE

Gorse is one of the remedies for people who suffer uncertainty. It is used for a very great feeling of hopelessness. The Gorse type may seek for help in order to please others but underneath they know that nothing can be done for them. They are resigned and have given up trying. This resignation is a response to some event or fear that made them give up hope. The Gorse type is stuck in a perpetual circle of negativity and suffering. Their future is clear. They do not complain. They have lost the heart to strive.

 METHOD

The Sun Method (see page 42)
Gorse starts flowering in the early spring. Pick the flowers by their hairy stalks. Pick from big, healthy clumps, taking flowers from the center and edges of many plants.

Lesson
Positive possibilities
Gorse helps open a door to possibilities and strengthens the heart to face them. Gorse can achieve remarkable results, although it may need to be given with Agrimony or Mimulus.

BELOW *Gorse is an evergreen bush, 2–8ft. (60cm.–3m.) high, spreading in habit, and armed with rigid, sharp branched spines. It grows abundantly on poor, stony soils, and heathlands.*

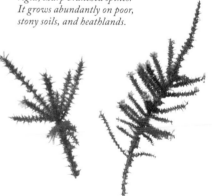

Slippery Elm *Ulmus fulva var. rubra, Ulmus rubra, red elm*

 HERBALISM

Use a decoction, powder, or tablets for any sort of inflammation or irritation in the digestive tract; nausea, indigestion, wind, food allergies, stomach ulcers, acidity, heartburn, hiatus hernia, abdominal distension, colitis, diverticulitis, and diarrhea. This is one of the most useful herbal medicines in this area. Slippery elm bark is often used to back up other remedies. Use as a nourishing drink during convalescence. The powder mixed with sufficient water to make a paste is helpful for drawing splinters and mixed with sage tea or witch hazel for weeping eczema. It makes a good base for poultices.

 PROPERTIES

• Soothing
• Mucilaginous

Notes and Dosages
• A level teaspoon of slippery elm powder stirred into a glass of water or milk, three times daily before meals.
• Tablets flavored with peppermint and other carminative herbs are especially useful. Take one or two tablets with a glass of water or milk before meals.
• For nausea, travel sickness, and nausea of pregnancy suck one tablet slowly.

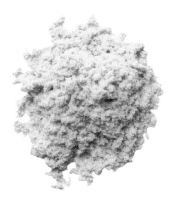

ABOVE *The bark of this small American tree is usually sold powdered to use in herbalism.*

Elm *Ulmus procera, English elm*

 FLOWER ESSENCES

Elm is one of the remedies for those who suffer despondency and despair. It is used for temporary feelings of inadequacy. Elm types are good workers, proud of themselves and their calling. They hope to do something important and to be of benefit to all humanity. They seek perfection, and this goal can be dauntingly overwhelming. Elm is for brief faltering moments of despair and lack of confidence, when the idealism within a task or its significance can seem too much to live up to.

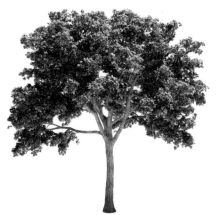

ABOVE *The elm is a majestic deciduous tree, 150ft. (45–50m.) tall with a strong and massive trunk. It was once a common and powerful presence in the English countryside. Since 1970, Dutch elm disease has killed millions of trees in Europe and North America.*

 METHOD

The Boiling Method (*see page 43*)
The elm flowers from the early spring on bare twigs before the leaves open. Pick twigs with flowering clusters, about 6in. (15cm.) long. Pick from as many trees as possible until the saucepan is three-quarters full.

Lesson
Balanced idealism
Elm helps us find the strength to balance idealism and practical reality, so that we do not strive for an unattainable external perfection but appreciate the perfection of our inner process. Balanced Elm people achieve much good.

Valerian Valeriana officinalis

 HERBALISM

The decoction or tincture is helpful for anxiety, confusion, headaches due to tension, migraines, depression with anxiety. It is useful on plane journeys. Valerian helps withdrawal from tranquilizers. Use with motherwort or hawthorn for palpitations; with thyme for irritable coughs and smoker's cough; with linden flowers, hawthorn, and yarrow for high blood pressure; with skullcap, linden flowers, or chamomile for insomnia; with dandelion root and chamomile for colic and nervous indigestion; or with cramp bark for menstrual cramps and intestinal colic.

 HOMEOPATHIC

Calming to overwrought, over-stressed, anxious individuals.

 PROPERTIES

- Sedative
- Nerve restorative
- Calms the heart
- Antispasmodic
- Carminative

 CAUTION

Do not take for long periods without examining why you are so tense.

Contraindications

- *The cold decoction is best:* soak 1 teaspoon in a cup of cold water overnight, dose ½ to 1 cup.

- *Tincture:* 20-60 drops three times daily. More may be needed to help tranquilizer withdrawal.

- Relaxing tablets containing valerian are widely available—follow dose on the package. They may not work right away, but be persistent.

Contraindications

- Safe, if you start low and increase.

- Large doses can cause headaches and excitability.

- May be counterproductive in insomnia from overstimulation—anxiety and nervous exhaustion are the best indications.

- Not physically addictive but people may become reliant on it.

- Tranquilizer withdrawal should only be undertaken with psychological support.

 SYMPTOM PICTURE

Mental and Emotional Symptoms
Tense and uptight, light-headed, not grounded.

Physical Symptoms
Cramps and constrictions, nervous asthma, rheumatism, and insomnia.

Remedy Picture
Their physical aches and pains and emotional state are worse when resting and during extreme exercise, better during gentle movement.

Dosage: 5-10 drops of mother tincture three to four times a day.

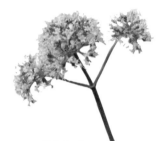

RIGHT *Valerian is a wild plant with pink or white flowers that grows in damp places. The valerian root is used in herbalism.*

Mullein Verbascum thapsus

 HERBALISM

A tea, tincture, and syrup of leaves or flowering spikes is helpful for deep and ticklish coughs and bronchitis. It is helpful in asthma, by clearing sticky mucus. To make mullein tobacco, rub honey water into the dried leaves, spread on a tray and allow to dry. One or two cigarettes daily help to reduce asthma attacks. Use mullein flower infused oil as eardrops for itchy ears and chronic earache and as a salve for itchy eyelids. Mullein and garlic infused oil soothe acute earaches.

 CHILDREN

2 drops of mullein flower infused oil, in a little juice, three times daily is helpful for bedwetting.

 METHOD

- A soothing expectorant, clears mucus
- Heals wounds

Notes and Dosages
- The tea gives the best results for coughs.
- Allow a long infusion and drink freely.

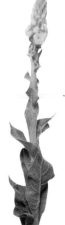

LEFT *Mullein is a beautiful wildflower with a tall, thick spike of yellow flowers. Both the leaves and flowers are used in herbalism.*

Vervain Verbena officinalis

 HERBALISM

Vervain is one of the most useful general tonics. The tea or tincture is helpful for weariness and postviral fatigue, ME. It helps us to let go of tension, including exhaustion from overwork; it is particularly useful for chronic nervous depression, fevers and flu, especially with headaches and nervous symptoms, insomnia, and excessive dreaming; also in depression and to relieve feelings of paranoia. It improves digestion and liver function and restores digestive function and appetite after intestinal infections. Use it for worms and parasites and for colicky pains. It is helpful in asthma with chest tension. Sip the tea throughout labor to encourage regular contractions. Continue after the birth to encourage milk flow. It may be helpful for postnatal depression. It can also be used for stopped periods (amenorrhea).

 CHILDREN

Digestive discomfort, especially associated with worms. Combines with meadowsweet to reduce irritability from itchy skin conditions.

 FLOWER ESSENCE

Vervain, one of the twelve healers, relates to overenthusiasm and tolerance. It is one of the remedies for those who overcare for the welfare of others. It is useful for those with strong, fixed ideas and principles they believe are right. They are strong-willed, rarely change their views, and obstinately maintain a stance when others would have conceded. They are great doers and wish to convert all those around them, sometimes with much fervor and enthusiasm. They believe this will bring harmony and happiness, but the effort of battling against the will of others is exhausting. The Vervain type of person strains with excess effort.

 PROPERTIES

- Tonic
- Fever herb
- Relaxing
- Nerve restorative
- Antispasmodic
- Carminative
- Promotes milk flow
- Emmenagogue

Notes and Dosages
Use freely in fevers, otherwise use the standard doses (*see pages 21-25*).

 METHOD

The Sun Method *(see page 42)*
The small pale mauve flowers grow on spikes and bloom throughout the summer. Pick the whole spike above any dead flowers. Gather from young plants so that there are not too many unopened buds or spent flowers on a spike. Float on the water, covering the surface completely.

Lesson
Will
Everyone has a will and purpose. Vervain types can be great teachers if they learn to do less and be more, and allow others to be and live their own truth. Vervain helps us bring our personal will into harmony with the greater will.

 CAUTION

Do not use in pregnancy, except during labor.

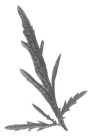

VERVIAN

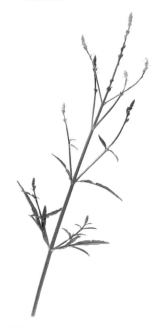

ABOVE *Vervain is a common wayside perennial growing 1-2ft. (30-60cm.) high in dry, sunny places. The leaves are deep and irregularly cut and covered with short hairs. The stem is square. It has an unprepossessing wild flower that is often missed. The whole plant is used in herbalism. Pick in full flower.*

Vetivert *Vetiveria zizanoides*

 AROMATHERAPY

The soothing properties of vetivert oil have been recognized for centuries. In India and Sri Lanka, where the plant grows, the oil it produces is known as the "oil of tranquility." In massage or in a bath, vetivert helps to balance the nervous system and is excellent for depression, mood swings, stress, and anxiety. Burned in a room, it helps insomnia. It is also a natural aphrodisiac, which may help to overcome some forms of impotence and frigidity. Massaged over the limbs, it is a great reliever of aching muscles, sports sprains, arthritis, rheumatism, and general stiffness. In a vaporizer or as an astringent, it is used to treat skin conditions such as acne, sores, oily skin, and blackheads. It combines well with other oils, such as patchouli, lavender, rose, jasmine, and ylang ylang.

 PROPERTIES

- Antiseptic
- Antidepressant
- Antirheumatic
- Fortifier of nervous system
- Circulatory
- Tonic
- Aphrodisiac

 CAUTION

- Use in a vaporizer if treating babies
- Avoid while pregnant

RIGHT *Vetivert essential oil is extracted by steam distillation from the rootlets of wild grass that originated in India; it is a cousin of lemongrass, citronella, and palmarosa. Vetivert is grown in South America, Indonesia, and the Caribbean. The oil is a rich dark brown or amber or a dark olive green color, and it has a distinctive earthy, woody, sweet aroma.*

Cramp Bark *Viburnum opulus*

 HERBALISM

A decoction, tincture, or capsules are useful for any sort of cramping pains including leg cramps, colic, period pains, muscle spasm, and shoulder and neck tension. Back pain usually involves an element of muscle spasm and it often improves dramatically. The cream is useful for the same symptoms when massaged in gently.

 CHILDREN

For bedwetting associated with tension and anxiety.

 PROPERTIES

- Relaxant
- Antispasmodic
- Mildly sedative

Notes and Dosages

- Best taken freely, 1 cup of the decoction or 1 or 2 teaspoons of the tincture four or five times daily. May be improved by the addition of a little ginger.

- For children, 30 drops of tincture, in fruit juice, three times daily.

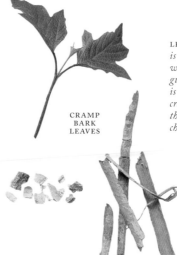

CRAMP BARK LEAVES

LEFT *Cramp bark is taken from the wild form of the guelder rose, which is a small tree with creamy flowers that grows on chalky soils.*

Agnus Castus Vitex agnus-castus

 HERBALISM

The decoction or tincture is useful for PMS, especially with irritability, mood swings, breast pain, and water retention. Use it for menopausal symptoms especially with mood swings and depression. Use it with sage for hot flushes. It is also good for early menopause and prolonged menstrual bleeding. It also helps restore a regular menstrual cycle when coming off the contraceptive pill or when the cycle has been disrupted by illness or prolonged stress. Use for excessive sex drive in both sexes. It is helpful in postnatal illness and for settling symptoms following terminations and miscarriages. It can also promote breast milk in nursing mothers. Use with burdock root and dandelion root for acne (which often has an hormonal component).

 PROPERTIES

- General tonic
- Balances hormones

Notes and Dosages

- The best time to take the berries is first thing in the morning, before breakfast. 1 cup of the decoction or 20-30 drops of the tincture in a little water, taken daily, will usually suffice.

- Women taking agnus castus for PMS and period problems may notice a change in the length of their cycle. The berries should be taken until the cycle settles down, usually for three to six months.

- Also available as tablets; follow the instructions on the package.

Contraindications

- Safe to use but may cause headaches in some people.

- Always have prolonged menstrual bleeding and absent periods checked by a health professional before you treat yourself.

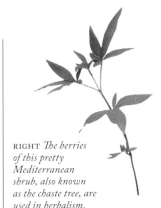

RIGHT *The berries of this pretty Mediterranean shrub, also known as the chaste tree, are used in herbalism.*

 CAUTION

Do not use without advice from your herbalist if you are taking hormone drugs.

Vine Vitis vinifera

 FLOWER ESSENCE

Vine is one of the remedies for those who overcare for the welfare of others. It is useful for capable, confident, and successful people "who would be king." They believe that being right confers an automatic authority over others. Being right, they believe they know better and that others would be happier if they did things the Vine way. They can bully and dominate, disabling others, and gaining authority at the expense of other people's confidence. They can be ruthless and dominating and even in illness can order their carers around.

 METHOD

The Sun Method *(see page 42)*
The small green flowers grow in dense clusters. Pick the entire cluster from as many different plants and parts of the plants as possible.

Lesson
Power and authority
Vine allows us to stand back and let others express their power and authority to make personal choices, and to respect their ability to do so. The positive Vine has authority and compassion and is of great value in an emergency.

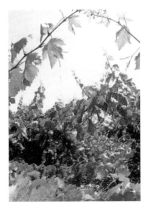

LEFT *The grape vine is a deciduous climber reputed to live for hundreds of years. It climbs by means of long curling tendrils. The large, palm size leaves are used to wrap food and cheeses. The fruit is eaten fresh, dried as raisins, pulped to make juice and fermented to make wine. The grape seed is crushed to extract an oil.*

Ginger *Zingiber officinale*

 HERBALISM

Ginger is a very useful remedy in herbalism. Its gentle warming, circulating and relaxing properties make it applicable to a wide range of conditions. A little ginger may be added to any recipes for nausea, stomach cramps, menstrual pains, chills, colds, and poor circulation. Apply fresh, grated ginger to the lower abdomen to ease menstrual pains.

 AROMATHERAPY

Used in massage or as an inhalation or burned in the room, ginger encourages immunity against colds and flu, bronchitis, catarrh, blocked sinuses, and headaches. Ginger also helps the circulatory system; used in a footbath, it is good for chilblains and poor circulation. Ginger generally helps rheumatic conditions. Massaging ginger oil, diluted in a carrier oil, over the kidney area will assist the body's vital force. Ginger acts on the digestive system, treating diarrhea, flatulence, and general eating problems. It is excellent for nausea and travel sickness. Ginger combines well with other essential oils, such as palmarosa, citrus oils, cedarwood, frankincense, and coriander.

 FOOD USES

Powdered ginger, ginger tea, and crystallized ginger are usually effective when taken for travel sickness. Ginger also has a calming effect on nausea in general. A poultice of fresh ginger may help to ease the discomfort of rheumatism. Chewing fresh ginger can relieve toothache. Ginger will expel mucus from the upper respiratory tract.

 PROPERTIES

- Anticatarrhal
- Aphrodisiac
- Digestive system
- Circulatory
- Stomachic

Properties

Ginger, which in Ayurvedic medicine is called "universal medicine," has a calming effect on the digestive system and a stimulating effect on the circulatory system. It is an antiseptic that can help in the prevention of ailments affecting the respiratory tract.

Special Notes

Ginger's stimulant properties prevent its use in some cases.

Contraindications

- Better not to use ginger essential oil in the bath since it may act as an irritant to sensitive mucous membranes.

- Use the oil with care, in half-measures for babies, infants, and children.

- Use half the normal amount of ginger oil when pregnant.

- People suffering from gastric or peptic ulcers should avoid ginger in all its forms.

THE TRAVELER'S FRIEND

Ginger has been statistically proved to reduce nausea and vomiting. This makes it one of the best natural remedies known for travel sickness. Drink ginger tea (take some with you in a thermos) or chew on fresh root or crystallized ginger to prevent or relieve symptoms.

 CAUTION

Do not use ginger in cases of hypertension.

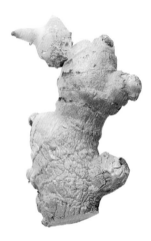

ABOVE *Ginger has been used since ancient times in cooking and in medicine. It is found in the Caribbean, West Africa, and the Far East. It is a warming and comforting herb with many medicinal uses. The root is used fresh or dried. Ginger essential oil is produced from the root by steam distillation. It is a pale greenish-yellow color and has an exotic, hot aroma.*

Elements, Compounds, and Minerals

$\mathcal{N}$ot all natural remedies come from plant or animal sources. Homeopathy in particular looks to chemical elements and compounds and minerals for remedies. In the following section, the remedy sources are grouped together thematically: calcium-based remedies, sulfur-based remedies, potassium-based remedies, and phosphorus-based remedies are followed by remedies made from dangerous substances: antimony, arsenic, mercury, and nitroglycerine. Then comes a group derived from metal (silver and lead), wood (charcoal), and water. The final twelve remedies are the biochemic tissue salts listed by Dr. Schuessler (*see page 31*).

Calcarea Carbonica (Calc. Carb.) Calcium carbonate

 HOMEOPATHIC

Calc. carb. is often needed by people who are physically slow, who have weight but no strength.
Constitutional type: Sluggish, pale, fat, and flabby with large head. Babies are late to teethe, sit up, crawl, and walk. Fontanels are late to close.

 SYMPTOM PICTURE

Mental and Emotional Symptoms
• Feel worthless and restless, disinterested, dull, fearful, and obstinate. Worry about silly things, academic plodders.

• Nightmares especially in children.

• Babies are unadventurous, sit where you put them.

• Averse to work.

Physical Symptoms
Head and chest: Catches cold at every change of weather, chronic catarrh, swollen glands in neck, recurrent throbbing ear infections, glue ear.

Gut: Constipated with large, hard stool, better for being constipated. Diarrhea from infections. Weak, sluggish gut.

Lungs: Dry cough at night, loose in morning, thick yellow mucus, breathing difficult lying down, painless hoarseness or with sore throat. Swollen glands in neck, pain between shoulder blades.

Rheumatism: Cold, puffy joints with cramping pains especially spine and knees. Weak back muscles cause backache.

Women's complaints: Sudden onset of profuse menstruation. Periods start too early or continue too long. Milky leucorrhea, itching, and burning.

Breast-feeding: Helps with too much or too little milk when woman is weak and sweaty from lactation.

Remedy Picture
• Head sweats especially at night.
• Slow digestion, better for being constipated.

• Soft and flabby with weak muscles. Adults have a limp, boneless, clammy hand-shake.

• Craves eggs, salt, chalk and coal. Dislikes coffee, milk, meat.

• Worse for exertion, walking uphill, cold weather, cold bathing, wet weather, full moon, standing.

• Better for dry warm weather, lying on painful side.

Dosages: 6c or 30c
Antidotes: Camphor, Ipecac. Nux vom.

Complementary Remedies: Belladonna, Rhus tox. Lycopodium, Silica

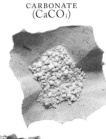

CALCIUM CARBONATE (CaCO₃)

RIGHT *The edible oyster, Ostrea edulis, provides the source for the Calc. carb. remedy. It is made from the crystalline deposits of calcium carbonate found in the middle layer of the shell.*

OYSTER

Hepar Sulfuris Calcareum (Hep. S.) Calcareum, calcium sulfide, flowers of sulfur

HOMEOPATHIC

Think of this remedy for unhealthy, infected skin and respiratory ailments.
Constitutional type: Extremely chilly. Hypersensitive physically and mentally.

SYMPTOM PICTURE

Mental and Emotional Symptoms
• Irritable with flares of violent anger, worries about health, anxious in the evening. Easily offended, hypersensitive.

Physical Symptoms
• Distended abdomen with foul wind, difficult to open bowels.

• Constipated with a soft stool.

Sore throat: Feels as though a fishbone is stuck, pricking pains shoot into the ears on swallowing. Swollen tonsils and neck glands.

Cough: Worse from a cold, dry wind. Dry, hacking, croupy, suffocating cough with thick, yellow phlegm. Sweats with cough.

Worse at night, on uncovering, in dry, cold weather. Better for moist air.

Croup: Worse at night or in the morning, with thick mucus that can be difficult to bring up, and relieved by warm, steamy air.

Skin: Cuts and wounds get infected and form pus instead of healing. Boils and abscesses with needlelike pricking pains, red and swollen. Hepar sulf. discharges pus and stimulates healing to take place.

Remedy Picture
• Hypersensitive to pain, to touch.

• Hurried—eats, drinks, walks, talks quickly.

• Even the smallest cut gets infected and forms pus, slow to heal.

• Offensive body odor and cold, sweaty feet—smell like old cheese.

• Extremely chilly, even in summer. Dislikes drafts, takes cold easily, better in warm, wet weather.

• Desires acidic, sour foods, vinegar, strong flavors.

• Splinterlike, pricking pains.

Dosage: 6c
Antidotes: Ars. alb., Belladonna, Chamomilla, Silica *Complementary Remedy:* Calendula

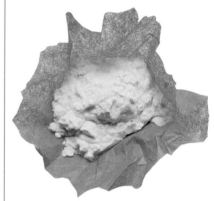

ABOVE *Hepar sulf. is made from Flowers of Sulfur (a form of calcium sulfide, or sulfurated potash).*

Magnesia Sulfurica (Mag. Sulf.) Magnesium sulfate, Epsom salts

HOMEOPATHIC

As epsom salt, it acts as a laxative and cleanser of the gut when taken internally, applied as a poultice externally it draws impurities out of the skin. As a homeopathic remedy, it removes heat and impurities by improving the function of the affected organs.

SYMPTOM PICTURE

Mental and emotional symptoms
• Apprehensive, weepy, uneasy and restless, gloomy.

Physical symptoms
Urinary tract: Copious bright yellow urine that becomes cloudy with red sediment when

left to stand. Urethra stitches and burns after passing urine (cystitis).

Women's complaints: Thick profuse burning discharge, heavy like a period with tired aching in small of back and down thighs. Worse for moving. Menstruation is too early, thick, black, profuse blood with a sick headache.

Skin: Extremely itchy pimples all over the body. Scratching makes them burn.

Remedy Picture
• Weak and trembly, lack of energy. Feels bruised and tired. Feels sick with tiredness.
• Sensitive to touch. Better for resting in bed or walking.

Dosage: 6c
Antidotes: None
Complementary Remedies: None

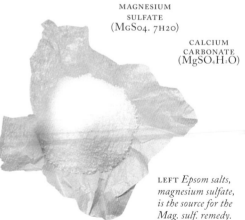

MAGNESIUM SULFATE
($MgSO_4 . 7H2O$)

CALCIUM CARBONATE
($MgSO_4H_2O$)

LEFT *Epsom salts, magnesium sulfate, is the source for the Mag. sulf. remedy.*

Sulfur (Sulf.) Sulfur

 HOMEOPATHIC

Sulfur is a great cleanser and should be used with caution in skin complaints. Be prepared to have an aggravation of the symptoms initially; if the condition is severe consult a homeopath.
Constitutional type: Tall, thin, hungry, lax with stooped shoulders, or ruddy and rotund, Likewise children can be thin and scrawny or fat and lazy. Whatever shape or size they have a dirty unkempt appearance and are prone to skin problems.

 SYMPTOM PICTURE

Mental and Emotional Symptoms
• Academic, philosophizes, unrealistic, selfish, and childish, untidy, lazy, forgetful, and irritable, very sensitive to smells.
• Children are lively, quick and full of curiosity.

Physical symptoms
Headache: With constant heat on top of head, throbbing in temples, and nausea, worse for stooping. Periodic headache.

• Colds, coughs, and flu: Catarrh chronic and dry, stuffed up nose indoors, nosebleeds.
• Earache that is stitching, burning pains, worse in left ear. Sensation of running water in ear. Glue ear with strong-colored offensive discharge. Humming, whizzing noises in ears. Sore throat, dry, red raw and burning. Cough—loose cough with green sweet-tasting phlegm, rattly chest, difficult to breathe, wants windows open. Heaviness of a weight on chest. Hot burning pains in chest and between shoulder-blades. Worse at night and for lying on back, must sit up.
Gastrointestinal tract: Acid stomach, worse for milk, a.m. Sour, hot burps, taste like rotten eggs. Stomach burns and feels heavy and full. Very thirsty. Diarrhea—urgent on waking. Painless, rumbling abdomen with foul wind, diarrhea is hot and burns anus. Worse at 5 a.m. Constipation—hard knotty stool, painful to pass.
Skin: Appears unwashed, dirty-looking, dry, rough, scaly, red, hot, very itchy, bleeds easily from scratching. Infected. Worse for washing. Worse for scratching—makes it burn. Dry itchy scalp. Eczema, red, rough, dry, hot, very itchy, especially in skin folds, worse at night, scratching makes it bleed. Eczema and asthma that alternate. Acne and boils that occur in recurrent crops, hot, red, angry looking, itch, and burn. Rashes of infectious childhood diseases such as chickenpox and measles where Sulfur symptoms predominate and the child is slow to recover.

Remedy picture
• Heat everywhere or in patches. Hands, feet and top of head burn.
• All complaints are hot, burn, intensely itchy.
• Orifices are red, hot and sore.
• Discharges are offensive, burning, itchy, bloody.
• Craves fatty and sweet foods.
• Very thirsty for cold drinks.
• Better for fresh air, moving, warm and dry weather, lying on right-hand side.
• Worse for rest, standing, stuffy room, overheating, damp cold, washing, warmth of bed, alcohol, morning, and night.
• Complaints occur periodically.
• Hunger at 11 a.m.

Dosage: 6c
Antidote: Nux vom.
Complementary Remedies: Aconite, Ars. alb, Nux vom.

SULFUR(S)

RIGHT *Sulfur is a nonmetalic element, usually found in crystalline form. It is the source for the homeopathic remedy Sulfur.*

Kali Bichromicum (Kali bich) Potassium bichromate, bichromate of potash

 HOMEOPATHIC

Kali bich. is used for ailments where the pain occurs in localized spots. The person can point to the pain, for example sinusitis causing pain behind the bridge of the nose.

 SYMPTOM PICTURE

Mental and Emotional Symptoms
• No strong mental indications.

Physical Symptoms
Catarrh: Thick, ropy, yellow-green. Nose blocked especially in chubby babies. Postnasal catarrh.

Sinusitis: With localized hot, tender pain.
Headache: Catarrhal, above the eyes in the forehead, is preceded by blurred vision, which passes off as headache worsens. Aching pain over one eye. Scalp sore and tender.
Throat: Dry, rough, hoarse.
Lungs: Croupy, dry, hard cough, pain extends to the back and shoulders. Yellow stringy phlegm. *Rheumatism:* Tearing pains, bruised and sore pain. Pain moves from joint to joint. Joints swell and are stiff and sore.
Measles: With catarrh.

Remedy Picture
• For chilly people prone to catarrh and rheumatism. They are worse in the morning, from hot weather, for undressing and for beer drinking; better for heat.
• Pains felt in localized spots, fleeting, shifting pains.

Dosage: 6c
Antidotes: Ars. alb., Lachesis, Pulsatilla
Complementary Remedies: Follows Ars. alb. well but does not follow well after Calcarea carb. Ant. tart, and Pulsatilla follow well.

RIGHT *Bichromate of potash is the source of Kali bich. It is made from chromium ore.*

BICHROMATE OF POTASH

Phosphoricum Acidum (Acid phos.) Phosphoric acid

 HOMEOPATHIC

Phosphoric acid is a remedy with a tonic effect on the nervous system. It is for weak, debilitated people who have become depressed from their circumstances or have become weakened from a severe chronic infection or the loss of body fluids—for example, nursing mothers, hemorrhage, heavy menstrual periods, diarrhea etc.

 SYMPTOM PICTURE

Mental and Emotional Symptoms
• Grief, sorrow, disappointed love, and homesickness cause an apathetic depression, the person is indifferent and listless. Thinking tires them and they become confused.

• Also for children who grow too fast, are studying hard at school and become exhausted and apathetic.

Physical Symptoms
Indigestion: Loss of appetite, craves juicy things, has sour belches, feels nausea in the throat.

Flatulence: After sour food and drink, abdomen is hard and distended, aches in umbilical region.

RIGHT *Acid phos. was first made by Dr. Hahnemann himself. He steeped animal bones in a mixture of sulfuric acid and brandy.*

Diarrhea: Watery diarrhea that does not debilitate, although may be weak afterward. Catching cold in the summer causes diarrhea.

Nocturnal enuresis (bedwetting): Children who wet the bed at night passing copious amounts of clear or cloudy urine.

Headache: Crushing headache in temples with pressure on top of head, worse for shaking head and noise.

Remedy Picture
• Not thirsty except for cold milk and beer, desire juicy fruits and foods, dislike bread and coffee.
• Easily rested by a short sleep and feel better for walking.
• Feel worse for sitting and standing, in the evening and at night, and for talking.
• Pale wan face, blue shadows under eyes.

Dosages: 6c or 30c
Antidotes: Camphor, Coffea
Complementary Remedies: None.

Phosphorus (Phos.) Phosphorus

 HOMEOPATHIC

Just as phosphorus ignites quickly, so complaints requiring Phosphorus tend to flare up quickly.
Constitutional type: Tall slender people with fine reddish-blond hair, look young for their age.

 SYMPTOM PICTURE

Mental and Emotional Symptoms
• Affectionate, likes company, sensitive; can become irritable and indifferent to companions.
• Fearful at night, of ghosts and imaginary things. They thrive on sympathy and reassurance.

Physical Symptoms
• Insomnia from cough, nausea, fears, and anxieties, better for sleeping on the right side. Have vivid dreams.

• Headache with violent, darting shooting pains, better for lying quietly in a cool, dim room.
• Sore throat. Burning pain.

Cough: Dry, tickling, hacking cough that causes headache and trembling. Tightness and weight on chest. Burning pains. Yellow, rusty, salty sputum. Worse laughing, talking, lying on left side, at night, for cold air. Wakes at night. *Gastrointestinal tract:* Very thirsty for long drinks of cold milk or water, which is vomited once warm in the stomach. Very hungry with burning pains in the stomach. Long, hard, thin stools. Profuse, painless, watery diarrhea. *Women's complaints:* Menstruation too early and scanty. Lasts too long.

Remedy Picture
• Chilly people with burning pains, better for cold things.
• Flush easily.
• Worse in thunderstorm.

• Thirsty for cold water.
• Desires salt, cold milk, ice cream, spicy food.
• Tires easily, becomes weak and trembly, refreshed by rest.
• Hemorrhages bright red blood.
• Is worse for light, warm food and drinks, lying on left or painful side, thunder, changes in weather.
• Is better for cold things, rest, sleep, lying on the right side.
• Better for massage, touch.
• Worse a.m. and p.m.

Dosages: 6c or 30c
Antidotes: Coffea
Complementary Remedies: Ars. alb., Carbo veg.

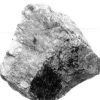

ABOVE *Phosphorus is a nonmetallic chemical element; it is poisonous and can burst into flames spontaneously at room temperature.*

Antimonium Tartaricum (Ant. Tart.) Tartrate of antimony and potash, tartar emeti

 HOMEOPATHIC

Antimonium tart. may be useful for someone who looks ill and suffering. The face is pale or dusky with dark shadows under eyes. There may be a cold, clammy sweat, especially on the head and forehead. Trembling.

 SYMPTOM PICTURE

Mental and Emotional Symptoms
• Not very marked in adults although they may feel hopeless and miserable about their condition.
• They are drowsy.
• Children do not want to be looked at or touched, they whine and cry pitifully. Will cough if they are angry.

Physical Symptoms
Cough: Loose rattly cough but very little phlegm is coughed up. Phlegm is white. Rapid, short, difficult breathing, has to sit up. Can be used for any chest complaint—asthma, bronchitis, pneumonia, if the symptoms fit. May alternatively cough and yawn.
Nausea and vomiting: Usually has no appetite but may desire refreshing foods and then feel sick and vomit. Vomit is sour and difficult with a lot of retching.
Chickenpox: For large, pustular spots that are slow to come out and slow to heal. May also have a cough.

Remedy Picture
• Drowsy, wants to lie completely still.
• Usually thirstless but may be thirsty for frequent small sips of cold water.
• Desires apples and juicy foods, acids, sour fruits, and refreshing foods.
• Dislikes milk, induces vomiting.
• Worse for heat, better for still fresh air.
• Worse for eating and drinking.

Dosages: 6c or 30c
Antidotes: Cocc, Ipecac, Pulsatilla, Rhus., Sepia

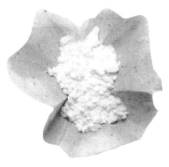

ABOVE *Tartar emetic is an extremely poisonous salt of tartaric acid. Its ability to induce purging vomiting is well known in orthodox medicine.*

Arsenicum Album (Ars. alb.) Arsenic trioxide, arsenic

 HOMEOPATHIC

Arsenicum album is an excellent remedy for people who are restless, anxious, despairing, oversensitive and at the same time fussy and overfastidious. It can be used when debility and weakness seem out of all proportion to the nature of the attendant physical illness. They may be obsessively clean and tidy and even slightly agoraphobic.

 SYMPTOM PICTURE

Mental and Emotional Symptoms
• May break out in a cold sweat. Restless sleep with fearful dreams.

Physical Symptoms
Gastrointestinal tract: Everything burns; stools dry and hard.
Food poisoning: Where the vomit and diarrhea smell foul and burn, feel worse for sight and smell of food. Weak, trembly, and exhausted. Thirsty.
Colds and flu: With burning watery eyes, burning nasal discharge, headache throbs and burns, better for cool facecloths, swollen, burning throat, difficult to swallow. Chest burns and wheezes. Cannot lie down, better propped up. Weak, trembly, worse for least effort.
Skin: May be fine or dry, rough and scaly, burns and itches but is better for warmth, worse for cold and for scratching.

Remedy Picture
For chilly people who sweat easily; they need warmth, hug the fire. Worse in wet weather, from cold things, except head, which is better for cold. All their discharges burn and excoriate. Very thirsty. Worse for vinegar, acid, ice cream, iced water, and watery fruits.

Dosages
Acute illness: 6c hourly until definite improvement, then three times a day if required.
Chronic ailments: 6c three times a day. Do not repeat if improvement is maintained.
Antidotes: Carbo veg., Hepar sulf., Nux vom.
Complementary Remedies: None.

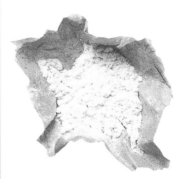

ABOVE *Arsenic, a white tasteless powder, is extremely poisonous.*

Mercurius Solubilis (Merc. Sol., Merc.) Mercurius solubilis, mercury or quicksilver

 HOMEOPATHIC

People who need Merc. are chilly, their discharges smell, and they are weak and trembly. Merc. sol. is the most commonly needed mercury-based homeopathic remedy. There is a range of mercury remedies: Mercurius vivus (known as Merc.), Mercurius cyanatus (Merc. cyan), Mercurius corrosivus (Merc corr.), Mercurius dulcis (Merc. dulc.), Mercurius iodatus flavum, and Mercurius iodatus ruber. All these must be ordered from a homeopathic pharmacist and should not be used by untrained people.

 SYMPTOM PICTURE

Mental and Emotional Symptoms
• Restless, discontented, suspicious, and depressed.
• Children are impish, naughty, enjoy being led or leading others astray.

Physical Symptoms
Colds with sneezing, sneezing in the sunshine, nose raw and smarting inside. Yellow-green smelly mucus.
• Earache, thick yellow glue, stitching pains worse at night, warmth. Boils in ear canal.
Mouth complaints: Mouth ulcers, abscesses, toothache -drools saliva. Stinging throbbing pains, pains spread up to ears and cheeks. Dirty mouth, flabby, yellow-coated tongue with toothmarks. Better for warmth.
Gastyointestinal complaints: Diarrhea, burning, slimy yellow or green stool. Sweats while passing stool.

Remedy Picture
• Foul, offensive breath, saliva, sweat.
• Moist mouth, lots of saliva, drools, yet intensely thirsty.
• Salty, sweet, metallic, bad taste in mouth.
• Drenching sweats without relief. The worse the sweat, the worse the complaint.
• Creeping chilliness, at onset of cold, and within sores.
• Worse at night, for warmth of bed, lying on right side, sweating. Damp weather.
• Weakness and trembling.
• Better from rest, mild weather.

Dosages: 6c
Antidotes: Ars. alb., Sulfur

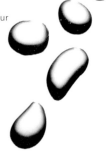

RIGHT *Mercury is a heavy white metallic chemical element. It is liquid at normal temperatures, and is poisonous to the touch.*

Glonoine (Glon.) Nitroglycerine, dynamite

 HOMEOPATHIC

Glonoine is a headache remedy. It is also good for migraine. Glonoine is indicated when headaches are sudden and violent, and is particularly useful for headaches brought on by exposure to the glare of the sun. It is the specific homeopathic remedy for sunstroke. In conventional medicine, nitroglycerine, the source for glonoine, is an ingredient in a heart drug. Since Glonoine is primarily a first-aid remedy there is no constitutional type.

 SYMPTOM PICTURE

Mental and Emotional Symptoms
Since it is primarily an acute remedy, used in short-term situations, there is no extensive mental and emotional picture for Glonoine.

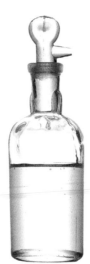

LEFT
Nitroglycerine is made by treating glycerine with nitric and sulfuric acid. It is extremely unstable and provides the explosive component of dynamite.

Physical Symptoms
Headaches: For sudden onset of strong, bursting, pulsating pain all over head or one-sided, usually the left. Brain feels too large for the skull as if it wants to burst out of the head. Face is congested, dusky-red. Headache is brought on by hot sun on the head, by looking into a dazzling light, or by getting overheated.
Sunstroke: Treats sunstroke with above symptoms.

Remedy Picture
• Relieved by sips of brandy and cold applications such as ice-packs.
• Made worse by hot sunshine, stooping, jarring, lying down.
• Worse in the morning from 6 a.m. to noon as the sun rises, and improves as the day goes on and the sun sets.

Dosages: 6c or 30c
Antidotes: Aconite, Camphor, Coffea, Nux vom.

Argentum Nitricum (Arg. Nit.) Silver nitrate

HOMEOPATHIC

Arg. nit. is often required by students and people facing an ordeal that fills them with dread and anxiety, causing trembling and diarrhea. It is excellent for stage-fright, exam nerves, fear of flying, vertigo, and driving test nerves. Choose it when people are at once anxious yet excitable.

SYMPTOM PICTURE

Mental and Emotional Symptoms
• Highly strung, lacks self confidence, has a fear of failure and suffers from diarrhea brought on by anticipation; for example, exam nerves.
• Claustrophobic and dislikes crowds.
• Fear of heights, fear of flying, irrational fears.

Physical symptoms
Headache: Boring pain, better for wrapping head up tightly. Feels cold and trembly.
Conjunctivitis: Eyes pink with purulent, bland discharge.
Gastrointestinal symptoms: Craves sugary foods that ferment into gas in the gut causing lots of belching, which gives relief. Green offensive diarrhea.

Remedy Picture
• Usually for thin and wiry people who look older than their years. They are hot, worse for heat, better for cold air, cold food and drinks.
• They have a sweet tooth but are the worse for sugar.

Dosages
Antidote: Natrum mur.
Complementary Remedies: None

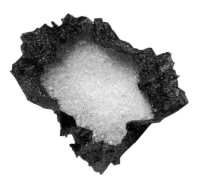

ABOVE *Silver nitrate is a colorless crystalline salt made by dissolving silver in nitric acid. It is used to make photographic plates as well as medicinally.*

Graphites (Graph.) Black lead, graphite

HOMEOPATHIC

Graphites is mostly used for skin problems characterized by thick, honeylike discharge.
Constitutional type: Overweight and flabby, sad, chilly, and constipated. Fair complexion, prone to skin problems.

SYMPTOM PICTURE

Mental and Emotional Symptoms
• Easily startled, disinclined to work, sad and despondent, weeps when listening to music.
• Children are cheeky and laugh when admonished.

Physical Symptoms
Gastrointestinal tract: Dislikes meat, sweet foods cause nausea. Poor digestion with burning pains and sour burps. Feels temporarily better for eating, for hot drinks and for rest. Full hard abdomen with foul wind that is difficult to expel. Must loosen clothing. Constipated with large knotty stools mixed with mucous threads.
• Diarrhea is brown fluid with undigested food, smells sour and offensive. Burns the anus.
Women's symptoms: Leucorrhea, which is white, profuse, burning with weak backache. Menstruation arrives late with pinky-red scanty blood.
• Constipated and nauseous.
• Nipples are cracked and sore with a honeylike discharge.
Skin: Unhealthy skin, cuts get infected, heal badly with scarring.
Eczema: Skin rough, hard, dry. Cracked and sore with honeylike discharge. On scalp, face, corners of eyes and nose, behind ears, palms of hands, in skin folds and joint creases, inside elbows, behind knees.

Remedy Picture
• Has honeylike sticky crusts on eyelids at lash margins.
• Sensation as if there is a cobweb on the face.
• Hears better in noisy places.
• Worse for getting chilled, at night, during and after menstruation.
• Improves from walking outdoors in the fresh air, hot drinks and for wrapping up.

Dosages: 6c
Antidotes: Aconite, Ars, alb., Nux vom.
Complementary Remedies: Ars, alb., Hepar surf., Lycopodium

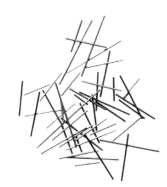

ABOVE *Graphite is not actually made from lead; it is a form of carbon and is used to make the "lead" in pencils.*

Carbo Vegetabilis (Carb. veg.) Wood charcoal

 HOMEOPATHIC

Carbo veg. has three main areas of use: acute heart failure or circulatory collapse and shock, following hemorrhage; poor recovery from infectious diseases; flatulence and indigestion.

 SYMPTOM PICTURE

Mental and Emotional Symptoms
Sluggish mentally, disinterested in current affairs, afraid of the dark, of ghosts.

Physical Symptoms
Heart and circulation: Blueness and pallor to face and nails, weak, thready pulse, cold sweats, cold breath, cold hands and feet, air-hunger. Think of it for acute heart failure, circulatory collapse following hemorrhage, or loss of body fluids, newborn babies that fail to breathe immediately, and give a 200c potency as an emergency remedy while waiting for medical help.

Poor recovery: For people who have never felt well since an infectious disease for example measles, whooping cough, influenza, and are weak, exhausted and sleepy.
Digestive symptoms: Indigestion and heartburn, worse for fatty foods, foods stagnate and putrefy in the gut causing a bloated, rumbling abdomen with sour, offensive wind. Better for burping. Worse in the evening.

Remedy Picture
• Must have fresh, cold air blowing on them, needs windows open and fans on, better for it.
• Worse for being overheated, for warm, humid weather.
• Better for burping.
• Worse for eating and drinking, dislikes meat, fat, and milk.
• Worse in the morning and evening.
• Dull, foggy mind, sluggish, dislikes the dark.

Dosages: 6c
Antidotes: Camphor, Ars. alb.
Complementary Remedies: Drosera

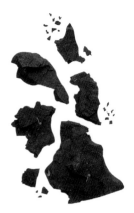

ABOVE *Charcoal is a form of carbon; it is made by partially burning wood in an oven from which air is excluded.*

Rock Water Hydrogen dioxide

 FLOWER ESSENCE

Rock water is one of the remedies for those who overcare for the welfare of others. It is useful for people who are very strict with themselves, who practice self-discipline, and deny themselves anything that might distract them from their goals. They take their goals seriously and have high ideals and expectations. They may martyr themselves in order to set an example. This is not the negative, manipulating martyrdom of Chicory. The Rock Water type will not ask others to do anything they would not do themselves.

 METHOD

The Sun Method (*see page 42*)
Look for a perfect, still, and sunny day, perhaps in summer when the sun is at its strongest. Fill a glass bowl to the brim with freshly drawn spring water. Leave it out in the open sunshine for three hours. Chose an open place away from grasses, contamination by pollen, overhanging shadows, and road pollution.

Lesson
Discipline
True self-discipline does not involve denial. Denial is necessary only when the person has a narrow view of their goal and is not truly in harmony with it. Rock water differentiates between the idea of discipline and self-denial. It helps us to understand the natural order.

> **WHAT IS ROCK WATER?**
> The water taken from a natural well or spring, preferably one with a traditional reputation to heal. There are many such half-forgotten springs and wells. Choose one that is open to the air and sunshine and is as natural as possible. Do not use water from a well dedicated to a saint or within a church or shrine. Do not use mineral-rich spa water.

Calcarea Fluorica (Calc. Fluor.) Calcium fluoride

HOMEOPATHIC

Calc. fluor. is a tissue salt, present in tooth enamel, bone surface, elastic fibers of the skin, muscles, and blood vessels. It works directly on the body at a cellular level. It has a particular affinity for connective tissue. It is an excellent remedy for swollen joints, varicose veins, hemorrhoids, and general lack of muscle tone.

SYMPTOM PICTURE

Mental and Emotional Symptoms
• General flabbiness.
• Slow development in all areas in children and infants.

Physical Symptoms
Colds: Stuffed-up nose, glue ear, hard swollen neck glands.

Backache: Worse on beginning to move, eases with continued movement.
Pregnancy: Helps to maintain skin-tone and prevent stretchmarks.
• Prevents and treats varicose veins and hemorrhoids.

Remedy Picture
• Flabby muscles, overstretched skin, varicose veins, teeth that crumble and decay.
• Worse for cold, damp weather, change of weather, rest.
• Better for heat and warm applications.

Dosages: 6c
Antidotes: None
Complementary Remedies: Calc. phos., Natrum mur., Silica

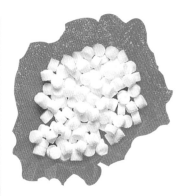

ABOVE *Calcium fluoride is the first of the twelve Schuessler tissue salts. It occurs in the body in the bones, teeth, blood vessel walls, and connective tissue.*

Calcarea Phosphorica (Calc. Phos) Calcium phosphate

HOMEOPATHIC

Calc. phos. is a tissue salt found in blood cells and plasma, saliva, stomach juices, bones, connective tissue, and teeth. Calc. phos. is one of the tissue salts, so works directly on the body at a cellular level.
Constitutional type: Dark hair and eyes, sallow complexion, may have a sweaty head, thin and anemic with cold, sweaty feet.

CHILDREN

Calc phos. is an excellent remedy in adolescence and during puberty. It helps with growing pains, with discontent, mood swings, and restlessness. It is also the remedy of choice for unrequited love, the bane of teenage years. It is also helpful for babies who cannot tolerate milk. People at the other end of life may also find it helpful as it helps bones to repair after fracture.

SYMPTOM PICTURE

Mental and Emotional Symptoms
• Mentally exhausted and dull from too much studying.
• Always wants to be somewhere else.
• Peevish, discontented, and restless.

Physical Symptoms
• Children who grow too fast and are left tired and wan.
• Who are mentally exhausted and dull from too much studying.
• Teething, especially back teeth, is slow and painful.
• Tummyache worse for eating, flatulent flabby abdomen, green, spluttering diarrhea. Stiff neck from cold drafts.
• Rheumatism of joints with cold, numb sensation, worse for cold weather, better for warmth.
• For fractured bones that are slow to heal (combine or alternate Calc. phos. with Calc. fluor. or Symphytum).

Remedy Picture
• Hunger with thirst.
• Desires salty bacon and ham.
• Worse for fruit, cold milk, ice cream.
• Better for warmth.
• Worse for cold and wet weather.

Dosages: 6x or 6c
Antidotes: None
Complementary Remedies: Symphytum to heal bones

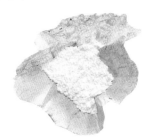

ABOVE *Calcium phosphate is the second of the twelve Schuessler tissue salts. It occurs in the body in the bones, teeth, and soft tissues.*

Calcarea Sulfuricum (Calc. Sulf.) Calcium sulfate, plaster of Paris

 HOMEOPATHIC

Calc. sulf. is a tissue salt that acts as a blood cleanser and speeds up healing of discharging wounds and abscesses. As one of the tissue salts, it works directly on the body at a cellular level.

 SYMPTOM PICTURE

Mental and Emotional Symptoms
Not very marked but may be sluggish, anxious, and weepy.

Physical Symptoms
Colds and coughs: Thick, lumpy, yellow, smelly mucus, often only one nostril is affected. Postnasal drip. Headache from catarrh. Cough with thick, yellow, lumpy phlegm, for croup.

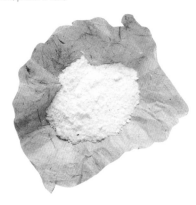

ABOVE *Calcium sulfate is the third of the twelve Schuessler tissue salts. It occurs in the body in the blood, liver, and connective tissues.*

Conjunctivitis: Inflamed red eyes with thick, yellow discharge.
Skin: Acne—the spots are red, hot, and tender with oozing yellow heads, discharge matter and bleed easily when touched. For discharging abscesses, weeping varicose eczema that takes a long time to heal.
• Calc. sulf. promotes the discharge initially so that the wounds can then heal effectively with minimal scarring.

Remedy Picture
• Thick yellow lumpy or watery discharges, may be blood streaked.
• Thick yellow lumpy catarrh.
• Warm-blooded people.
• Better for cool fresh air and uncovering.
• Worse for milk, drafts, heat, cold, wet.
• Burning and itching of soles of feet.

Dosages: 6x or 6c
Antidotes: None
Complementary Remedies: None

Ferrum Phosphate (Ferr.phos.) Iron phosphate

 HOMEOPATHIC

Ferr. phos., homoeopathic tissue salt, carries oxygen to the tissues. It is beneficial in the first stage of inflammations where there is congestion, pain, high temperature, and a fast pulse. Use it before discharges start. As one of the tissue salts, it works directly on the body at a cellular level.
Constitutional type: Pale and anemic people who are easily flushed. Ferrum phos. is the remedy to choose for complaints that come on after excess exertion. People who need Ferr. phos. feel very weak and want to lie down; they may even faint. They may have bright pink cheeks, caused by flushing.

 CHILDREN

Ferr. phos. is an excellent children's remedy, especially in childhood diseases such as measles.

 SYMPTOM PICTURE

Mental and Emotional Symptoms
Talkative, complaining, listless, depressed.

Physical Symptoms
Colds and influenza: At onset, before discharges start. Face flushed, skin hot and dry. High temperature, nose stuffed up, sneezes, dry, red, sore throat, croup, hoarseness. Tickly, hard dry cough.
Women's complaints: Profuse menstruation, bright red blood, anemia.
Rheumatism: Red, puffy sore joints, pains move from joint to joint.

Remedy Picture
• Thirsty.
• Prone to hemorrhage -nosebleeds, menstrual flooding, bleeding stomach ulcers. May feel weak but better in themselves after the bleed.
• Better for sleep, lying down, gentle movement, cold applications.
• Worse at night, 4 to 6 a.m., suppressed sweat, touch.

Dosages: 6c
Antidotes: None
Complementary Remedies: None

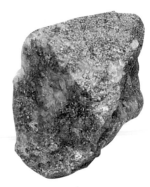

ABOVE *Ferrum phosphate is the fourth of the twelve Schuessler tissue salts. It occurs in all the cells of the body, particularly the red blood cells.*

Kali Muriaticum (Kali Mur.) Potassium chloride

 HOMEOPATHIC

Kali mur. is a tissue salt that resolves the second stage of inflammation when the tissues have begun to secrete. As one of the tissue salts, it works directly on the body at a cellular level. It is particularly useful for earache caused by a blocked Eustachian tube.

 CHILDREN

Kali mur. is effective given before immunization to help eliminate side effects.

 SYMPTOM PICTURE

Mental and Emotional Symptoms
There are no significant mental or emotional patterns to this remedy.

Physical Symptoms
Catarrh: Thick, grayish white. Stuffy head cold.
Glue ear: Glands around ears swollen, snapping noises in ear.
Cough: Loud stomach cough or short and paroxysmal, like whooping cough—has thick, white expectoration.
Women's complaints: Menstruation too early or too late with dark, clotted, or tarry blood. Morning sickness, vomits white phlegm.
Gastrointestinal tract: Indigestion from starchy foods.
Skin: Blisters of chicken pox. Eczema with blisters filled with white matter. Raised rash of measles. Warts.

Remedy Picture
Is generally worse for motion and from starchy, fatty foods.

Dosages: 6x or 6c
Antidotes: None
Complementary Remedies: None

Combination Remedies
Tissue salt combination remedies are available commercially Combination S, with Kali mur, Nat. phos., and Nat. sulf., is good for queasy stomach upsets.

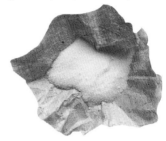

ABOVE *Potassium chloride is the fifth of the twelve Schuessler tissue salts. It occurs in the body in fibrin, an elastic insoluble protein formed when blood clots.*

Kali Phosphoricum (Kali Phos.) Potassium phosphate

 HOMEOPATHIC

Kali phos. is a tissue salt that strengthens and revitalizes the body, especially the nerves. It works directly on the body at a cellular level. It is particularly useful where the brain is either sluggish or overactive, and is a very good remedy for insomnia. It can also help with postnatal depression.

 CHILDREN

Kali phos. is useful for hyperactivity in children and for sleepwalking caused by bad dreams.

 SYMPTOM PICTURE

Mental and Emotional Symptoms
• Complaints are caused by excitement, worry, overwork -especially mental work.
• Irritable, depressed and anxious with a nervous dread, jumpy, averse to company.
• Night terrors, sleepwalk.
• Insomnia from excitement or mental stimulation.
• Often suited to children and young people.

Physical Symptoms
• Postviral exhaustion with muscular weakness.
• Back aches, is sore and bruised, better for movement.
• Nervous headache in back of head with empty feeling in stomach.
• Nervous indigestion, fluttering sensation in stomach.
• Nervous diarrhea, putrid odor when frightened, depressed, and exhausted.
Women's complaints: Menstruation too late, too scanty, or too profuse with deep red, thin blood.
Insomnia: With an empty feeling deep in stomach.

Remedy Picture
• Weak, easily exhausted from physical and mental work.
• Profuse sweats when tired.
• Humming and buzzing in ears.
• Worse for excitement, worry, mental, and physical exertion, eating, early morning, cold.
• Better for warmth, rest, nourishment.

Dosages: 6x or 6c
Antidotes: None
Complementary Remedies: None

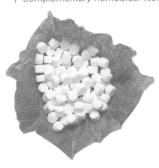

LEFT *Potassium phosphate is the sixth of the twelve Schuessler tissue salts. It is an excellent remedy for nervous and neurotic complaints.*

Kali Sulfuricum (Kali sulf.) Potassium sulfate

 HOMEOPATHIC

Kali sulf. is a tissue salt that carries oxygen to the cells, especially the skin and the mucous membranes. It works directly on the body at a cellular level.

 SYMPTOM PICTURE

Mental and Emotional Symptoms
Vague anxieties, irritability, and sadness.

Physical Symptoms
• Colds with yellow, slimy mucus that lingers.
• Coughs with yellow, slimy phlegm that is difficult to cough up and spit out—whooping cough, bronchitis, pneumonia.

• Rheumatism and neuralgia where the pains flit around
• Skin complaints with yellow slimy discharges, irritating spots, weeping eczema, psoriasis.

Remedy Picture
• Yellow slimy discharges and catarrh.
• Yellow coating at back of tongue.
• Alternate hot and cold sensations.
• Weariness and heaviness.
• Worse in the evening and for warmth.
• Better for cool fresh air.

Dosages: 6x
Antidotes: None
Complementary Remedies: None

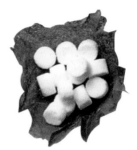

ABOVE *Potassium sulfate is the seventh of the twelve Schuessler tissue salts. It occurs in the body in the external layers of the skin.*

Calcarea Sulfuricum (Calc. Sulf.) Calcium sulfate, plaster of Paris

 HOMEOPATHIC

Mag. phos. is a tissue salt found in blood cells, bones, teeth, brain, nerves, and muscles. Mag. phos. is indicated for cramp, spasms, neuralgic shooting pains. It works directly on the body at a cellular level. Mag. phos. is the specific homeopathic remedy for menstrual cramps; it is also useful for general abdominal cramp and spasmodic pains in general, particularly about the eyes. Consider Mag. phos. for repetitive stress injuries such as writer's cramp.

 CHILDREN

Mag. phos. is indicated for babies suffering from colicky pain with accompanying diarrhea; the pain is on the right side and the baby draws up his or her legs for relief.

 SYMPTOM PICTURE

Mental and Emotional Symptoms
Miserable from pain.

OATS, A SOURCE OF
MAGNESIUM PHOSPHATE
(MGHPO$_4$. 7H$_2$O)

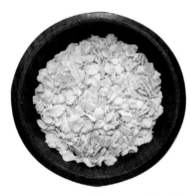

ABOVE *Magnesium phosphate is the eighth of the twelve Schuessler tissue salts. It occurs in the body in the bones, teeth, nerve tissues, blood vessels, and muscles. It also occurs plentifully in grain cereals such as oats.*

Physical Symptoms
• Writer's cramp and other cramps after excessive exercise, or cramp generally.

• Colic and wind with Mag. phos. indications.

• Teething and toothache with shooting, stabbing pains, better for heat, warm drinks.
Women's symptoms: Severe period pains, cramping, better for firm pressure, warmth, bending double.

Nervous asthma: Tight, constricted, difficult breathing.

• Spasmodic cough, worse for lying down..

Remedy Picture
• Worse on right side, cold, night.

• Better for firm pressure, warmth, bending double.

• Similar to Colocynth, but with Mag. phos. the complaints do not follow anger.

Dosages: 6x
Antidotes: None
Complementary Remedies: None

Natrum Muriaticum (Nat. Mur.) Sodium chloride, salt

 HOMEOPATHIC

Natrum mur. is a tissue salt that carries water into all the cells. It works directly on the body at a cellular level. A lack of Natrum mur. causes edema by holding water in the spaces between cells, dry skin, excessive thirst, anemia. For more information about the therapeutic properties of salt *see page 238.*

 HOMEOPATHIC

Mental and Emotional Symptoms

• Irritable, broods over old insults, dislikes company.
• Weeps in private, hates sympathy, which makes him or her feel worse.
• Laughter with tears.
• Difficulty in passing urine if people are close by.
• For complaints from suppressed grief.

Physical Symptoms

Skin: Greasy, unhealthy Very dry. Herpes (cold sore) blisters that itch and burn. Raw inflamed eczema worse at the beach. Crack on lower lip.
Gastrointestinal tract: Indigestion from lack of stomach acid. Hungry, sweats while eating. Very thirsty. Constipated with dry crumbling stool.
Headaches: One-sided headache from repressed emotion. From sunrise to sunset, as if little hammers were knocking on the brain. May see zigzags and flashes of light before headache.
Fever: Thirst before and during chill, thirstless with fever. Hammering headache as fever subsides.
Anemia: Cold and exhausted, if other symptoms fit.

Remedy Picture

• Craves salt.
• Loathes fat, bread.
• Profuse watery white discharges.
• Has cold legs and feet, numbness and tingling.
• Worse for heat and cold, at the beach.
• Better for open air.
• Wind makes eyes water.
• Worse at 10-11 a.m.

Dosages: 6x, 6c, 30c
Antidotes: Ars. alb., Phosphorus, Nux vom.
Complementary Remedies: Apes, Ignatia, Sepia

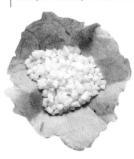

LEFT *Sodium chloride is the ninth of the twelve Schuessler tissue salts. It is common salt.*

Natrum Phosphoricum (Nat. Phos.) Sodium phosphate

 HOMEOPATHIC

Natrum Phos. is a tissue salt that neutralizes acidity in the body. It works directly on the body at a cellular level.

 SYMPTOM PICTURE

Mental and Emotional Symptoms

Nervous exhaustion, apathetic, and indifferent. Nervous at night.

Physical Symptoms

• Headache in forehead and on top of head from mental strain with sour stomach.
• Itchy skin with redness, general acidity.
• Rheumatism with stiffness, pain, and swelling of joints.

Gastrointestinal tract: Acid stomach. Creamy yellow coating at back of tongue, sour heartburn (pain to back), sour burps, sour vomit. Colic with sour burps and vomit in babies. Morning sickness with sourness. Gallstone colic, with sour vomit.

Remedy Picture

• Sourness of all discharges: sweat, stool, urine, vomit, flatulence.
• Thick creamy yellow mucous discharges.
• Worse in the evening, sugar, fats.
• Better for cold things.
• Feet icy cold by day, burning hot at night.

Weakness: Weak, acidic digestion, weak, acidic, rheumatic joints.

• Creamy yellow coating at back of tongue.

Dosages: 6x
Antidotes: None
Complementary Remedies: None

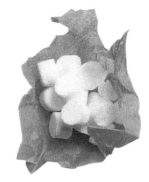

ABOVE *Sodium phosphate is the tenth of the twelve Schuessler tissue salts. It occurs in the body in the tissues generally, where it controls acid and fat intake.*

Natrum Sulfate (Nat. Sulf.) Sodium sulfate, Glaubers salt

HOMEOPATHIC

Natrum sulf, one of the twelve original tissue salts, helps to balance body fluids by stimulating the kidneys to eliminate excess water and by stimulating the digestive organs to secrete properly.

SYMPTOM PICTURE

Mental and Emotional Symptoms
Melancholy and sad, sensitive to music, tired of life, jumpy, sensitive to noise.

Physical Symptoms
Warts: Soft warts singly or in crops. Whitlows.
Headaches: Violent throbbing pains on top of head with vertigo and bilious nausea, bitter taste in mouth, dislikes light.
• Sallow complexion.
• Never well since a head injury, pains or vertigo persist.
Gastrointestinal tract: Indigestion with bloated, rumbling abdomen, sour belches, sour bilious yellow-green vomit. Sour wind with stool. Feels better for passing wind and after stool. Smelly, watery diarrhea in the morning on waking. *Chest:* Asthma and chest infections with loose, rattly, thick ropy green mucus on chest. Chest feels sore as if there's a heavy weight on it. Worse for coughing, wet weather, night.

Dosages: 6x, 6c, 30c
Complementary Remedies: Arnica for head injury

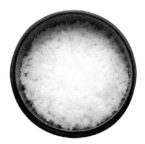

ABOVE *Sodium sulfate is the eleventh of the twelve Schuessler tissue salts. It is important in the regulation of the body's water balance.*

Silica(Sil) Silicon dioxide, flint, sandstone, quartz

HOMEOPATHIC

Silica is a tissue salt found primarily in the blood, skin, hair, and nails. Silica helps to bring boils and infected wounds "to a head," expel pus and foreign bodies, for example, splinters from the skin, aid healing with minimal scarring. It promotes a healthy, clear skin.
Constitutional type: Frequently needed for children who "fail to thrive," cannot utilize the nutrients in their food, and despite a good diet remain malnourished. Slow physical, mental, and emotional development, biggish heads, fontanels slow to close, pale skin, weak hair and nails with puny pot-bellied bodies.

SYMPTOM PICTURE

Mental and Emotional Symptoms
• Lacks self-confidence, shy, anxious, poor concentration.
• Stubborn and self-willed.
• Irritable, jumpy, restless.
• Complaints from mental strain or shock, sensitive to noise.
• Dislikes consolation.
• Lacks stamina (grit), tires easily.

Physical Symptoms
Headache: Rises up from the neck, over the top of the head and settles behind the right eye. Violent, hammering, throbbing pain as if head would burst.
Colds and coughs: Cold develops slowly, lasts a long time. Blocked sinuses, dry hard crusts in the nose with a loss of sense of smell. Often goes to the chest and produces an irritating cough. Middle ear infection.
Gastrointestinal tract: Constipation: hard, shy stool—difficult to expel, slips back. Women's complaints: Heavy menstrual periods. She feels icy-cold all over, always constipated before and after her period.
Skin: Hard, dry, unhealthy. Cuts fester, heal slowly with lumpy scars. Boils form slowly in crops. Acne is characterized by pustular sore spots. Dryness and cracks at fingertips, nails split and flake.
Infectious diseases: Mumps—parotid glands swell, feel cold, better for heat, wearing a scarf.
• Convalescence after any illness, where extreme tiredness persists along with swollen glands, and other silica symptoms.

Remedy Picture
• Complaints come on slowly, with slow recovery.
• Glands (specially neck) swell.
• Very cold, easily chilled.
• Discharges are yellow-green and smell offensive, sour, cheesy.
• Sour head sweats at night.
• Feet icy-cold, sweaty.
• Very thirsty for cold drinks.
• Hungry for cold foods.
• Dislikes meat, warm foods.
• Upset by milk.
• Has splinterlike sticking-pains.
• Worse for getting chilled, at new and full moons, cold, wet weather, milk, mental exertion, movement, light, noise, drafts.
• Better for heat, wrapping up warmly, pressure, closing eyes, and lying in a quiet room.

Dosages: 6x, 6c, 30c
Antidote: Camphor
Complementary Remedies: Calc. carb., Pulsatilla

RIGHT *Silica is the last of the twelve Schuessler tissue salts. It occurs in the body in the connective tissue and the coverings of nerve fibers.*

Food and Drink

Many products we might define as food, or whose natural domain is the kitchen cupboard or the fruit bowl, have a healing energy of their own. Citrus fruit is dealt with on pages 121-125 in the Plant and Animal section, but orchard, soft, and tropical fruits, vegetables, spices, cereals, together with other foodstuffs are described here. The material is arranged thematically: fruit and vegetable; spices and seeds; cereals; eggs and dairy products; natural sweeteners; and liquids. Within each theme group, the items are listed alphabetically.

Almond Prunus amygdalmus (bitter almond) P. amygdalmus dulcis (sweet almond)

 FOOD USES

Almond oil soothes and lubricates the skin. It is a particularly safe and effective remedy for cradle cap: massage the oil gently into the baby's scalp. Finely ground almonds mixed to a paste with warm water can be used to exfoliate and cleanse facial skin.

 PROPERTIES

Almonds have cleansing and moisturizing properties. They contain good amounts of vitamin E, calcium, iron, magnesium, phosphorus, and potassium.

Special Notes
• No safe dosage has been established for almonds.
• Almonds contain large amounts of salicylates—aspirinlike compounds also found in foods such as oranges and berries and in some painkillers.
• Like all nuts, almonds may trigger an allergic reaction.

Contraindications
It is best to avoid eating almonds in any quantity if you are allergic to aspirin. If symptoms appear after eating, seek medical advice. If symptoms are severe, get medical help immediately.

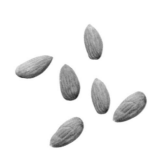

ABOVE *Almonds are the kernels of a stone-fruit produced by the bitter and sweet almond trees. Almonds and the oil that is extracted from them are used for culinary, cosmetic, and therapeutic purposes.*

! CAUTION

Do not eat almonds in any form without medical advice if you have previously had an allergic reaction to any other nut.

Apple Malus species, including Malus pumila

 FOOD USES

Eating one or two fresh, uncooked apples a day provides good amounts of pectin, which helps prevent constipation. Eating an apple after a meal will aid digestion. Apples can help lower cholesterol levels when eaten in quantities of two to three a day. As a treatment for intestinal infections, hoarseness, rheumatism, and fatigue, increase your daily intake to about 21b. (1kg.). For curative purposes, as an alternative to eating the whole fruit, drink 1pt. (5001.) of naturally sweet apple juice a day. Grated apple, mixed with live yogurt, may be helpful in cases of diarrhea. Apples may aid in the elimination of dietary fats from the body. Apples offer slow release carbohydrate energy and so are very good for a lunchtime snack if you are planning an energetic afternoon.

 PROPERTIES

Mental and Emotional Symptoms
Apples are an excellent source of fiber, vitamins, amino acids, and minerals—they have a higher proportion of phosphates than any other fruit or vegetable. Apples can also be used as a curative for problems arising in the digestive tract, for rheumatism, mental and physical fatigue, and hoarse throats. They are said to be beneficial in cases of urine retention and reputedly combat high levels of cholesterol in the blood. The whole fruit, minus the seeds, is used.

Special Notes
Apple seeds can be toxic when taken in large amounts since they contain a substance called amygdalin, which breaks down into prussic acid (hydrogen cyanide) during digestion.

Contraindications
De-seed apples before giving them to babies and young children.

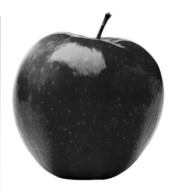

ABOVE *According to tradition, apples are one of the best foods for preventing illness. Modern nutritionists and practitioners of naturopathy concur with this long-held belief.*

Apricot Prunus armeniaca

 FOOD USES

Apricot kernel oil protects and softens the skin. It may help prevent the formation of fine lines in aging skin. Apricots can help promote healing of the lungs following infection. Three to six fresh apricots a day can help prevent bronchitis and asthma. A little warm apricot kernel oil applied to absorbent cotton and placed in the outer ear may relieve earache. Apricots have been used by some alternative therapists in the treatment of cancer. Laetrile, extracted from the apricot stone, is used. At present there is no scientific evidence to support this treatment.

 PROPERTIES

Apricots are a rich natural source of vitamin A, vitamin B2, and iron; the fresh fruit also supplies some vitamin C. The dried fruit contains twice the amount of vitamin A as the fresh fruit, and ten times the amount of iron. Apricot kernel oil is an excellent source of vitamin E. The fruit aids resistance to infection and strengthens the mucous membranes.

Special Notes
• Apricot kernels can be toxic when eaten since they contain a substance called amygdalin, which breaks down into prussic acid (hydrogen cyanide) during digestion.

• Dried apricots are often treated with sulfur dioxide to prevent discoloration. This may cause a severe allergic reaction in anyone who is sensitive to sulfites.

Contraindications
Choose only untreated dried apricots (brown in color, rather than orange) to avoid possible allergic reaction. When purchasing apricot oil look for products marked "FFPA" (free from prussic acid).

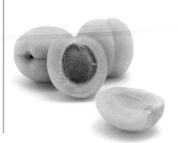

LEFT *Apricots are a popular summer fruit but are available all year round as dried fruit. The whole fruit is used for both culinary and therapeutic purposes.*

 CAUTION

Do not give whole, fresh fruit to young children; remove the stones first.

Avocado Persica americana gratissima

 FOOD USES

The flesh of a ripe avocado soothes sunburned skin. Cut in half and rub gently over the affected area. Vitamin B6 is known to be effective in the treatment of PMS. It promotes a healthy immune system since it is essential for the production of antibodies. Avocados are rich in carotene, vitamin E, the B vitamins, vitamin C, potassium, and iron. They are nourishing for convalescents and teenagers going through a growth spurt. Some naturopaths claim that they can soothe the pain of cystitis. Avocado makes an excellent face mask and moisturizer for dry skin. It is often a constituent of natural skincare products available from stores.

 PROPERTIES

Avocados contain good amounts of vitamins A and C, and are an excellent source of vitamin B6 (pyridoxine). They also provide fairly good levels of potassium.

Special Notes
• Because avocado is high in fats it should be avoided by those on a low-fat or calorie-controlled diet.
• Avocados may cause adverse reactions when taken with certain drugs.

 CAUTION

Do not eat avocados or take any product containing avocado if you have been prescribed an antidepressant of the MAOI (Monoamine-oxidase inhibitor) type.

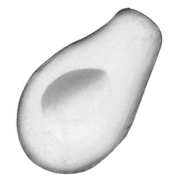

ABOVE *Avocados are the fruit of a small, subtropical, bushlike tree. They are well known for their high fat content—the highest of any fruit or vegetable (22g. per 100g.). Of the fats, 79 percent are monounsaturates and 9 percent polyunsaturates. The whole fruit, including the oils, is used.*

Banana Musa sapientum

 FOOD USES

The potassium present in bananas may be useful in reducing hypertension and preventing stroke. Vitamin B6 (pyridoxine) is known to be effective in the treatment of PMS. It promotes a healthy immune system since it is essential for the production of antibodies. Banana powder may help in the healing of ulcers and prevent gastric ulcers that are caused by aspirin.

 PROPERTIES

Bananas are a good source of fiber and have high amounts of vitamin B6 and vitamin C. They are also rich in potassium, contain good amounts of magnesium, are low in fat and sodium, and high in carbohydrates. Both fresh and dried bananas can be used for culinary and therapeutic purposes.

Special Notes
• The fruit should be eaten ripe. Unripe (green-skinned) fruit contain proteins that inhibit the digestion of starch and other complex carbohydrates.

• Dried bananas are often treated with sulfur dioxide to prevent discoloration. This may cause a severe allergic reaction in anyone who is sensitive to sulfites.

• Bananas may cause adverse reactions when taken with certain drugs.

Contraindications
• Choose only untreated dried bananas to avoid any possible allergic reaction.

RIGHT *Bananas are the fruit of a large herbaceous semitropical and tropical plant. Nutritionally, they are one of the most important of all fruit. They also have very valuable therapeutic applications.*

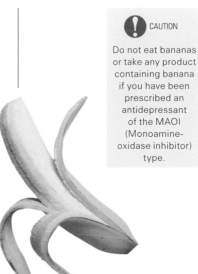 CAUTION

Do not eat bananas or take any product containing banana if you have been prescribed an antidepressant of the MAOI (Monoamine-oxidase inhibitor) type.

Cranberries Vaccinium oxycoccos var. palustris

 FOOD USES

Pure cranberry juice drunk frequently throughout the day is used as a treatment for cystitis and other infections of the urinary tract. Cranberries have a cleansing effect on the whole of the gastro-urinary system.

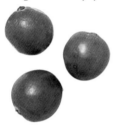

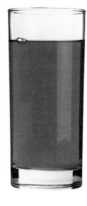

LEFT *Cranberries are the fruit of a small shrub. The bright red berries are very acidic and benefit from the addition of sugar to make them more palatable.*

 PROPERTIES

• Cranberries are a source of carbohydrates in the form of sugars, and have some vitamin C, iron, and potassium. Almost 90 percent of the fruit is water.
• Cranberries have an antiseptic effect on the urinary system.

Special Notes
Cranberry drink and cranberry sauce are high in sugar and therefore may not be as beneficial as pure cranberry juice.

Figs Ficus carica

 FOOD USES

Figs are recommended for constipation, hemorrhoids, abscesses, and chilblains. For constipation, soak dried figs in water overnight and eat for breakfast prior to other food. Drinking the water gives added benefit. Figs relieve chest complaints and can be used as part of the treatment for colds and throat infections. Dried figs contain more vitamins and minerals than fresh ones and are a good source of natural sugars. They contain a lot of folic acid, which is good for pregnant woman and those who are planning to become pregnant. However, diabetics should avoid dried figs, as should people who have a problem digesting sugar.

 PROPERTIES

Figs have high amounts of sugars and fiber. They are an excellent source of iron (4.2mg. in 100g. fresh figs), potassium, and calcium.

Special Notes
• Figs may cause adverse reactions when taken with certain drugs.
• Dried figs are often treated with sulfur dioxide to prevent discoloration. This may cause a severe allergic reaction in anyone who is sensitive to sulfites.

Contraindications
• Choose only untreated dried figs to avoid any possible allergic reaction.
• Treated dried figs should also be avoided by those on a low sodium diet.

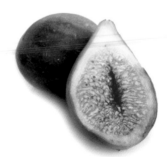

LEFT *Figs are the fruit of a variety of trees native to the Middle East. They provide valuable nutrients when eaten fresh or dried.*

! CAUTION

Do not eat figs or take any product containing figs if you have been prescribed an antidepressant of the MAOI (Monoamine-oxidase inhibitor) type.

Grapes Vitis vinifera

 FOOD USES

Grapes may be helpful to people suffering from rheumatism, liver, and gallbladder complaints. Grapes are astringents that help to clear toxins from the body. They may contribute to the healing of varicose veins and help to control heavy bleeding during menstruation. Grapes may also play an important role in the prevention of heart disease by lowering blood pressure. The fruit is sometimes recommended to improve poor liver function. The great therapeutic value of grapes is their ability to cleanse the blood, liver, and digestive system. They are high in vitamins and minerals and easy to digest, which is why they are good for the elderly or convalescent. Dried grapes, or raisins, pack more energy than grapes. They are particularly useful when you are working hard physically, and so make good snacks for walkers and sports-people. Raisins are also good for dry coughs. However, they should be avoided by diabetics. Made into wine, grapes retain their excellent tonic properties. A moderate amount of red wine in the diet can help keep blood pressure low.

 PROPERTIES

• Grapes are rich in bioflavinoids, vitamin C, phosphorus, and potassium; raisins are good sources of potassium, calcium, magnesium, iron, and copper.
• Grapes contain small amounts of fiber, and fats.
• They also contain tannin.
• Unripe grapes have high amounts of malic acid.
• Grapes are cleansing, and have a beneficial action on the skin, circulatory and reproductive systems.

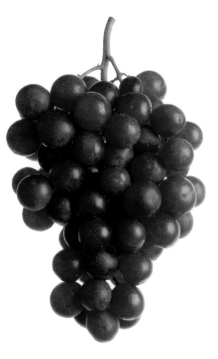

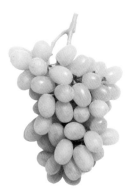

ABOVE *Grapes are the fruit of the vine; green and red varieties are equally nutritious although some people may find the skin of red grapes indigestible.*

Kiwi Fruit Actinidia deliciosa

 FOOD USES

Because of its vitamin C content, kiwi fruit may be included in a cancer-prevention diet. Kiwi fruit is recommended for circulatory and digestive disorders, and because of its very high potassium levels, helps to reduce stress.

 PROPERTIES

Kiwi fruit provides good supplies of vitamin C, fiber, vitamin E, and potassium.

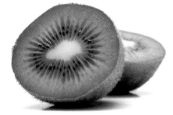

LEFT *The kiwi fruit, or Chinese gooseberry, is a relatively recent introduction to the mass-produced fruit market. It is usually eaten fresh in salads or used as a garnish for other dishes.*

Pineapple Ananas comosus

 FOOD USES

Because of its high vitamin C content, the fruit and juice of pineapple may form part of a cancer-prevention diet. Fresh pineapple provides relief from indigestion and heartburn. Fresh pineapple juice is excellent for relieving the pain and inflammation of a sore throat. It is also useful in fevers, where the sufferer is sweating profusely and is extremely hot. It is best given as juice in these circumstances. Fresh pineapple juice is also useful for bruising, as the enzyme (bromelin) in it helps to digest the debris (the blue and yellow marks under the skin) left as the body repairs itself. Pineapple is also good, either eaten as fruit or drunk as fresh juice, for excessive menstruation or painful periods.

 PROPERTIES

Pineapples contain some thiamine and potassium and are a good source of vitamin C (25mg. per l00g, of pineapple juice). They are low in fiber and sodium. They also contains a substance called bromelin, which breaks down proteins.

Special Notes
• The bromelin in pineapple may cause an irritating skin rash after handling the fruit.
• Dried pineapple is often treated with sulfur dioxide to prevent discoloration. This may cause a severe allergic reaction in those who are sensitive to sulfites.

Contraindications
Choose only untreated dried pineapple to avoid possible allergic reaction.

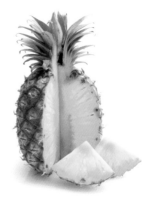

ABOVE *Pineapple is a tropical fruit used mainly as a food. Its therapeutic uses are based on its vitamin content and the enzyme bromelin.*

Strawberries Fragaria vesca

 FOOD USES

Strawberry leaves and roots are used to treat diarrhea, gout, and stomach complaints. Strawberries are recommended for treating high blood pressure and for helping to eliminate kidney stones. Strawberries replenish the intestinal flora. The juice is applied to the skin to treat blemishes and sunburn. Rubbing the teeth with the juice may help to whiten them. Because of their high vitamin C content, strawberries are often recommended in a cancer-prevention diet.

 PROPERTIES

Strawberries are rich in vitamin C and are a good source of fiber, iron, and potassium. They contain natural sugars, a trace of fat, and have a low sodium content. The roots and leaves contain tannins.

• Strawberries are astringent, act on the digestive system, and are beneficial to the skin.

Special Notes
Strawberries may cause hives and other allergic reactions.

Contraindications
Symptoms associated with a strawberry allergy include upset stomach, swelling of the face, eyes and lips, hay-feverlike symptoms, and skin rash. Should any of these occur, seek medical advice as soon as possible.

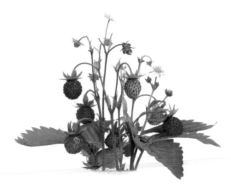

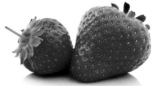

RIGHT *Both the wild strawberry and its cultivated varieties are popular summer fruit, traditionally used for therapeutic purposes as well as food. The fruit, roots, and leaves are used.*

Globe Artichoke Cynara scolymus

 FOOD USES

The essential oils in globe artichokes may help the body's metabolic processes. Globe artichokes may be of some help in the treatment of rheumatism and arthritis. They are sometimes recommended for lowering cholesterol levels and may be of some benefit to a congested liver. Globe artichokes can act as a diuretic in cases of water retention. They are also an effective laxative. The high mineral content in artichokes helps combat anemia and other deficiency symptoms such as brittle nails, split ends in the hair, and lassitude.

 CHILDREN

Nursing mothers should not overindulge in artichokes, because they can reduce lactation.

 PROPERTIES

Globe artichokes contain valuable nutrients. They are a low-fat source of vitamin C, potassium, and calcium.

Special Notes
This vegetable must be cooked since the raw plant contains a substance that prevents the body from adequately digesting and absorbing proteins.

Contraindications
The whole plant may cause contact dermatitis when handled by those who are sensitive to its essential oils.

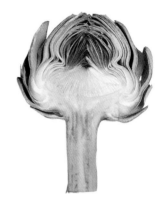

ABOVE *Globe artichokes belong to the thistle family of plants. They are totally unrelated to the Jerusalem artichoke, which belongs to the sunflower family and has no therapeutic application. The flowerheads of globe artichokes are used mainly for culinary purposes, although they do have some therapeutic effects.*

Asparagus Asparagus officinalis

 FOOD USES

Asparagus may be of use in the treatment of kidney complaints, rheumatism, gout, and edema caused by heart disease. It is a gentle diuretic. The B vitamins in asparagus include folic acid, which is particularly beneficial to pregnant women because it aids in fetal development and can prevent birth defects. Vitamin C, ascorbic acid, helps prevent and fight infection and aids the absorption of iron in the body. It also acts as an antioxidant, helping to rid the body of free radicals, which are believed to encourage cancer growth. Vitamin A helps prevent night blindness and respiratory infections and is important in the formation of bones and teeth.

 PROPERTIES

Asparagus is a good source of the vitamins A and C, and some vitamin B. It also contributes a small amount of iron. Eating 3.5oz. (100g.) fresh, cooked asparagus provides an adult with about 30 percent of their recommended daily vitamin C requirement and 20 percent of their vitamin A requirement.

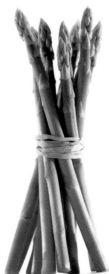

RIGHT *This is a plant of the lily family. In England it was once commonly known as "sparrow grass." Both the young shoots and rhizomes are used medicinally. For culinary purposes only the shoots are used.*

Special Notes
• Pregnant and breast-feeding women require additional amounts of folic acid in the form of supplements recommended by their physician. They should not exceed the appropriate dose.
• After eating asparagus, the harmless sulfur compound methyl mercaptan, which has a strong, unpleasant smell, is excreted in the urine.

Beets Beta rubra

FOOD USES

Eat raw, grated beets daily to improve liver function and treat bladder infections. Eating the whole, cooked vegetable will help prevent and treat constipation and hemorrhoids. Fresh beet juice is reputed to be a good cure for hangovers. Drinking the juice regularly can help restore health during convalescence. Mix beet juice with cucumber and carrot juice as an additional treatment for kidney stones and to improve the blood.

PROPERTIES

Beets are an excellent source of carbohydrates. They contain some C and B vitamins and are a good source of potassium. Beets aid digestion, cleanse the liver, and are good for the blood

and skin diseases such as eczema. They can be used effectively to improve general weakness. Some therapists consider beet juice to be among the most beneficial of vegetable juices.

Special Notes
Beets are best eaten fresh and young; the root can be eaten raw or cooked. Cook beets in their skin, then remove the skin before eating. Pickled beets have little nutritional value and should not be used for therapeutic purposes.

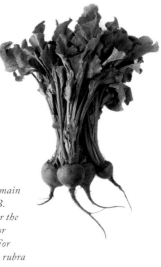

RIGHT *Beta rubra is the popular red root vegetable that is the main ingredient in borscht (soup). Of the two other species of beets, B. vulgaris and B. cicla, the former is the sugar beet and the latter the vegetable variously known as chard, or Swiss chard, and leaf or spinach beet. Only the leaves and midribs of chard are eaten. For culinary purposes both the leafy green tops and the root of Beta rubra are used; for therapeutic purposes, the root and its juices are used.*

Broccoli Brassica oleracea italica

FOOD USES

Broccoli makes an important contribution to a cancer-prevention diet. Broccoli, as a regular part of the diet, may be of use in the treatment of breast cancer. Eat broccoli regularly to supplement any deficiencies of vitamins A and C, and the important minerals calcium and potassium.

PROPERTIES

Broccoli is an excellent source of vitamin a and vitamin C (100g. of broccoli has about l00mg. of vitamin C), calcium, and potassium. It is low in sodium, fat, and proteins and provides reasonable amounts of fiber. Broccoli also contains sulforaphanes. (Sulforaphanes are part of a group of chemicals called phytochemicals that promote good health.) These stimulate certain enzymes in the body, which in turn aid in the removal of carcinogenic molecules in the cells. Experiments have shown that sulforaphanes have inhibited the growth of tumors in certain animals.

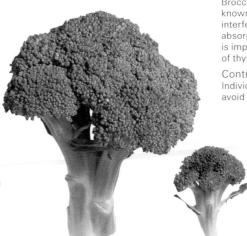

Special Notes
Broccoli contains substances known as goitrogens that interfere with the body's absorption of iodine. Iodine is important for the prevention of thyroid goiter.

Contraindications
Individuals with goiter should avoid eating broccoli.

LEFT *Broccoli is a valuable nutritious vegetable that has proven to be effective in the prevention of disease.*

Cabbage Brassica oleracea

FOOD USES

Cabbage is an important contributor to a cancer-prevention diet. Red and green cabbage may be of use in the treatment of cancer. A cabbage poultice is helpful for boils, bruises, and swelling. A warm compress of cabbage may help to relieve headaches, rheumatic pains, neuralgia, and eczema. Cabbage juice is valuable for gastric ulcers, bronchial infections, and hoarseness. Rinsing the mouth with cabbage juice may help in the treatment of mouth ulcers. A cabbage leaf, lightly pounded, can be placed directly on the breast to relieve mastitis.

> ## ! CAUTION
> Do not eat cabbage or take any product containing cabbage if you have been prescribed an antidepressant of the MAOI (Monoamine-oxidase inhibitor) type or are taking an anticoagulant.

PROPERTIES

Cabbage contains high amounts of vitamins A and C. The vitamin C content is most useful when green cabbage is eaten raw. The mineral content of cabbage is low; of the minerals, calcium is present in the highest amounts. Red cabbage should always be cooked since raw red cabbage contains an enzyme that locks in the thiamine molecule and thus prevents its use by the body. Like broccoli, cabbage also contains the group of chemicals called phytochemicals that are effective in preventing cancer. It also contains various other substances that may reduce the risk of this disease.

Special Notes
• Cabbage may cause adverse reactions when taken with certain drugs.
• Cabbage contains substances known as goitrogens that interfere with the body's absorption of iodine. Iodine is important for the prevention of thyroid goiter.

Contraindications
Individuals with goiter should avoid eating cabbage.

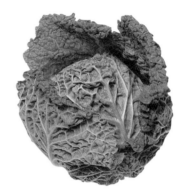

ABOVE *Cabbage has traditionally been used for medicinal purposes as well as culinary ones. It is a valuable nutritious vegetable that has proved to be effective in the prevention of disease.*

Carrots Daucus carota

HERBALISM

In herbal medicine, grated carrots are used as a compress for sore and cracked nipples. Carrot leaf tea is a serviceable diuretic used for chronic cystitis, kidney stones, and gout. Wash the leaves well.

FOOD USES

Carrots make an important contribution to a cancer-prevention diet. They may be particularly protective against cancer of the lung. A regular supply of carrots will prevent night-blindness, caused by a deficiency of vitamin A. Carrots may be helpful in the prevention of cataracts. The vegetable and its juice act as a diuretic and can be helpful in the treatment of cystitis. Carrots can have a beneficial effect on the respiratory and circulatory systems.

PROPERTIES

Carrots are an excellent source of beta-carotene, which the body converts into vitamin A. They have significant levels of sodium and fiber and are fat- and cholesterol-free. They are of great benefit to the eyes and appear to be beneficial in the prevention of cancer as a result of their large amounts of beta-carotene.

Special Notes
One raw carrot per day will provide the necessary vitamin A to maintain good night sight.

Contraindications
• Eating carrots or drinking the juice in excess over a long period can be dangerous and can cause vitamin A poisoning.
• An excess may also cause the skin to turn yellow.

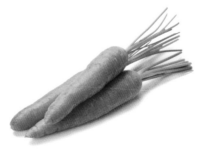

LEFT *Carrots are such a common part of the diet that they can be too easily dismissed. In fact they make very important contributions to good health.*

Celery Apium graveolens

 HERBALISM

Celery seeds are used in herbalism for treating arthritis and rheumatism. They are often combined with willow bark. Drink three cups of the combination tea a day. Celery seeds help increase the milk flow in nursing mothers.

 FOOD USES

Use grated, raw celery mixed with linseed as a poultice for swollen glands. Take celery seeds as an antioxidant. Drink celery juice sweetened with a little honey if you have high blood pressure. Drinking the juice before meals helps to suppress the appetite. The juice is also recommended as a digestive and for this purpose should be taken after meals. Celery root is said to be an aphrodisiac.

! CAUTION
• Do not use in pregnancy
• Do not use seeds from seed packages since they are usually treated with chemicals

 PROPERTIES

Celery provides good amounts of potassium, chlorides, and sodium. It helps to reduce high blood pressure, spasm in smooth muscle, and gas in the intestinal tract. It may also be helpful in the treatment of arthritis, rheumatism, gout, and sleeplessness. Claims have been made for its action as an antioxidant.

Special Notes
• No safe dosage has been established.

• Celery has no harmful effects when eaten in small quantities as part of the normal diet, but commercially prepared celery products can be dangerous in a few circumstances. Follow the manufacturer's directions for use. If ill-effects occur stop taking immediately and seek medical advice.

Contraindications
Celery can cause uterine contractions in both pregnant and nonpregnant women.

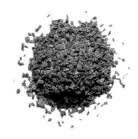

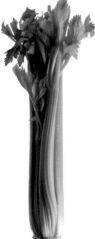

ABOVE *Celery is a popular salad vegetable and cooking ingredient. The whole celery plant and its seeds have culinary and medicinal uses. Commercially prepared celery products are available in several forms for therapeutic purposes, although some benefits can be obtained by using the vegetable in its natural state.*

Cucumber Cucumis sativus

 HERBALISM

In herbal medicine, cucumber juice is used to soothe irritable bladders and cystitis. Peel the cucumbers and pass them through a liquidizer. Take 2 teaspoons of the resulting juice every three hours for acute conditions.

 FOOD USES

Drinking cucumber juice may be of some benefit in the treatment of eczema. It is also recommended for skin blemishes. Cucumber juice is a tonic for the kidneys. Slices of cucumber will cool and clear tired, sore eyes

and skin damaged by sun and scalding. Ground cucumber seeds are used as an effective remedy for tapeworm. A cucumber and apple poultice relieves swellings under the eyes and inflammation of the joints.

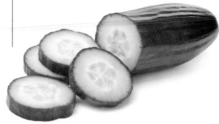

 PROPERTIES

Cucumber is a source of vitamin C and small amounts of iron and potassium. It has cooling and cleansing properties, with primarily external applications.

Special Notes
Cucumber may cause the accumulation of gas in the gut in some people.

LEFT *The cucumber is used mainly as a salad vegetable although it has cosmetic and medicinal applications. Both the whole fruit and the seeds are used.*

Lettuce Lactuca sativa

 FOOD USES

Lettuce may be beneficial as part of a cancer-prevention diet. It has a calming effect on the nervous system and is sometimes prescribed for palpitations. It also curbs excessive libido. Lettuce may help to relieve intestinal spasms. Use lettuce leaves to make a poultice for swollen joints and bruises. Simply tie the leaves onto the affected area, and change them every few hours or so for fresh ones.
Lightly steamed, lettuce is useful for irritable bowel syndrome, ulcers, and gastric problems.

 PROPERTIES

Lettuce contributes good supplies of vitamins A, C, B9 (folic acid), and potassium. It also contains some iron, copper, and calcium and is low in fat, fiber, and sodium. It acts on the nervous system and may offer some protection against cancer. Lettuce contains a mild, nonaddictive narcotic called lactucarium. The amounts are almost negligible in salad lettuce.

RIGHT *Lettuce is one of the most frequently used salad vegetables, but it also has some therapeutic applications. It is particularly well known for its soporific qualities.*

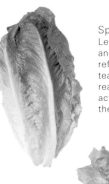

Special Notes
Lettuce is best eaten fresh and should be stored in the refrigerator. Do not cut or tear the leaves until you are ready to eat them since this action will destroy much of the vitamin C content.

Nettles Urtica dioica

 HERBALISM

Nettles are one of the most useful remedies in herbal medicine not only for their high iron content but also for their ability to clear the skin of allergic rashes and eczema due to nervous stress. The tea may be taken freely. It is useful when breast-feeding. The ointment soothes psoriasis.

 HOMEOPATHIC

Nettles are the source of the homeopathic remedy Urtica urens (Urtica). It is indicated when there is any kind of nervous rash that looks like the reaction caused by brushing against stinging nettles (white spots on a red skin). It can also be used for bee stings, breast pain during nursing, and gout.

 FOOD USES

Drink nettle tea or the juice of nettles to treat chilblains, cystitis, and high blood pressure.

Nettle acts as a tonic on the kidneys and liver, helping to rid the body of wastes and toxins. It may give relief to sufferers of hay fever and other allergies. A compress made by steeping a cloth in nettle tea will soothe burns. Nettles can be of some benefit in the treatment of psoriasis because they improve the circulation and contain minerals that can ease inflammation and pain. They are also used to treat nettle rash. The "stings" (hairs) of stinging nettles contain histamine and formic acid, both of which may be helpful in the treatment of arthritis. Nettle tea can be used as a hair rinse to help remove dandruff.

 PROPERTIES

Nettles contribute good amounts of vitamins C and A; they also contain some iron, potassium, and silica. Nettle is a diuretic, astringent, a tonic, and detoxifier. It helps to control bleeding.

Special Notes
The irritating rash caused by handling stinging nettles can be relieved by rubbing the skin with crushed dock leaves, which are usually found growing near nettles.

RIGHT *Nettle, including stinging nettle, is used in cooking (most notably as a soup and pasta sauce) and as a treatment for ailments. The whole plant and its leaves are beneficial.*

Onions Allium cepa

HERBALISM

Crushed onions are used in herbalism as a compress to clean infected wounds and draw splinters. Onion syrup, made by mixing chopped onions with an equal amount of honey, is a useful home remedy for colds and coughs. Use 1 teaspoon for children and 3 or 4 for adults, repeat every four hours.

FOOD USES

Onions are thought to be beneficial in lowering blood pressure and blood sugar levels. They may give some protection against cancer. Mix onion juice with honey to relieve the symptoms of a cold. Onion poultices are used to treat bronchitis and can also help in the treatment of acne and boils. Onions are often recommended for gastric infections.

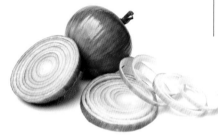

PROPERTIES

Onions contain small amounts of vitamins A and B, and some potassium. They also contain some sugars. They are low in fat, fiber, sodium, and carbohydrates. Onions help prevent infection, can relax muscles in spasm, and are used as an expectorant and diuretic.

LEFT *The bulb of the onion plant and its juices are used to treat ailments and maintain health.*

Red and Green Peppers Capsicum annuum var. annuum

FOOD USES

Peppers increase perspiration and therefore have a cooling effect on the body. They may be effective in the treatment of varicose veins, asthma, and digestive complaints. Peppers reduce sensitivity to pain by irritating the tissues and increasing blood supply to the affected area, which effectively numbs the pain. Cayenne acts as a tonic for those suffering from tiredness and cold. It can also induce a feeling of well-being. It is an expectorant and has been effective for treating catarrh and sinus problems. Peppers also help to eliminate toxins from the body.

PROPERTIES

Peppers are an excellent source of vitamin C (100mg. per 100g. in a fresh green pepper). All peppers also contribute small amounts of iron and vitamin A. The largest amounts of vitamin A are found in fresh red peppers, while paprika and chilli powder are also very rich in this vitamin. Peppers are a good source of potassium, and have low levels of sodium and fiber. They act as a tonic, have antiseptic effects, and are stimulating to the circulatory and digestive systems. Peppers also have anesthetic properties.

Special Notes
• Pungent peppers such as chili peppers may cause skin irritation and painful inflammation when used in excess or when in contact with the eyes and broken skin. The seeds are particularly powerful.

• Strong peppers may also temporarily irritate the urinary system since the oils are excreted in urine.

Contraindications
Care should be taken when preparing very hot peppers, which contain large amounts of a chemical called capsaicin. This may burn or irritate the skin. Some authorities recommend wearing protective gloves when handling these peppers since the chemical will not dissolve in water (it is soluble in milk fat or alcohol). Always wash your hands carefully after handling green or red chilis and never rub or touch your eyes, nose, or sensitive parts of the body before washing your hands.

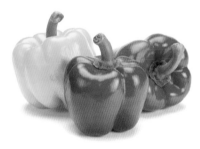

ABOVE *The fruits, when ripe, range in color from yellow to deep red. There are two general types of peppers: the mild and the hot varieties. Most of the mild peppers have relatively large fruits—red, green, or yellow—that are rich in vitamins A and C. Green bell peppers are picked before they are ripe. The term pimiento, from the Spanish for pepper, is applied to certain varieties of mild peppers. These include paprika, obtained by drying and grinding the bright red fruits. Hot peppers are often ground into a fine powder for use as spices. Hot peppers include the Tabasco pepper, the long chili, and cayenne peppers.*

Pumpkin Seeds Cucurbita maxima

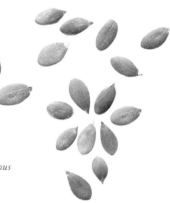

 FOOD USES

Pumpkin seeds may be included in a cancer-prevention diet. The zinc in pumpkin seeds can be beneficial in the treatment of prostate problems. As they are rich in zinc, they may help boost male fertility. Pumpkin seeds are soothing to irritated tissues. They are often recommended as a diuretic. Ground seeds mixed with an equal amount of honey expel intestinal worms. Take 5 or 6 teaspoons of the mixture before breakfast for three weeks.

 PROPERTIES

Pumpkin seeds are rich in protein and unsaturated vegetable oils, which supply vitamin E. They are also rich in B vitamins, zinc, and iron, contain some fat and contribute fiber to the diet. Pumpkin seeds act on the urinary tract and may help to expel intestinal worms.

RIGHT *The pumpkin is a valuable vegetable, containing good amounts of vitamin A and B. The seeds are also highly nutritious and have medicinal as well as culinary uses.*

Radish Raphanus sativus

 FOOD USES

Radishes are effective against bacterial and fungal infections. They are beneficial in the treatment of indigestion, flatulence, and bloating caused by intestinal gases. Radish seeds are used to treat bronchitis. Raw radishes are particularly useful in dispelling phlegm and clearing blocked sinuses. They are also diuretic. Avoid radishes if you suffer from gastritis or ulcers.

 PROPERTIES

Radishes contain some starch and sugar and low amounts of fiber. They are an exceptionally good source of vitamin C and contribute B vitamins, iron, and potassium. Radishes are antibiotic (they contain the antibiotic raphinin), antifungal, and act on the urinary tract. The black radish is used in homeopathy to treat the liver.

Special Notes
Radishes contain substances known as goitrogens that interfere with the body's absorption of iodine. Iodine is important for the prevention of thyroid goiter.

Contraindications
Individuals with goiter should avoid eating radishes.

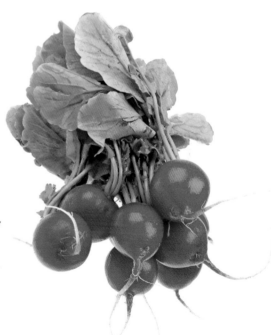

RIGHT *The radish belongs to the same family as the cabbage. It is the red root that is used for culinary purposes; the leaves, roots, and seeds have medicinal uses. The red radish is closely related to the mooli, or daikon (R. sativus var. macropodus).*

Corn Zea mays

 HERBALISM

Do not throw away the fine silk hairs that cover the corn; dry them and keep them for making herbal tea. They make an excellent soothing and healing diuretic, which is especially effective when the kidneys have been damaged by disease or drugs. Corn silk and chamomile tea is helpful in cases of gastritis.

 FOOD USES

A tea made by infusing corn silk in hot water may help in the treatment of kidney stones. Drink three times a day. Corn silk is also a good cleanser of the urinary tract. A little of it eaten raw, with or without the corn kernels, will benefit the whole urinary system. Corn flour is used as a substitute for wheat flour by people who are allergic to gluten and gliadin, such as those with celiac disease. Corn and its products may be beneficial in the treatment of bedwetting in children, disorders of the prostate, cystitis, and inflammation of the urethra. Cornstarch, manufactured from the inner part of the corn kernel, makes a fine powder suitable for use as a face or bath powder.

 PROPERTIES

Corn provides good supplies of carbohydrates, B vitamins (thiamine and riboflavin), vitamin A and C, potassium, and zinc. It is low in fat (2.4g. per 100g.) and contributes some protein. Corn also contains iron, but it is in the form of nonheme iron, which is difficult for the body to digest. Corn is stimulating and cooling. It is much used in Chinese medicine for urinary and kidney problems.

Special Note
Corn and its products may have adverse effects in certain circumstances.

Contraindications
• People suffering from pellagra (a niacin-deficiency disease) may be advised to eliminate corn and corn products from the diet.
• Corn can cause a classic allergic response in some people. Symptoms include swollen facial tissues, hives, and upset stomach. Seek medical advice if an allergic reaction occurs.

LEFT *Corn, or maize, is known primarily as a summer vegetable, but it also has therapeutic properties. The corn silk (stigmas and styles of female flowers), fruit, seeds, and oil are used.*

Watercress Nasturtium officinale

 FOOD USES

Watercress may help in the treatment of edema. It is used to treat respiratory ailments such as coughs, catarrh, and bronchitis. Watercress benefits the skin and may help skin eruptions when it is eaten regularly. It may strengthen the whole system in cases of debility caused by chronic illness, and help to relieve stress. Watercress is sometimes recommended for gallbladder complaints and anemia. It is also good for diabetes and rheumatism. To stimulate hair growth, especially for those losing their hair, make a paste of pounded watercress leaves and let it remain on the hair for a couple of hours before washing it off. Alternatively, use watercress infusion as a rinse after shampooing. Watercress is best avoided if you have cystitis.

 PROPERTIES

Watercress provides good supplies of the vitamins A, B (thiamine and riboflavin), and C, iron, and calcium. It contains a volatile mustard oil and other compounds that account for the slight burning taste on the tongue. Watercress is a stimulant that benefits digestion, a diuretic, and an expectorant. It has antiseptic properties and makes an effective tonic.

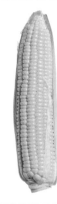

RIGHT *Watercress is a bitter, pungent herb used in cooking and for medicinal purposes. Only the leaves of the plant are used.*

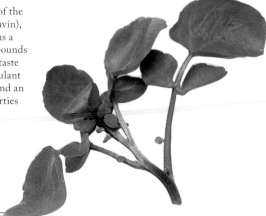

Black Pepper *Piper nigrum*

 FOOD USES

Black pepper is useful for treating indigestion and flatulence, and for respiratory problems. Pepper is an effective emetic and expectorant. In Ayurvedic medicine, black pepper mixed with ghee is used to treat nasal congestion, sinusitis, and inflammation of the skin.

 AROMATHERAPY

Its essential oil eases muscular aches and pains and is used to treat colds and flu.

 HOMEOPATHIC

When used as a homeopathic remedy for fever, pepper can help to lower the body temperature. If you have liver problems, avoid too much black pepper in your diet.

 PROPERTIES

Black pepper has stimulating, expectorant, anesthetic, and tranquilizing properties. It contains a chemical called piperine, which helps to relieve pain.

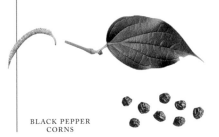

BLACK PEPPER
CORNS

Special notes
The essential oil may irritate the skin of those with sensitive skin. Large amounts of black pepper used regularly may result in overstimulation of the kidneys.

Contraindications
When using black pepper for medicinal purposes, follow the recommended dosage.

LEFT *Black pepper, a traditional seasoning for food, is a warm, aromatic, and comforting spice with therapeutic uses. The fruit, or corns, of the vine and the essential oil extracted from them are used. Black pepper is the whole, sun-dried, unripened fruit of the vine; white pepper is the ripe fruit from which the skins have been removed.*

Cardamom *Elettaria cardamomum, Amomum cardamomum*

 AROMATHERAPY

Cardamom oil, diluted in a carrier oil, can be rubbed on the abdomen to stimulate digestion.

 FOOD USES

Cardamom is beneficial for expelling gas from the bowels. The seeds may have some use as a laxative. Cardamom stimulates the appetite and helps relieve feelings of nausea. It is an excellent remedy for indigestion. Chewing the seeds will sweeten the breath. They can also help to counteract the formation of mucus.

 PROPERTIES

As well as its culinary uses, cardamom has important therapeutic uses for the body. It has beneficial effects on the digestive and respiratory systems. Both the whole seed and the kernel are used, and an essential oil is extracted from the seed.

Special Notes
Taken in excess cardamom may cause watery diarrhea.

Contraindications
• It is best to avoid cardamom if you have a chronic disease of the digestive system such as diverticulosis, spastic or ulcerative colitis, duodenal ulcer, or esophageal reflux.
• Cardamom tincture is a controlled substance in some countries.

RIGHT *Cardamom, an aromatic spice, is the fruit (or seed) of a large plant that belongs to the ginger family. Cardamom's is warm, spicy characteristics make it a popular ingredient in curries, desserts, and baked goods.*

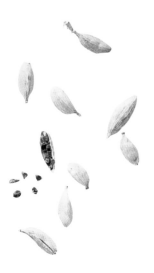

Cinnamon Cinnamomum zeylancium

 FOOD USES

Cinnamon tea can be useful in stopping heavy uterine bleeding and bleeding from the nose. The hot tea can cause sweating and stimulate the flow of blood around the body. It is beneficial to colds and influenza. Cinnamon temporarily raises the temperature of the body, and so helps to promote weight loss by using up energy. Cinnamon can be useful in expelling gas from the intestines and in easing diarrhea, nausea, and vomiting. It is sometimes used to treat high blood pressure, rheumatism, and arthritis.

 PROPERTIES

Cinnamon is a warming aromatic that can help to strengthen the immune system and the digestive system.

Special Notes
Commercially prepared natural products containing cinnamon are available for promoting weight loss. When taking

commercially prepared health products, follow the manufacturer's directions for use. If ill-effects occur, stop taking immediately and seek medical advice.

Contraindications
When taken in large doses cinnamon can have very serious effects. If symptoms occur (dizziness, nausea) seek medical help immediately.

 CAUTION

- Overdoses can cause kidney damage or coma
- Do not use if you are pregnant or breast-feeding

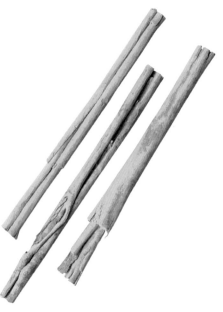

RIGHT *Cinnamon, the inner bark of a small tree, is used as a spice to flavor foods. Both the bark and the leaves have some therapeutic properties.*

Sesame Seeds Sesamum indicum

 FOOD USES

Sesame oil used in massage during pregnancy may help to prevent stretch marks. Use after bathing. The leaves are recommended as an internal treatment for cystitis, diarrhea, and catarrh. The seeds are taken to treat constipation, osteoporosis, and stiff joints. They may also be of benefit in the treatment of tinnitus, weak eyesight, and dizziness. Burns, boils, and ulcers may be relieved by applying the oil directly to the affected site. Sesame is beneficial for patients suffering from liver and gallbladder problems.

 PROPERTIES

Sesame seeds are rich in unsaturated oil (54.8g. of fat per 100g.), vitamins A, B (thiamine and riboflavin), and E, potassium, magnesium, and calcium. They have rejuvenating properties, are a soothing liver and kidney tonic, and act as a mild laxative. They also strengthen bones and teeth.

Special Notes
Because of their high fat content, sesame seeds and oil may best be avoided by those who are overweight.

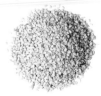

SESAME SEEDS   SESAME OIL

LEFT *Sesame seeds are used for culinary purposes and in the manufacture of the creamy paste known as tahini. The leaves, seeds, and the oil extracted from them are used for therapeutic purposes.*

Salt Sodium chloride

 FOOD USES

Salt is sometimes recommended as an emetic. Salt is used in the form of saline solution or salt tablets to treat salt depletion resulting from excess production of sweat in very high temperatures, from excessive vomiting and diarrhea and as a result of shock and hemorrhage. Saline solution is usually administered intravenously. A small bag of salt, previously warmed, pressed against the ear may help to relieve earache. Dissolving a pinch of salt in the mouth before going to bed is sometimes recommended for the prevention of night cramps. A warm water and salt gargle can ease inflammation of the throat. To exfoliate the skin, put a little salt on a facecloth and rub gently over the face and body. Rinse well.

 PROPERTIES

The body needs salt to maintain water in the body and help distribute carbon dioxide through the blood. Salt has cleansing and antiseptic properties and acts as a digestive and a laxative.

Special Notes
Too much salt in the diet may lead to fluid retention and hypertension. Some authorities recommend a daily intake of no more than 5g., but in the U.S. the average daily intake is between 10 and 12g. On average, about 70 percent of our salt intake occurs naturally in our food, or we add it while cooking or preparing food in the home. The remaining 30 percent is added in manufacturing or preserving.

Contraindications
• People with high blood pressure should restrict their intake of sodium chloride. Substituting potassium salts, available commercially as products marked "low" or "lo" salt, can help. People on low-sodium diets must restrict their salt intake as advised by their general practitioner or dietitian.

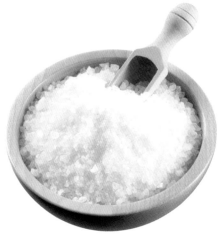

ABOVE *Salt has been used traditionally as a preservative—for example, to salt beans and salt cod—and as a seasoning for food. It also has therapeutic uses, some of which are based on folk medicine.*

Baking Soda Bicarbonate of soda

 FOOD USES

To cure flatulence, drink a solution of ½ teaspoon baking soda dissolved in a glass of hot water. Baking soda mixed to a paste with water eases the pain of a bee sting. Remove the sting from the skin before applying. Sour breath can be sweetened by gargling with a solution of baking soda and water. It can also be used as an efficient toothpaste. The juice of half a lemon mixed with 1 teaspoon of baking powder and warm water will help ease headache if taken every fifteen minutes. A baking soda poultice will help to soothe diaper rash.

 PROPERTIES

The chemical name of baking soda, an alkaline salt, is sodium bicarbonate ($NaHCO_2$). When used medicinally it is soothing to the skin, can neutralize offensive odors, and ease pain.

Special Notes
No safe dosage for baking soda has been established.

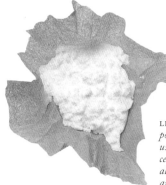

 CAUTION

Use only externally on babies and children, as a treatment for stings and rashes.

LEFT *Baking soda is a white powder that is traditionally used as a raising agent for certain baked goods. It also has useful therapeutic applications.*

Barley *Hordeum vulgare*

FOOD USES

Barley may help to prevent heart disease since it promotes the normal functioning of the heart and stabilizes blood pressure. To ease vomiting, drink some barley water made by boiling 1 teaspoon of barley in 2pts. (1l.) water and then simmer for 10 minutes. Drinking barley water may help in the treatment of cystitis. Barley water reduces acid in the spleen if drunk twice a day for a month. Make a poultice of barley flour to reduce inflammation of the skin. Barley's soothing properties also aid inflammations of the digestive tract, respiratory systems, urinary systems. Drinking barley soups and water can be helpful for flatulence, diarrhea, constipation, and colic.

PROPERTIES

Barley is an excellent source of vitamin B9 (folic acid), potassium, phosphorus, and magnesium. It also contains iron and calcium. A large proportion of these minerals cannot be made available to the body because barley contains phyric acid, which forms insoluble compounds that cannot be digested.

Special Notes

Use whole barley rather than pearl or milled barley since it contains more nutrients. Barley contains gluten.

CAUTION

Do not eat barley or products containing barley if you have a gluten allergy.

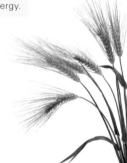

RIGHT *Barley is a member of the grass family and an important cereal, grown as a food for humans and animals. Large quantities of barley are made into malt, which is used in the manufacture of alcoholic and nonalcoholic beverages.*

Bread *Hordeum vulgare*

FOOD USES

Wholewheat bread is a useful source of dietary fiber, which keeps the digestive tract functioning efficiently. A traditional folk remedy for pleurisy was a drink made from toasted wholewheat breadcrumbs, a pinch of salt, a knob of butter, and hot boiled water.

PROPERTIES

Yeast breads are an excellent source of carbohydrates and the B vitamins—folic acid (B9), niacin (B3), pantothenic acid (B5), pyridoxine (B6), riboflavin (B2), and thiamine (B1). Wholewheat breads have additional amounts of pyridoxine, pantothenic acid, and thiamine. All breads, including unleavened bread, have a high sodium content and are a good source of iron, potassium, and calcium. In addition to the valuable nutritional benefits to be gained from eating bread, its main therapeutic use is as a poultice.

Special Notes

Avoid eating bread if you are on a low-sodium or low-fiber diet. In certain cases bread can provoke an allergic reaction.

Contraindications

• Anyone on a gluten-free diet should not eat breads made with barley, rye, wheat, oats, or buckwheat.

• Bread enriched with milk should be avoided by anyone on a lactose-free diet.

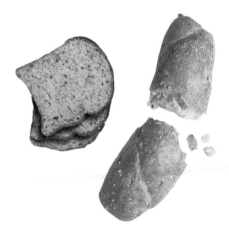

ABOVE *For nutritional purposes dietitians recommend eating wholegrain yeast breads in preference to white bread.*

Oats *Avena sativa*

 HERBALISM

Oats are the basis for a specific herbal remedy for nervous exhaustion and depression.

 FOOD USES

Oats may give some protection against cancer of the bowel. They lower the amount of cholesterol in the blood, so helping to protect against heart disease. Oatmeal may be of benefit to women suffering from menopausal symptoms, and men suffering from impotence or sterility. Oatmeal is a gentle, effective tonic for the nerves and may help those trying to overcome an addiction. An oatmeal bath moisturizes the skin and gives relief to eczema sufferers.

 CHILDREN

Oatmeal may be recommended to calm hyperactive or highly strung children.

 PROPERTIES

Oats are high in carbohydrates, most of which are starch; the sugar content of oats is low. Oats are a good source of fiber, contain some protein, and have a higher fat content than rye and wheat flours. They also contain sodium (33mg. per 100g.) and are an excellent source of B vitamins (thiamine and pantothenic acid), iron, phosphorus, and potassium. Oats have laxative properties and act as a tonic on the heart, uterus, nervous system, and thymus gland. They also affect the reproductive system.

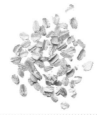

LEFT *Oats are a cereal plant, the grains of which are usually made into oatmeal. Oatmeal is the product of rolling or grinding oats and then steaming them. Milled oats are found in muesli, granola, and other breakfast cereal products. Oats have therapeutic properties. Products based on wild oats are available commercially.*

Special Notes
• Oats contain gluten.
• People on special diets, and those suffering from certain diseases, may be advised to avoid eating oats and products containing oats.

Contraindications
• People with celiac disease cannot tolerate gluten or gliadin.
• These substances are also found in wheat and rye. All three cereals should be avoided by those with the disease, as well as any others on a gluten-free diet.
• Oats should also be avoided by people on low-carbohydrate, low-fiber, and low-sodium diets.

Rice *Oryza sativa*

 FOOD USES

The seeds are used to treat urinary ailments. The water poured off from boiled rice helps to overcome stomach upsets and rehydrate someone suffering from fluid loss through diarrhea. Rice and rice flour are used as substitutes for wheat and some other cereals by people who cannot tolerate gluten and gliadin, such as those with celiac disease. Germinated rice seeds may help in the treatment of abdominal bloating, lack of appetite, and indigestion.

 PROPERTIES

Rice contains high levels of carbohydrates (87g. per 100g. of white, uncooked rice). It contributes B vitamins - folic acid and pyridoxine—iron, and potassium. Brown rice also contains the B vitamin thiamine, which is present in the bran. White rice has 1g. of fat per 100g.; in brown rice the amount of fat is higher. Rice has low amounts of sodium and is cholesterol-free. It is a tonic, a diuretic, and a digestive. It also controls sweating.

Special Notes
• White rice contains fewer vitamins than brown, unpolished rice. If possible, use brown varieties for rice dishes.

• Rice contains proteins that lack the essential amino acids lysine and isoleucine and are therefore known as incomplete proteins (complete proteins, such as those found in animal protein, have their full complement of amino acids). To make up for this lack, eat rice with legumes such as peas or beans. These foods lack the essential acids tryptophan, cystine, and methionine, so when the two foods are combined the body benefits from complete proteins. Protein is necessary for the growth and repair of tissues, and provides energy. Incomplete proteins are of relatively little use to the body.

RIGHT *Rice is the cereal that is a staple food to more than half of the world's peoples. It also has important medicinal uses, for which the rhizomes, seeds (the grains), and germinated seeds are used. White rice is the grain that is left after the bran and germ have been removed; brown rice retains the bran and germ. Rice is available as a breakfast cereal (the grains are "puffed" during manufacture) and is fermented to produce rice wine, called saki by the Japanese.*

SHORT-GRAIN
RICE

Eggs Hordeum vulgare

FOOD USES

The white of eggs act on the mucous membranes of the digestive tract and may help in the treatment of digestive ailments. Egg white, whisked to a froth with a drop of vinegar or milk, makes a soothing face mask. Whisked egg white also provides relief for diaper rash, and sore, cracked nipples. Egg yolk makes an excellent tonic for the hair and can be used in both shampoos and conditioners.

PROPERTIES

Eggs are an excellent source of protein, B vitamins (thiamine and riboflavin), vitamin D, vitamin A, and the minerals calcium, phosphorus, potassium, and iron. About 74 percent of the weight of an egg is water. Most of the nutrients are in the yolk, although the white does contain thiamine. An egg provides twice as much fat as it does protein and almost the maximum amount of cholesterol that is currently recommended for daily consumption.

Special Notes
• Under certain circumstances eggs can cause salmonella poisoning.

• A significant number of people, particularly children, may develop an allergy to eggs. Symptoms of an adverse reaction include swollen eyes and lips, abdominal pain, nausea and subsequent vomiting, and skin reactions.

• Viruses grown in egg culture to make vaccines can occasionally cause an allergic reaction.

• The iron in eggs is more easily made available to the body if foods containing vitamin C—such as orange or grapefruit juice—are eaten with the egg.

• To relieve the irritation of chilblains, make a paste with egg white, honey, and flour; smear over the chilblains and cover with aclean bandage.

Contraindications
• If any of the above symptoms occur after eating eggs, seek medical attention immediately. Should similar symptoms occur following vaccination for mumps, measles, or flu, you should also seek immediate medical advice.

• Pregnant women, elderly and ill people should avoid eating raw eggs. Because of the high cholesterol content of eggs, people with a history of heart disease should confine their consumption of eggs to the whites only, or restrict their consumption to two or three whole eggs a week.

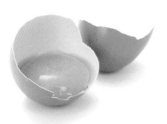

ABOVE *Egg yolk can be used in shampoos and conditioners and makes an excellent hair tonic.*

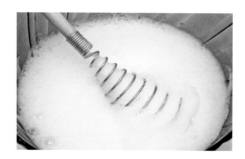

ABOVE *Whisked egg white can provide relief for diaper rash and sore nipples.*

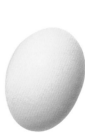

ABOVE *Eggs arc rich in nutrients and easily digested. They have valuable therapeutic properties with external and internal applications.*

Honey

 FOOD USES

Honey's long recognized antiseptic properties can be utilized to advantage for coughs and sore throats. It is particularly effective when mixed with lemon or vinegar. Apply a honey compress to cuts and bruises. Set honey can be helpful in the treatment of ringworm. Smear honey on the affected area as many times throughout the day as possible. Do not cover. Repeat again at bedtime. Honey is extremely useful for moisturizing the skin and is often a constituent of natural skincare products. To relieve the irritation of chilblains, make a paste with honey, egg white, and flour; smear over the chilblains and cover the area with a clean bandage. As a preventive to hay fever, eat a little of the local honey.

 PROPERTIES

Honey is comprised mainly of the sugars glucose and fructose. It has a very high nutritional value, although it does contain small amounts of minerals—among them calcium, phosphorus, and potassium—and several vitamins: the B complex, C, D, and E. It also contributes some amino acids. Honey is used for both culinary and therapeutic purposes. It is an antiseptic, which recommends it for the treatment of both internal and external infections, and is reputed to be an excellent food for promoting general good health. A small

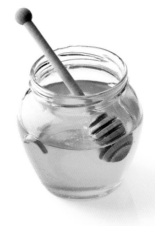

amount of pollen is usually present in honey. Pollen, unlike honey, is a very rich source of nutrients and therefore can be of benefit in itself when taken in large enough quantities.

Special Notes
Honey is a healthy alternative to refined sugars.

 CAUTION

Diabetics must avoid honey at all times.

LEFT *Honey has traditionally been regarded as having therapeutic properties. Certainly, pure honey is one of the few foods that can be eaten today in its near-natural form. Pure honey by its very nature does not contain any additives and is almost always free of herbicides and pesticides.*

Molasses

 FOOD USES

Blackstrap molasses is a very effective laxative. It is also a good source of iron and other essential minerals. It can be eaten as it comes from the jar, one teaspoonful a day, or it can be used as an ingredient in cakes and puddings. It was once used as the sweetener for the folk remedy that is known as Brimstone and Treacle, which mixed sulfur with molasses or black treacle.

 PROPERTIES

Molasses is a rich source of minerals, especially potassium, which the body requires for healthy muscles and for maintaining cells and nervous tissue. It also contributes the mineral alumina, necessary for the growth of bones and teeth, calcium, chromium, iron, zinc, and magnesium.

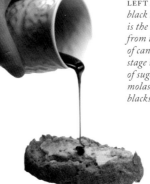

LEFT *Also known as black treacle, molasses is the residue that is left from the manufacture of cane sugar. The final stage in the extraction of sugars produces the molasses known as blackstrap molasses.*

Alcohol

 FOOD USES

Some types of alcohol are used in therapeutic practice as carriers or preservatives for other healing substances; for example, vodka or brandy are often used to make a herbal tincture. Wine tonics stimulate the appetite. Digestives made from red wine and certain herbs aid digestion when taken after a rich or heavy meal. Alcohol taken in small quantities may help guard against heart disease, diseases of the arteries, and the formation of gallstones caused by cholesterol. Red wine is a rich source of flavonoids, which help protect the body from viruses and allergens.

 PROPERTIES

Alcohol has culinary, cosmetic, and therapeutic uses. It relaxes and warms the body, acts as an antiseptic and diuretic, and is a depressant.

Special Notes
• Safe levels of alcohol consumption are around 10-20g. per day, that is, around two glasses (4fl. oz./125ml.) of wine or just under one pint of beer a day.

• Alcohol can be toxic in large amounts, and under certain circumstances it should be avoided altogether.

Contraindications
• If you are taking any other prescription or over-the-counter drugs—including vitamin and mineral supplements—seek advice from your pharmacist or general practitioner before drinking alcohol.

• Alcohol is best avoided by people who suffer from migraine.

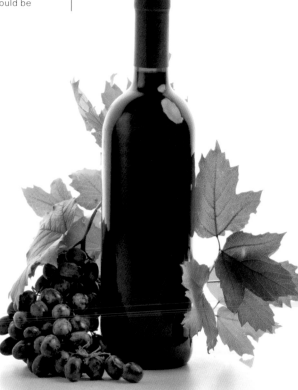

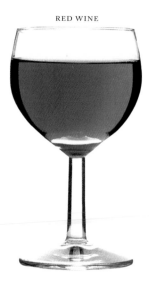

RED WINE

 CAUTION

Do not drink alcohol if you are pregnant, are taking antibiotics or aspirin, or have gout. Never give alcohol to someone who is suffering from shock, or someone who is or has been unconscious.

RIGHT *Alcohol is a drug that affects the nervous system— altering mood and perception, for example—and in excessive amounts it can seriously, sometimes fatally, damage the body. However when taken in small amounts it can have a positive effect on health.*

Vinegar *Acetic acid*

FOOD USES

Vinegar's antiseptic properties make it beneficial in the treatment of urinary infections, such as cystitis, and bowel infections. Vinegar is used to reduce swelling and pain produced by wasp stings. Cider vinegar sweetened with honey will counteract stomach acidity, treat coughs, hay fever, and nasal congestion. Vinegar and honey may be beneficial in the treatment of arthritis and asthma. A daily drink made by mixing one tablespoon of vinegar in a glass of water may help in the treatment of thrush. Dab neat cider vinegar on the skin to treat athlete's foot, ringworm, and eczema. A drop of vinegar added to the bathwater can soothe skin irritations, including those caused by eczema.

PROPERTIES

Vinegar acts on the urinary tract; it is antiseptic, astringent, and antifungal.

RIGHT *Vinegar is used as a preservative, a flavoring, and a remedy for ailments. It is produced by the action of bacteria that oxidize alcohol. Red and white wines, apple cider, perry, and malt are used to make vinegar. Apple cider vinegar is particularly beneficial to health.*

RED WINE VINEGAR

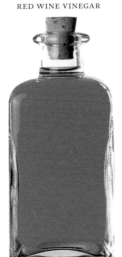

Yogurt

FOOD USES

Eat live, plain yogurt after completing a course of antibiotics. This will replenish supplies of the beneficial bacteria (flora) that live in the gut and are depleted by repeated use of antibiotics. In cases of oral or vaginal thrush, apply plain, live yogurt to the area. Repeat two or three times a day until the condition has improved. Live yogurt may help to reduce blood cholesterol and therefore has a role to play in the prevention of heart disease.

PROPERTIES

Yogurt is a rich source of protein and provides good supplies of vitamin A, the B vitamins thiamine and riboflavin, and calcium. Yogurt made from skimmed milk is relatively low in cholesterol and fats (1.0g. per 100g.). Yogurt is beneficial to the digestive system and the urinary tract. It is antifungal and soothing.

Special Notes
• People on special diets may be advised to avoid yogurt.
• Anyone with a lactose intolerance may experience adverse effects from eating yogurt.
• Like milk, yogurt promotes the production of mucus and should therefore be avoided by those with a cold or catarrh.

Contraindications
• People with a lactose intolerance lack the enzyme lactase, which is needed to break down lactose into glucose and galactose. However, they may be able to tolerate acidophilus yogurt because it seems to supply the missing enzyme.
• Anyone on a low-fat or low-cholesterol diet may be advised to avoid full-fat yogurt.
• Women who are carriers of the disease galactosemia may have to avoid yogurt and other milk products during pregnancy.

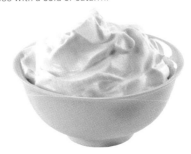

LEFT *Yogurt is milk that has been curdled, or "cultured," by the action of bacteria. These may include Lactobacillus acidophilus, which can be of particular benefit to people who cannot tolerate milk and other milk products. "Live" yogurt contains active bacteria.*

Water Hydrogen dioxide

 FOOD USES

Water prevents dehydration. It can help to prevent tooth decay when sufficient fluoride is present. Water acts as a diuretic and a mild laxative—it adds water to stools and may stimulate muscle contraction in the digestive tract. Hard water may play a role in preventing hypertension and heart disease. Ice reduces swellings and is particularly beneficial for sprains. Ice packs help to relieve backache. Swallowing cracked ice may be beneficial in relieving morning sickness. Bathing in warm water can induce relaxation. Hot baths may help to soothe muscular aches and pains. A cool bath can be soothing for sufferers of prickly heat. A hot compress can help to reduce skin inflammations caused by infection. Dip a facecloth or other thick cloth in hot water and wring out before applying. Cold compresses placed around the throat may ease croup.

 CHILDREN

Children suffering from croup will get relief when placed in a steamy bathroom. This is best achieved by running the hot water faucet or the shower.

PROPERTIES

Water has very few nutrients except for the minerals calcium and magnesium, and these vary according to whether the water is hard or soft (hard water contains more minerals than soft water). Other substances may be added to water, for example chlorine to purify it, and fluorides to help prevent dental caries, although fluorine may occur naturally in some cases. Water also contains some sodium; the amount varies from one area to another. Bottled waters may be particularly high in sodium.

Special Notes
• Water should be filtered before it is drunk if it contains impurities.

• Bottled mineral waters may be high in sodium.

Contraindications
• If contaminants such as excess chlorine are present, avoid drinking the water and notify the appropriate authority.

• Those on a low-sodium diet may need to avoid some bottled waters. Check the label before drinking.

• Check sodium levels before serving bottled water to infants and children.

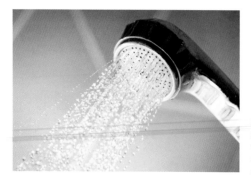

LEFT *Children suffering from croup will feel better when they're in a steamy bathroom.*

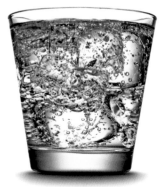

ABOVE *Water makes up about 75 percent of the human body. It is not just essential for health; it is essential for life. Water is necessary for maintaining the correct osmotic pressure in cells and is needed for many other body processes, such as transporting nutrients and waste products around the body in the blood (blood is about 80 percent water). Water that has been cooled to form ice, or heated to form hot water or steam, can be used to treat minor complaints.*

Tea Camellia sinensis

FOOD USES

The fluoride in tea may be beneficial in the prevention of dental caries. Tea may help in the treatment of diarrhea, dysentery, hepatitis, and gastroenteritis. The flavonoids in tea may help to destroy harmful bacteria and viruses. Cold, steeped tea bags placed over the eyes will soothe soreness and irritation. Their astringent properties also make them useful for treating minor injuries and insect bites. The leaves of green and black tea may be beneficial in the prevention of heart disease and stroke. Raspberry-leaf tea (*see page 195*) is a well-known tonic when taken during pregnancy. It also helps prepare the breasts for breast-feeding.

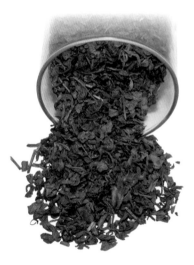

ABOVE *Studies have shown that green tea may contribute to the prevention of cancer, particularly stomach cancer.*

PROPERTIES

Tea provides folic acid (vitamin B9), and some potassium and magnesium. It contains fluoride (0.3-0.5mg. per cup), tannins, and methylxanthines—stimulants that include caffeine. Tea acts on the area of the nervous system that controls the respiratory and digestive systems. It is a diuretic and astringent. Antioxidants called polyphenols have beneficial effects on the circulatory system, while flavonoids act on the immune system.

Special Notes
• Studies have shown that green tea may contribute to the prevention of cancer, particularly stomach cancer. Green tea capsules are commercially available but benefits may also accrue from drinking freshly made green tea.

• Always allow the tea to cool slightly before drinking. Do not drink it very hot.

• The caffeine content of tea is much higher than that of coffee.

• Tea may cause adverse reactions in people who are undergoing medical treatment.

Contraindications
• Drinking tea to excess can cause constipation, indigestion, dizziness, palpitations, irritability, and insomnia.
• Tea can interfere with the effectiveness of drugs such as allopurinol (for the treatment of gout), antibiotics, antiulcer drugs, and the drug theophylline, prescribed for asthma. It can prevent the absorption of iron and interfere with the effectiveness of sedative drugs.

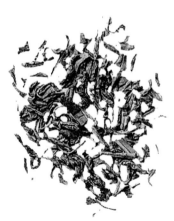

LEFT *Green tea is made from the tips of shoots of the shrub Camellia sinensis; black tea is made from the fermented, dried leaves. An essential oil, called tea absolute, is distilled from black tea. Both the leaves and oil are used for medicinal purposes. Fruit teas can also be beneficial to the health.*

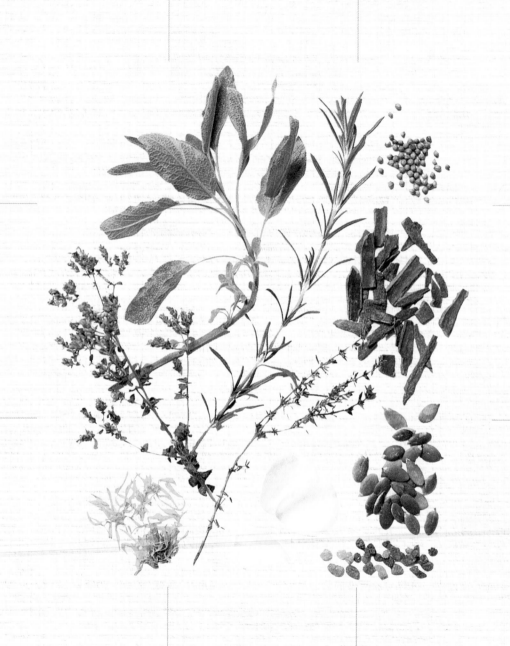

PART FOUR

Practical Matters
& Useful Information

This part includes sections on first aid, suggestions for what remedies to buy or make for a natural home medicine chest, data on the recommended daily allowances of vitamins and minerals, and an exhaustive directory of healing plants cross-referencing common, local, or traditional names with the Latin botanical name. There is also a glossary of terms, pointers toward further reading, useful addresses, and a general index.

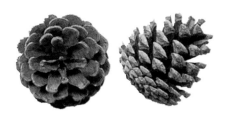

First-Aid

*T*his section covers the minor injuries and common mishaps that occur in most households at some time or another. Natural remedies are given, and a suitable home medicine chest suggested. In the case of serious accidents, make sure that you get qualified help immediately.

Bites and Stings

Bites and stings should always be treated immediately. Stings from a bee, wasp, or hornet are not usually dangerous unless you suffer from an allergy. Bites may be more serious, partly because germs from the animal's mouth can be injected deep into the flesh, causing infection, and partly because a bite may break bones and damage tissue.

 CAUTION

Multiple stings or stings to the eyes, ears, or mouth should be treated at all hospital. Animals bites that cause bleeding should be seen by a doctor—particularly if there is any possibility of contracting rabies.

 HERBALISM

• Marigold petals are useful on a bee sting. Calendula cream reduces swelling.

• Wormwood or sage leaves can be macerated and applied to spider, scorpion, or jellyfish stings.

• Cover bites and stings with a wet, macerated plantain leaf. When dry, replace with a wet leaf.

• Witch hazel is useful on mosquito bites.

 HOMEOPATHY

• Clean wounds with tincture of Hypericum.

• Ledum can be taken for all puncture wounds.

• Take Apis for bee stings, after removing the sting with a pair of tweezers.

• Arnica is useful if there is bruising from a bite.

• Take Aconite for shock.

 FLOWER ESSENCES

• Apply Rescue Remedy directly to bites or stings, or take a few drops internally.

 AROMATHERAPY

• Use neat lavender oil on stings to reduce swelling.

• Rub one drop of tea tree oil into an insect bite or sting.

• Use a few drops of geranium oil in water to clean a bite and encourage it to heal.

 FROM THE LARDER

• A slice of onion or a paste of bicarbonate of soda and water will reduce the discomfort of a bee sting.

• Apply garlic and onion to ant bites, and cucumber juice to ease the discomfort.

• Apply a compress of cotton batting soaked in lemon juice to a wasp sting.

• Apply a poultice of sugar to a bite wound (*see page 259*).

 SELF-HELP

• Always remove a sting before beginning treatment. Wash animal bites with soap and warm water.

• Prevent insect bites by diluting eucalyptus or citronella oils in half a mug of water and then applying to exposed areas, avoiding the eyes and mouth. Use cider vinegar in the same way.

Cuts and Grazes

Small cuts and abrasions will usually heal without treatment, but any wound to the skin presents a risk of infection, so it is important that you clean and dress the wound to prevent this from happening. Deeper wounds may require sutures and should be seen by a physician.

 HERBALISM

• A few drops of marigold tincture in fresh, warm water can be used to clean the wound. This will help to prevent infection and encourage healing.

• Ecinachea can be diluted and used directly on the wound to prevent infection. Reapply when bandages are changed.

• Comfrey ointment can be used on wounds that have become inflamed.

• Use a witch hazel compress on wounds and swellings.

• Tincture of myrrh is an excellent antiseptic. Apply a few drops to bandages before dressing a wound.

 HOMEOPATHY

• The wound can be cleaned with Calendula or Hypericum tinctures. Put a few drops on a little clean gauze; never use absorbent cotton on an open wound.

• Arnica should be used in the case of all injuries, to encourage healing and reduce the risk of bruising.

• Hypericum is useful for wounds accompanied by shooting pains.

• Try Ledum for most wounds, particularly when there is a risk of tetanus.

 FLOWER ESSENCES

• Rescue Remedy can be applied neat to a cut to encourage healing and reduce pain, or applied to the temples and pulse points to calm.

 AROMATHERAPY

• A few drops of tea tree oil, in clear, warm water, can be used to clean a wound and act as an antiseptic.

• Geranium oil can be dropped onto a dressing to encourage healing.

• Lavender oil, applied directly to the nostrils or massaged in a light carrier oil into the temples, will provide relief from any accompanying shock or pain.

 FROM THE LARDER

• Lemon juice is an excellent styptic and can be diluted and applied directly to a clean wound. Dress as normal.

• A compress made of peach pit tea can be used on infected wounds.

• Sugar is said to prevent scar tissue; press a few teaspoons of granulated sugar into a clean wound and dress with gauze. Rinse the wound carefully and redress. Repeat up to five times daily, but take care not to disturb the clotting action.

• Cayenne pepper is a very useful styptic, and a minute quantity can be applied directly to a clean wound to stop any bleeding.

 SELF-HELP

• Wash all wounds with warm, soapy water to prevent infection.

• Minor abrasions should be allowed to dry in the air, so leave open or apply a single layer of gauze bandage.

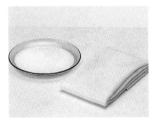

1 You need a sterile piece of gauze dressing, about 4oz. (100g.) granulated sugar and a sterilized teaspoon. Clean the wound thoroughly before you begin.

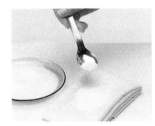

2 Sprinkle 2 to 3 teaspoonfuls of sugar either directly on to the wound or on to the gauze. If you choose the second method, carefully place the gauze over the wound, making sure that the sugar covers the wound.

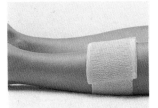

3 Bind the gauze firmly on top of the wound with a crepe bandage. Change the dressing regularly. Do not disturb the healing action of the sugar. A sugar dressing is particularly useful for ulcerations or wide, shallow wounds where the skin cannot knit together on its own.

 CAUTION

If you have been bitten, or the wound has been caused by a rusty nail or tool or object that has been in contact with soil, a tetanus shot is recommended.

Bruises

A bruise occurs when the blood is released into the tissues as a result of a blow. It is characterized by a blue-black mark, which changes color as the bruise heals and blood is reabsorbed into the body. Occasionally a bruise can occur without an injury—this is a feature in some diseases.

RIGHT *Arnica is the homeopathic remedy of choice for bruises; apply it as a cream, or take internally as a tincture.*

(!) CAUTION

If bruising appears spontaneously and is not caused by a blow, see your physician.

Most bruises should heal within a week or two; if yours has not, see your physician.

 HERBALISM

• Use a cold compress of lavender or fennel on the bruise in order to reduce swelling and help to disperse the blood.

• Rosemary, used as a compress, can encourage healing.

• The crushed roots and leaves of agrimony can be applied to bruises.

• Comfrey, used as a compress or poultice, will work to heal bruising. Comfrey cream works well, especially in the early stages of bruising.

• Witch hazel in the form of a compress will relieve swelling and inflammation.

• Yarrow is also useful, crushed and applied to new bruises.

 HOMEOPATHY

• Arnica, taken internally, will help to relieve symptoms. Arnica cream can be applied to any bruise, as long as the skin is not broken.

 FLOWER ESSENCES

• Rescue Remedy encourages healing and reduces the effects of shock.

 AROMATHERAPY

• Essential oil of lavender in a sweet almond oil carrier can be gently applied to the bruised site to reduce swelling and encourage healing.

 FROM THE LARDER

• Cabbage, lightly macerated, dipped in boiling water and slightly cooled, can be applied to bruising to discourage swelling.

• A compress made from cider vinegar may be applied to all bruises, but avoid the eye area.

• Onions, cut into slices and applied to the bruise, will encourage the blood to disperse.

• Caraway seeds, heated and gently pounded, can be administered to bruises.

(ii) SELF-HELP

• An ice pack, placed directly on the bruised area, will reduce swelling.

• A vitamin C deficiency may make you susceptible to bruising. Ensure that you have an adequate intake (*see page 276*).

Blisters

Blisters are small pockets of blood serum that appear as raised bumps or bubbles on the skin. They are usually the result of friction, but they can be caused by injury, such as a burn or scald, or appear as a symptom of diseases such as chickenpox, herpes, eczema, impetigo, among others. Some insect bites produce blisters.

(!) CAUTION

Try not to burst a blister, which will leave the skin open to infection.

LEFT *Constant pressure on skin unused to it can cause painful blisters; weekend gardeners are often afflicted.*

 HERBALISM

• Marigold (calendula) cream can be applied to a blister to promote healing.

• Witch hazel, applied neat to a bruise, will quickly relieve pain and swelling, and encourage healing.

 HOMEOPATHY

• Urtica urens ointment can be applied to blisters caused by infection or burns.

• Hypericum ointment will encourage healing of blisters.

• Cantharis is useful for itching, burning blisters.

• Try Rhus tox. for red and itchy blisters, particularly those caused by the chicken-pox virus (herpes).

• Punctured blisters can be cleansed with a few drops of tincture of Calendula in clean water.

 AROMATHERAPY

• Neat lavender oil can be applied to blisters.

• Benzoin applied to areas susceptible to blisters can prevent as well as heal them.

• Roman chamomile has antiseptic properties. Use a few drops in half a mug of water to cleanse punctured blisters and the area around.

 FROM THE LARDER

• Peach pit tea is recommended to heal blisters.

• Ice will also reduce inflammation and any itching or pain.

• Boiled and mashed carrots can be applied to blisters to help to heal the area. This treatment is ideal when a punctured blister has become infected.

• Use roasted onions, applied as a poultice, to blisters, particularly those that have become infected.

 SELF-HELP

• Apply surgical spirit and then petroleum jelly to areas that may be susceptible to blisters caused by chafing.

• Cover blisters in the daytime to prevent them from being punctured and infected.

• Remove bandages at night to allow them to dry out. Replace any bandage that becomes damp.

Sprains and Strains

A sprain is caused when a ligament becomes overextended. It is characterized by pain and usually restricted movement, and there will be swelling, bruising, and occasionally some bleeding.

 HERBALISM

• A compress or ointment of comfrey leaves can help to heal the ligament.

• Burdock can be taken internally in the form of a tea, or applied as a poultice to the affected area.

• Ginger added to bathwater, or a footbath, or applied as a compress encourages healing.

• Chamomile can be taken internally to calm and reduce pain.

 HOMEOPATHY

• Arnica should be taken internally, until the injury has healed.

• Ruta can be taken after the first day.

• A cold compress with Arnica tincture should be applied hourly for the first eight hours to reduce swelling.

 FLOWER ESSENCES

• Rescue Remedy can be taken internally to reduce shock and to calm. A few drops on a cold compress, applied to the injury, can help to reduce pain. When the swelling has gone down, a little Rescue Remedy cream can be massaged into the joint area.

 AROMATHERAPY

• Use a little lavender oil in a footbath or on a cold compress applied to the area. Avoid massaging the area, which will increase inflammation.

• A compress with essential oils of sweet marjoram and rosemary can be used to heal and to reduce the inflammation.

 FROM THE LARDER

• Cider vinegar can be used as a compress in order to relieve the pain and swelling.

• A poultice of raw onions can be applied to the sprain.

 SELF-HELP

• Raise the affected limb and apply a cold compress as soon as possible.

• Strains should be bandaged with an elastic bandage to provide support, but take care not to bind too tightly and cut off circulation.

• Keep the limb elevated until the swelling goes down and there is some normal movement possible.

 CAUTION

If you suspect a fracture, see your physician immediately.

If the sprain is accompanied by any bleeding, or other symptoms not listed above, seek medical attention.

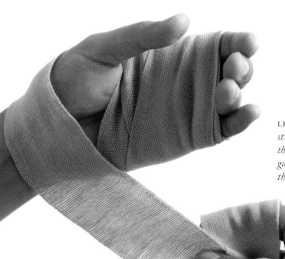

LEFT *Sprains and strains that occur in the excitement of the game are painful off the court.*

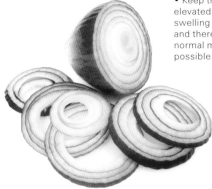

ABOVE *A poultice of raw onions can be applied to a sprain for relief.*

Nosebleeds

The lining of the nose is very thin, and even heavy blowing or a minor jolt can rupture a capillary and cause bleeding. Unless there is an accompanying blow to the head or intense pain, nosebleeds are not usually serious.

 CAUTION

See your physician if you suffer from chronic nosebleeds, or if bleeding is profuse or accompanied by pain.

 HERBALISM

• A cold compress of witch hazel can be applied externally to the nose.

• Tincture of yarrow, held under the nostrils, may also be useful.

• Marigold tincture, on a cotton swab, may be placed in the nose to stop the bleeding and encourage healing.

 HOMEOPATHY

• Arnica should be taken, particularly if there has been a blow to the nose.

• Phosphorus is recommended when the nosebleed is caused by blowing too hard.

• Ferrum phos. can be used when there is nausea or faintness.

 FLOWER ESSENCES

• Rescue Remedy can be applied neat into the nose to provide some relief. Apply to pulse points if there is accompanying shock or injury.

 AROMATHERAPY

• Apply a few drops of essential oil of lemon on a cotton swab and gently apply to the affected nostril.

• A compress of lavender oil or Roman chamomile oil can be placed across the bridge of the nose to provide relief.

• Gently massage the head with essential oil of lavender in a peach kernel carrier oil to reduce accompanying headache.

 FROM THE LARDER

• Apply lemon juice to a cotton swab to dab inside the nose and staunch the bleeding.

• Juniper berries can be crushed, wrapped in one layer of gauze, and placed in the nose to stop bleeding.

 SELF-HELP

• During a nosebleed, gently pinch together the nostrils and lean forward. Hold for several minutes, until the bleeding stops. Avoid blowing the nose for several hours after a nosebleed.

• Chronic nosebleeds may indicate poor capillary health. Ensure that your intake of vitamin C and zinc are sufficient (*see pages 276-277*).

STOPPING A NOSEBLEED
To stop the flow of blood, lean forward slightly and pinch the top of the nose, just where the bone ends, so that the nostrils are closed.

Toothache

Toothache can be caused by many things, including an abscess, gum disease, neuralgia, or simply sensitive teeth. There may also be referred pain from the sinuses or ears.

 HERBALISM

• Echinacea, myrrh, and golden seal are useful to treat gum infections, abscesses, and cankers. They may used as a poultice, mouthwash, or dabbed neat, in tincture form, on the affected area.

• Comfrey tea bags or ointment can be applied to a painful tooth or gum area to reduce swelling and pain.

• Fennel can be applied as a poultice to the cheek, to help relieve pain.

 HOMEOPATHY

• Use Chamomilla for pain.

• Use Belladonna for throbbing pain, particularly that accompanied by swelling and flushed cheeks.

• Use Aconite when the pain comes on suddenly.

• Use Coffea when there are shooting pains.

• Hepar sulf. may be useful to bring out an abscess.

 FLOWER ESSENCES

• Rescue Remedy can be applied to the affected tooth or gum, or taken internally to calm.

 AROMATHERAPY

• Oil of clove is useful, if applied directly to the tooth or gum area. Soak a cotton ball and tuck it into the cheek to provide relief, and to act as an antiseptic.

• A hot compress with lavender or chamomile may ease the inflammation and encourage the healing process.

 FROM THE LARDER

• Peach pit tea can be used when the gums are infected. Use as a mouth rinse, several times daily.

• Chew whole cloves for their antiseptic and analgesic properties.

• Chew juniper berries to provide relief from the paid of neuralgia.

• Rub lemons on the affected tooth or gum to reduce the pain and prevent any bleeding.

• Cayenne is a natural anesthetic and can be daubed on the painful site.

 SELF-HELP

• Dental problems should always be seen by a dentist in the first instance, but there are many treatments that can provide relief until you are able to see one. A cold compress, applied to the cheek, will reduce pain and swelling.

ABOVE *Chew juniper berries to relieve the pain in the face that sometimes accompanies toothache.*

 CAUTION

If there is profuse bleeding or swelling, seek emergency treatment.

Burns and Scalds

Minor burns and scalds can be quite safely treated at home, but more extensive burns can cause damage to the nerves and lead to a condition called "surgical shock," which can be fatal. Always cool a burn before undertaking any other treatment—that means allowing cool running water to flow over it for about ten minutes. Try to avoid applying anything to the burn until it is cooled and you can see the extent of the damage. "Wet" burns should be dressed with a fabric, such as gauze, that will "breathe." Change regularly.

 CAUTION

Any burn that is larger than about 2 inches across should be seen by a physician.

 HERBALISM

Aloe can be applied directly to a burn in order to soothe and seal it from infection. It will also encourage healing.

A few drops of echinacea tincture in 2pt. (1l.) of water poured over the burn will help to prevent infection.

Marigold tincture applied sparingly to a dressing is a useful healing agent.

 HOMEOPATHY

Arnica can be taken to promote healing.

Cantharis can help to relieve pain, when taken immediately after the accident.

Urtica can be used if the burn continues to be painful.

Aconite should be taken for shock.

Urtica urens ointment may help to soothe a burn.

Use Hypericum ointment or Calendula to prevent infection and encourage the burn to heal.

 FLOWER ESSENCES

Rescue Remedy will help to calm. A little bit of diluted tincture can be applied directly to a burn.

AROMATHERAPY

Lavender oil is ideal for burns and can be applied neat (use sparingly).
A few drops of geranium oil in 2pt. (1l.) of cooled, boiled water can be poured over a burn or scald to encourage healing.

RIGHT *Run cold water over the injured part as soon as you can after a minor scald or burn. Keep it there for as long as you can, to cool the skin below the site of the burn.*

FROM THE LARDER

Honey can be applied directly to a burn to facilitate healing and to help prevent infection. Crush and extract the juice of blueberries and keep in the refrigerator or freezer to use on emergency burns or scalds. Raw potatoes can be placed on a burn to provide instant relief.

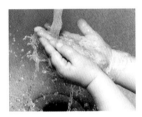

Travel Sickness

It is believed that travel sickness occurs in susceptible individuals because of a disturbance of the balancing mechanisms in the inner ear. Common symptoms of travel sickness are nausea, dizziness, tiredness, pale, clammy skin, and vomiting.

 CAUTION

You may feel unwell for several hours after traveling, but if symptoms persist, see your physician.

 HERBALISM

• Angelica root, hung in the car or boat cabin, is said to relieve nausea.

• Ginger infusions, tablets, or roots may be taken to relieve symptoms.

• Small sips of peppermint tea will reduce nausea.

 HOMEOPATHY

• Sepia is useful, when the symptoms become worse with the smell of food, but better upon eating it.
• Arnica may help when symptoms come on through fatigue.
• Nux vom. is useful for vomiting when there is a feeling of chilliness and an accompanying headache.

• Tabacum may help nausea and a feeling of faintness.

 FLOWER ESSENCES

• Rescue Remedy can be applied to the pulse points for relief of symptoms. Apply several drops an hour or so before the journey.

 AROMATHERAPY

• A few drops of aniseed, fennel, or ginger essential oils on a handkerchief, placed near to the sufferer, will help ease symptoms.

• Massage a few drops of peppermint essential oil, diluted in a little sweet almond oil, into the chest and upper back a few hours before traveling.

 FROM THE LARDER

• Chew ginger root to reduce feelings of nausea.

 SELF-HELP

• Ensure that you have lots of fresh air while traveling.

• Take care to eat a light, complex carbohydrate-based meal before you go. Avoid sugary, greasy foods and alcohol.

• There are acupressure points on the wrist that are said to prevent the symptoms of travel sickness when stimulated. You can now purchase slim bands to affix to your wrists to do this for you.

RIGHT *Natural remedies for travel sickness (and for the fear of travel sickness) get the family vacation off to a good start.*

Food Poisoning

Food poisoning is usually caused by inadequate hygiene or cooking. The two main types of bacteria that cause food poisoning are staphylococci and salmonella. Hepatitis A may also be passed through food, if one of the handlers has not exercised care in handling the food. Symptoms include abdominal cramps, headache, nausea, vomiting and diarrhea, and fever.

 CAUTION

Any case of food poisoning that lasts longer than forty-eight hours should be seen by a physician.

All cases of salmonella should be reported to the medical authorities.

 HERBALISM

• The best treatment is to take mustard powder and warm water to induce vomiting, dock root to flush out the toxins, and ginger to settle the stomach.

• Comfrey root, decocted and taken internally, will help to relieve symptoms.

• Golden seal and meadowsweet can also be drunk as teas.

• Licorice tea will help to flush out the toxins.

• Chamomile, drunk as a tea, will help to ease digestion and reduce inflammation.

 HOMEOPATHY

• Arsenicum is excellent for many cases, particularly when there are burning pains and diarrhea.

• Nux vom. will help when the pain improves upon passing stools and there is a feeling of chilliness.

• Baptisia is useful for salmonella infections.

• Use Pulsatilla when the symptoms are worse at night and the sufferer feels tearful.

• Use Phosphorus when there is diarrhea with a burning sensation, vomiting, and a craving for cold drinks.

 FLOWER ESSENCES

• Rescue Remedy provides some relief from symptoms and any accompanying distress.

 AROMATHERAPY

• Essential oil of lavender or chamomile dropped on a handkerchief and placed by the sufferer should provide some relief from discomfort and help to calm.

FROM THE LARDER

• Drink warm water with a little lemon juice to cleanse the system.

• Chew ginger root to help ease the nausea.

• Cider vinegar, drunk with warm water, encourages vomiting to expel the poisons.

• When the vomiting has ceased, eat ripe bananas to help restore the bacterial balance in the gut. Live yogurt has a similar effect.

• Fresh garlic, or garlic capsules, should be taken to reduce infection.

SELF-HELP

• Drink plenty of cool fresh water and avoid any food for at least twenty-four hours.

• Avoid dairy produce for forty-eight hours.

• Some herbalists believe that strong spices such as cayenne, curry, and turmeric have preventive properties against food poisoning.

• When traveling in countries where food poisoning is common, ensure that you do not drink the local water or eat any food that has been in contact with it (including ice cubes in drinks). Take care to use bottled water even for brushing teeth.

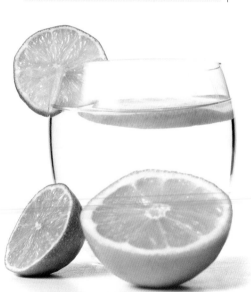

LEFT *Drinking warm water with a little lemon juice will help cleanse the system after food poisoning.*

Sunburn

Sunburn is caused by exposure to the ultraviolet rays of the sun and is a type of radiation burn. People with less melanin in their skin, which is a pigment produced to protect the skin from burning, are more susceptible; fair-skinned people have the least melanin. Sunburn is characterized by painful, reddened skin, occasionally accompanied by blisters. In some cases, minor fever may occur. It is often accompanied by sunstroke, which is a type of heat exhaustion and brings on dizziness, vomiting, headache, fever, and occasionally collapse.

 CAUTION

Direct exposure to sunlight is not recommended for children under the age of three. Use high SPF factor sunscreens (25) for small children, and ensure that they wear a hat. People of all ages should avoid the midday sun, when the rays are the strongest and most damaging.

Repeated sunburn can lead to premature aging and skin cancer.

 HERBALISM

• Use the juice of an aloe vera plant directly on the burn to reduce pain and encourage healing.

• Chamomile and witch hazel can be applied externally to reduce the pain and help promote healing.

• Sorrel tea may be taken internally to ease the effects.

• Use calendula or chamomile ointment for healing and pain relief.

 HOMEOPATHY

• Calendula ointment and Hypericum tincture may be used on sunburn.

• Internally, try Arnica for the pain of burns and to encourage healing.

• Use Cantharis immediately after exposure to the sun, when the pain of sunburn begins to make itself evident.

• Use Kali bich. and Urtica for pain.

 AROMATHERAPY

• A few drops of lavender oil, with an oil dispersant, can be used in the bath to encourage healing and reduce the pain.

• Essential oil of bergamot, in a little grapeseed oil, can be very gently massaged into the burned skin. Avoid the eye area.

• Chamomile oil, in a bath, or used in a light massage, may help to soothe the burn.

 FLOWER ESSENCES

• Rescue Remedy can be diluted in a little water and splashed on the burn, or applied in the form of a cream and gently massaged into the affected area. Where there is shock and pain, take a few drops internally, or apply to the pulse points for relief.

 FROM THE LARDER

• Grate a little raw potato and apply directly to the worst affected areas.

• A little honey, heated and mixed with a few teaspoons of petroleum jelly, can be gently massaged into the affected area to soothe.

 SELF-HELP

• Always use a sunscreen before going into direct sunlight, and wear a hat.

• Cool a sunburn with plenty of fresh running water (showers and lukewarm baths are effective). Wear light clothing and take care not to burst blisters (see page 260).

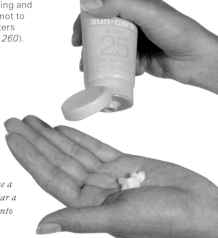

RIGHT *Always use a sunscreen and wear a hat before going into direct sunlight.*

A Home Medicine Chest

$\mathcal{T}$he best way to learn about natural medicines is to try them out on yourself, your family, and friends. Assemble a stock of home medicines. Keep them in a box or cupboard along with a thermometer, scissors, an eye bath, absorbent cotton, and a selection of bandages, bandaids, and sterile dressings. Use them for first-aid and to treat minor ailments. The more you use them the easier it becomes.

The lists that follow include remedies that most people will find useful. Check through the rest of the book and add remedies that are more specific to your own needs.

Make a checklist. What are the most common medical conditions that arise in your family? Make or assemble suitable remedies so that they are always available. Try to deal with illnesses as soon as they arise. Do not

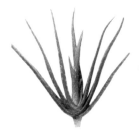

ALOE VERA
for burns and scalds

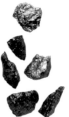

for splinters

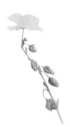

ROCK ROSE
for panic attacks

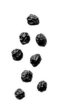

BLACK PEPPER
for aches and pains

HONEY
for sore throats

ABOVE *It is easy and economical to make up a medicine chest tailored to your household's specific needs. Some suggestions for practical remedies from herbalism, homeopathy, Bach Flower Remedies, and aromatherapy are shown above, together with a standby from the larder.*

wait for a runny nose to turn into sinusitis or bronchitis. Try to develop a general awareness of health and the patterns of health in your household. The aim of home treatment should always be to prevent minor illnesses from becoming major—to avoid visits to your practitioner.

Keep a notebook with the remedies to record your successes for future reference. A data file of indications and uses is given with each remedy. Use this as a guide and consult the body of the book for more detailed information. The various remedies below can be used alone or in combination, but decide which is to be your main internal remedy for a specific situation and use other suggestions as support. For example, use homeopathic Drosera for coughing attacks in children and back up with eucalyptus essential oil in a burner and chamomile tea at night.

Herbal Medicines

For most purposes keep either the dried herbs or their tinctures. Tinctures will keep, in dark-glass bottles in a cool place, for two or three years. Keep dried herbs in clean screw-top jars and replace them every year. Be sure to label all bottles and jars with the date and contents. Pills can be substituted where available and appropriate. They are especially useful for traveling and for unpleasant-tasting medicines. The creams and lotions can be bought or made at home. See the appropriate entry in the remedies section (Part Three) for methods of use.

Agrimony	*Diarrhea.*	**Elderflower**	*Colds, runny nose, hay fever, dust allergy. Children's fevers.*
Chamomile	*Headaches, tension, stress, insomnia, restlessness in children. Compress for sore eyes.*	**Fennel seeds**	*Infant colic. Indigestion and mild depression.*
Devil's claw	*For arthritic flare-up.*	**Peppermint**	*Indigestion, wind, colic, cramps, blocked nose.*
Echinacea	*Influenza with aches and pains. Recurrent infections.*		

Sage	Sore throat and mouth, early colds, and flu. Exhaustion.	**Yellow dock**	Constipation. Food poisoning.	
Slippery elm	Powder or tablets for all digestive upsets. Paste for drawing splinters and poison from bites and stings.	**Wild oat tincture**	Exhaustion. To keep going under stress.	

Creams and Lotions

Aloe vera juice	Sunburn, burns, infected rashes.	**St. John's wort tincture**	As lotion for cold sores and herpes.
Comfrey cream	Early bruising, sprains, deep cuts, and cracked skin.	**Witch hazel lotion**	Bites, stings, bruises, sprains, and swellings.
Marigold cream	Cuts and grazes.		

Herb Combinations for Specific Purposes: Make up specific combinations for regular and recurring problems in your household. With time you will figure out particularly good combinations of your own. The list below is offered as a starting point. All mixtures are equal parts, unless otherwise stated. These combinations are best taken freely for acute problems. See Part Three for more information about herb combinations.

Heartburn tea	Meadowsweet, chamomile, and comfrey.	**"Pick me up" tea**	Sage 2 parts, basil 1 part. Brings quick energy.
Cold and flu tea	Peppermint, elderflower, and yarrow.	**Cough syrup**	Thyme, mullein, and licorice.
Indigestion tea	Meadowsweet, chamomile, and fennel seed.	**Migraine tincture**	Valerian and feverfew.
Relaxing tea	Chamomile, linden, and skullcap.	**Period pain tincture**	Cramp bark 10 parts, ginger 1 part.
Headache tea	Chamomile and rosemary. Applicable to most types of headache.	**Spot lotion**	4fl. oz. (100ml.) of marigold tincture with 15 drops of tea tree essential oil and 5 drops of lavender essential oil.
Cystitis tea	Thyme, mallow, plantain, and uva ursi.		

Homeopathic Remedy

Buy your remedies from a reputable source. Keep them in the original bottles. Keep away from essential oils. Replace supplies before the sell-by date. Homeopathic remedies work best when they fit the full symptom picture. Try to find the remedies that especially suit the individual. Remember that they do not work so effectively if the person taking them has just drunk coffee or alcohol, or eaten spicy food.

Shocks and Wounds

Aconite	Sudden symptoms following exposure to cold. Frights and shock to the emotions. Anything that comes on suddenly.	**Arnica cream**	Apply to bruises, sprains, and aching muscles.
		Hypericum	Painful cuts and wounds. Falls injuring the spine.
Apis	Stings, bites, and swellings. Burning pains.	**Rhus tox.**	Sprains and strains from overexertion.
Arnica	Lessens shock after any injury. Bruising. After tooth extraction.	**Silica**	Thorns, splinters, boils, and abscesses.

Colds and Fevers

Belladonna	Sudden fevers with flushed face and pounding pulse. Throbbing pains, toothache, and earache.	**Ferrum phos.**	Raised temperature with bright red complexion.
		Gelsemium	Influenza, colds, and tight, nervous headaches. Examination nerves.

Irritability and Indigestion

Argentum nit.	Acidity and indigestion from worry and anticipation.	**Chamomilla**	Irritability and restlessness. Teething in children. Pains "out of proportion."
Arsenicum alb.	Food poisoning. Burning pains in stomach and restlessness.	**Merc. sol.**	Bad taste in mouth. Mouth ulcers. Feverish head cold.
		Nux vom.	Nausea, morning liverishness and nervous indigestion.

Coughs

Bryonia	*Hard, dry cough. For when colds go to the chest.*	Drosera	*Coughing attacks with retching. Whooping cough.*

Flower Remedies

Rescue Remedy is helpful for any kind of shock or distress. The important thing about Rescue Remedy is to remember to use it. Always take it yourself when you give it to others, and if you drive, carry a bottle in the car.

Walnut is worth keeping if you have children. It helps at any time of change in life.

Buy and keep other remedies according to your pattern.

Essential Oils

Keep essential oils in their original bottles. They last well but remember to screw the tops back on tightly or the oils will slowly evaporate. If you buy them with the eyedropper attached, remember to keep them upright or the oil will eat away at the rubber top and leak.

Lavender	*Relaxing and healing. The most generally useful oil. Apply directly to burns. Add a few drops to a glass of water to clean cuts and deep wounds. Massage, bath oil, and inhalant for restlessness, tension, insomnia, anxiety, and headaches.*	Thyme	*Antiseptic and expectorant. Inhalant and chest rub for coughs.*
		Eucalyptus	*Antiseptic and decongestant. Inhalant for colds and coughs. A few drops in water sprayed around the sick room to clear the air and keep down infection.*
Rosemary	*Warming and stimulating. Morning bath before a hard day. Bath or massage for muscle aches and pains.*	Chamomile	*Soothes irritation. Bath and massage for irritability, itchy skin, headaches, and period pains.*

| Rose | Cheering and relaxing. Expensive but worth it. Massage and bath for depression, grief, feeling unloved, broken heart. | Tea tree | Antiseptic and antifungal. Bath and cream for cuts, bites, itchy skin, athlete's foot, and thrush. Inhalant for lung and sinus infections. |
| | | Clove | Analgesic and antiseptic. Toothache. Massage oils for painful joints. |

Do-It-Yourself Remedies

One of the real pleasures of learning about home remedies is rediscovering the lost arts of making medicines for yourself. Try some of the simple recipes below.

St. John's wort infused oil: The method is explained in the herbalism section (*see page 27*). Use it neat on inflamed skin or as a base for making massage oils. Add 20 drops of lavender essential oil to 4fl. oz. (100ml.) of St. John's wort oil to make an excellent massage oil for back pain and neuralgia.

Warming oil: Make an infused oil with 1oz. (25g.) cayenne pepper powder, 1oz. (25g.) ginger powder, and 1pt. (500ml.) sunflower oil. Heat in a double boiler for two hours, strain, bottle, and label. For aches and pains, muscle knots, spasms, and unbroken chilblains. Massage in well twice daily. Do not use over large areas of the body.

Marigold cream: Follow the instructions in the herbalism section (*see page 27*). Excellent for use as a lip balm and for very dry skin.

Ginger tincture: Fill a small jar with grated, fresh ginger root, cover with vodka, and leave for two weeks. Strain, bottle, and label. Add 4 or 5 drops to any herb tea for chills, nausea, travel sickness, spasmodic pains, and aches and pains due to cold.

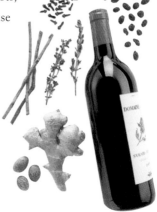

BELOW *The ingredients for a homemade tonic wine. White wine can also be used.*

GARLIC SYRUP AND INFUSED OIL

GARLIC SYRUP

Blend finely chopped garlic with an equal amount of honey for coughs and colds.
Garlic syrup will keep for a week or so in a cool place. Make it in batches to last
for three days.

1 *Finely chop between six and eight fresh, skinned garlic cloves. You need 6 tablespoons of chopped garlic for this mixture.*

2 *Put the garlic in a screwtop jar and add 6 tablespoons of clear honey. Mix together thoroughly. This should be enough for a three day supply.*

DOSAGE

ADULT STANDARD DOSE
• 2 teaspoons three or four times a day

CHILDREN OVER THE AGE OF FIVE
• 1 teaspoon three or four times a day

GARLIC INFUSED OIL

Half fill a clean jar with finely chopped garlic. Pour olive oil over, to fill the jar. Stand
overnight, strain off, bottle, and label. Use two or three drops in the ear, for acute
earache. Use as a chest rub, diluted with four parts of olive oil. This is also excellent
for coughs and colds and worth putting up with the smell. Keep in a cool place.

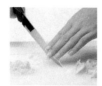

1 *Finely chop five or six cloves of fresh garlic. Put the garlic in a small, 5 fl. oz. (125 ml.) glass jar with a screw top.*

2 *Add 3.5 fl. oz. (85 ml.) olive oil to the garlic. Screw the top on and leave to stand overnight in a cool place.*

3 *Strain the infused oil into a dark bottle and put the lid on. Label and date the bottle. This oil should keep for several months.*

Tonic wine: To 1pt. (500ml.) of reasonable red wine add a sprig of fresh rosemary, 4 teaspoons grated fresh ginger, 4 teaspoons chopped fresh thyme, 1 cinnamon stick, ½ teaspoon powdered nutmeg, 1 teaspoon cloves, and 12 raisins. Stand for two weeks and strain off. Take half a wine glass for flagging spirits and lethargy. This is a traditional aphrodisiac mixture.

From the Larder

Many useful remedies can be made from common household items. These will not be kept in the medicine chest, but don't forget them. The most useful are listed below. More information on how to use common household ingredients "from the larder" can be found in Part Three.

• Barley decoction with a squeeze of lemon juice for digestive upsets, sore throats, and cystitis.

• Black pepper, a small pinch as snuff for congested head colds. Use twice daily for two or three days.

• Cabbage leaves can be crushed and wrapped around hot swollen joints. Tie on with a light bandage and replace every few hours. Also for mastitis when breast-feeding. Results can be dramatic.

• Cinnamon sticks chewed for colds.

• Carrot soup or juice for stomach pains and children's diarrhea.

• Garlic rubbed on infected spots.

• Honey for weeping eczema and infected cuts. Apply and cover with a light bandage. Honey and lemon for sore throats and colds.

• Mustard footbaths for tired and aching feet and at the beginning of colds.

• Salt water for sore gums, sore throats, and as eye drops. Baths for aches, pains, and stiffness of the joints.

• Cold tea for diarrhea.

CINNAMON

Vitamins and Minerals

$\mathcal{T}$he recommended daily allowance (RDA) of foods and supplements has traditionally been set by government health bodies in the USA, UK, and Europe. In the USA, RDA stands for "Recommended Daily Dietary Allowance," which is established for each vitamin and mineral by the Food and Nutritional Board of the National Academy of Sciences and the Food and Drug Administration (FDA). The US figures quoted here are from the FDA. In the UK the Department of Health gave the RDA for Vitamins A, C, and D, three of the B vitamins, and three minerals in 1979. However, in 1993 the European Union (EU) issued a directive on food labeling for its members, which included RDAs for twelve vitamins and six minerals. As a result, UK food labels are being revised to include the EU recommendations, although it may be some time before they appear.

In addition, the government of the UK issued a report in 1991 suggesting new guidelines for daily requirements of vitamins and minerals, which would replace the RDAs. These are called, collectively, Dietary Reference Values (DRVs), and consist of these terms:

Estimated Average Requirement (EAR), which should meet the requirements of half of the population.

Reference Nutrient Intake (RNI), which replaces the former RDA, is meant to represent the nutrient requirements of some 97 percent of the population. The amount recommended is higher than most people actually need.

NOTES

1. Fat-soluble vitamins dissolve in fat and any excess can be stored in the body Water-soluble vitamins dissolve in water and any excess is excreted.

2. iu=international unit. Old way to express vitamins in terms of their biological activity rather than weight; vitamins A, D, and E are still measured this way.

3. μg=microgram. It is sometimes written mcg. One million micrograms are equal to one gram.

Lower Reference Nutrient Intake (LRNI) is the nutritional requirement for those whose needs are low. Most people will need more than this amount in order to maintain their health. Anyone who is getting less than the LRNI might be in danger of nutritional deficiency.

Daily Intake The following list describes those vitamins and minerals that should be present in the daily diet. The descriptions include the RDAs for the USA, UK, and the EU. The amounts given are those that should be taken to prevent a vitamin or mineral deficiency, not those needed to improve health or prevent non-deficiency diseases.

Vitamins

VITAMIN A	is necessary for healthy skin and the ability to see in poor light conditions. The body manufactures vitamin A (retinol) from plants containing beta-carotene, but vitamin A is directly available from a few animal foods (e. g., liver and some fish). This vitamin is fat-soluble.[1]	RDA is: 5000 iu[2] (US); 750µg[3] (UK); 800µg (EU).
VITAMIN B1 (*thiamine*)	is necessary for healing and maintaining the nervous system and for the metabolism of carbohydrates. This vitamin is water-soluble.	RDA is: 1.2-1.5mg (US); 1.2mg (UK); 1.4mg (EU).
VITAMIN B2 (*riboflavin*)	is required for metabolizing foods, manufacturing and repairing tissues, and maintaining healthy mucous membranes. This vitamin is water-soluble.	RDA is: 1.7mg (US); non current (UK); 6mg (EU).
VITAMIN B3 (*niacin*)	belongs to the vitamin B complex. It is necessary for the efficient functioning of the digestive and nervous systems. It also helps in metabolizing foods. This vitamin is water-soluble.	RDA is: 1.3-1.8mg (US); non current (UK); 8mg (EU).

VITAMIN B5
(pantothenic acid)

is needed to release energy from fats and other foods, and to promote normal growth and development. This vitamin is water-soluble.

RDA is: 4.7mg (US) (new figures give 10mg); non current (UK); 6mg (EU).

VITAMIN B6
(pyridoxine)

is necessary for metabolizing the amino acids in proteins, the formation of antibodies and red blood cells, and for maintaining a healthy digestive and nervous system. This vitamin is water-soluble.

RDA is: 2mg (US); non current (UK); 2mg (EU).

VITAMIN B9
(folic acid)

is necessary for maintaining the digestive and nervous systems and works with B12 in the formation of red blood cells and genetic material. This vitamin is water-soluble.

RDA is: 400μg (US); 200μg (UK); 300μg (EU).

VITAMIN B12

is necessary for maintaining the nervous system, red blood formation, cell division during growth, and the development of genetic material. This vitamin is water-soluble.

RDA is: 3μg (US); 1μg (UK); 2μg (EU).

BIOTIN

is necessary for energy release from fats. It is water-soluble.

RDA is: 300μg (US); non current (UK); 0.15mg (EU).

VITAMIN C
(ascorbic acid)

is required for healthy skin, teeth, gums, and blood vessels. It assists in the absorption of iron, in healing wounds and broken bones, and is necessary for the prevention of scurvy. This vitamin is water-soluble.

RDA is: 60gm (US); 30gm (UK); 60mg (EU).

VITAMIN D

is required for the absorption of calcium and phosphorus. This vitamin is fat-soluble.

RDA is: 400iu (US); 2.5μm (UK); 5μg (EU).

VITAMIN E

helps to protect body tissues and is important for the prevention of anemia, although the precise role that this vitamin plays in the body is not clear. This vitimin is fat-soluble.

RDA is: 10mg (US); non current (UK); 10mg (EU).

Minerals

CALCIUM | is needed for the growth and development of healthy bones and teeth.

RDA is: 800mg (US); 500mg (UK); 800mg (EU).

IRON | is vital for the formation of the oxygen-carrying red blood cells.

RDA is: 10-30mg/18mg for pregnant women (US); 12mg (UK); 14mg (EU).

IODINE | is necessary for regulating the thyroid gland.

RDA is: 150µg (US); 140µg (UK); 150µg (EU).

MAGNESIUM | is necessary for strong bones, the release of energy from food, and the transmission of nerve impulses and muscular movements.

RDA is: 350mg (US); non current (UK); 300mg (EU).

PHOSPHORUS | is required for maintaining body functions, the production of energy, and, with calcium and magnesium, the maintenance of healthy teeth and bones.

RDA is: 300-400mg (US); non current (UK); 800mg (EU).

ZINC | helps to develop a healthy immune system and is necessary for growth and development, including that of the reproductive system.

RDA is: 15mg (US); non current (UK); 15mg (EU).

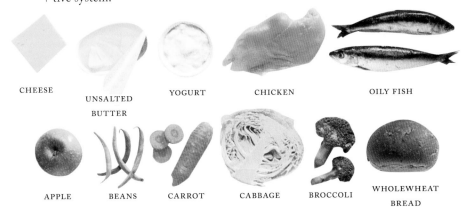

CHEESE   UNSALTED BUTTER   YOGURT   CHICKEN   OILY FISH

APPLE   BEANS   CARROT   CABBAGE   BROCCOLI   WHOLEWHEAT BREAD

LEFT *The most palatable way to get your daily vitamin and mineral requirement is to eat a balanced nutritious diet.*

Glossary

A

ABORTIFACIENT Agent that causes the early expulsion of an unborn baby

ABSCESS A lump of pus caused by inflammation or bacteria

ABSOLUTE A highly concentrated viscous, semi-solid, or solid perfume, usually obtained by alcohol extraction from the concrete

ACUTE Of sudden onset and brief duration

ADAPTOGEN Agent that modulates hormones

ADENOIDS Lymphatic tissue at the back of the nose

ADRENALIN Substance secreted by part of the adrenal gland that increases the heart rate in response to stress

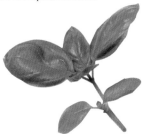

AGGRAVATION The exacerbation of symptoms that can occur when taking homeopathic remedies, particularly in the case of chronic ailments

AGORAPHOBIA Fear of open or crowed places

-ALGIA (suffix) "Pain in..." for example, arthralgia, pain in the joints

ALLERGEN Substance that causes an allergic reaction

ALLERGY Abnormal response by the body to a food or foreign substance

ALTERATIVE Corrects disordered bodily function

AMENORRHEA Absence of menses (periods)

ANALGESIC Remedy or agent that deadens pain

ANAPHRODISIAC Reduces sexual desire

ANEMIA Deficiency in either quality or quantity of red corpuscles in the blood

ANNUAL A plant that completes its life cycle in one year

ANODYNE Pain-killing

ANOREXIA NERVOSA Psychological problem causing extreme loss of appetite and drastic weight loss

ANTHELMINTIC A vermifuge, destroying or expelling intestinal worms

ANTIALLERGIC Agent that reduces allergic reactions

ANTIARTHRITIC Agent that combats arthritis

ANTIBACTERIAL Agent that prevents bacteria forming (e. g. penicillin)

ANTIBILIOUS Agent that helps remove excess bile from the body

ANTIBIOTIC Agent that prevents the growth or, or destroys, bacteria

ANTIBODY Chemical produced by the body's immune system to attack what it considers to be an invader (e. g. a bacteria, virus, or an allergen)

ANTICATARRHAL Agent that helps remove excess catarrh from the body

ANTICONVULSANT Agent that helps arrest or prevent convulsions

ANTIDEPRESSIVE Agent that relieves depression

ANTIDIARRHEAL Agent that is efficacious against diarrhea

ANTIDOTE In homeopathy the term used to describe other remedies or substances that cancel or nullify the effect of a prescribed remedy

ANTIEMETIC Agent that reduces the incidence and severity of nausea or vomiting

ANTIHEMORRHAGIC Agent that prevents or combats hemorrhage or bleeding

ANTIHISTAMINE Agent that treats allergic conditions; counteracts effects of histamine (which produces capillary dilation and, in larger doses, hemoconcentration)

ANTI-INFLAMMATORY Agent that alleviates inflammation

ANTILITHIC Agent that prevents the formation of a calculus or stone

ANTIMICROBIAL Agent that resists or destroys pathogenic microorganisms

ANTINEOPLASTIC Agent that helps prevent abnormal growths

ANTINEURALGIC Agent that relieves or reduces nerve pain

ANTIOXIDANT Agent used to prevent or delay oxidation or deterioration, especially with exposure to air

ANTIPRURITIC Agent that relieves sensation of itching or prevents its occurrence

ANTIPYRETIC Agent that reduces fever; see also **FEBRIFUGE**

ANTIRHEUMATIC Agent that relieves rheumatic problems

ANTISCLEROTIC Agent that helps prevent the hardening of tissue

ANTISEBORRHEIC Agent that helps control the products of sebum, the oily secretion from sweat glands

ANTISEPTIC Agent that destroys and prevents the development of microbes

ANTISPASMODIC Agent that prevents and eases spasms or convulsions

ANTITOXIC An antidote or treatment that counteracts the effects of poison

ANTITUSSIVE Agent that prevents coughing

ANTIVIRAL Agent that prevents viruses attacking the body

APERIENT A mild laxative

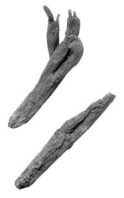

APERITIF A stimulant to the appetite

APHRODISIAC Increases or stimulates sexual desire

AROMATHERAPY The therapeutic use of essential oils

AROMATIC A substance with a strong aroma or smell

ARTERIOSCLEROSIS Hardening of the arteries

ARTICULATION Range of movement of the joints

ASTHMA Spasm of the bronchi in the lungs, narrowing the airwaves

ASTRINGENT Constricts the blood vessels or membranes in order to reduce irritation, inflammation, and swelling

AUTOIMMUNE DISORDER Occurs when the body creates antibodies against itself

B

BACTERICIDAL An agent that destroys bacteria (a type of microbe or organism)

BALSAM A resinous semi-solid mass or viscous liquid exuded from a plant, which can be either a pathological or physiological product. A "true" balsam is characterized by its high content of benzoic acid, benzoates, cinnamic acid, or cinnamates.

BALSAMIC Soothing medicine or application having the qualities of a balsam

BIENNIAL A plant that completes its life cycle in two years, without flowering in the first year

BILE Thick, oily fluid excreted by the liver; bile helps the body digest fats

BILIOUSNESS Disorder of bile production (to excess)

BITTER A tonic component that stimulates the appetite and promotes the secretion of saliva and gastric juices by exciting the taste buds

C

CALMATIVE A sedative agent

CANDIDA Candida albicans, fungus affecting the mucous membranes and skin; causes thrush

CARCINOGENIC Agent that can cause cancer

CARDIAC Pertaining to the heart

CARDIOACTIVE Agent that stimulates heart activity

CARDIOTONIC Having a stimulating effect on the heart

CARMINATIVE Settles the digestive system, relieves flatulence

CATHARTIC Agent that purges the body, usually the intestine, and cleanses the system

CENTESIMAL SCALE (c) In homeopathy, the scale that measures the potency of remedies in hundredths. One drop of mother tincture is mixed with ninety-nine drops of water or alcohol to make a remedy of 1 c potency. This remedy is then diluted with a further ninety-nine drops of water or alcohol to make a remedy of 2c potency. The sequence is repeated: 200c is usually the highest dose. The more the remedy is diluted, the more powerful it becomes.

CHOLAGOGUE Agent that stimulates the secretion and flow of bile into the duodenum

CHOLESTEROL A steroid alcohol found in nervous tissue, red blood cells, animal fat, and bile. Excess can lead to gallstones.

CHRONIC Persisting for a long time, a state showing no change or very slow change

CICATRIZANT An agent that promotes healing by the formation of scar tissue

COMPRESS A lint or substance applied hot or cold to an area of the body, for relief of swelling and pain, or to produce localized pressure

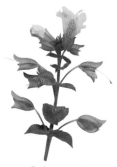

CONCOMITANT In homeopathy, a symptom coming at the same time, but not directly related to, the main complaint

CONCRETE A concentrate, waxy, solid, or semi-solid perfume material prepared from previously live plant matter, usually using a hydrocarbon type of solvent

CONGESTION Abnormal accumulation of blood

CONSTITUTIONAL Homeopathic term relating to the physical and mental constitution of a person, including hereditary factors and underlying health issues

CONTRAINDICATION Any factor in a patient's condition that indicates that treatment would involve a greater than normal degree of risk and is therefore not recommended

CORDIAL A stimulant and tonic

CORYZA Profuse discharge from the mucous membranes of the nose—"common cold"

COUNTER-IRRITANT Applications to the skin that relieve deep-seated pain, usually applied in the form of heat; see also **RUBEFACIENT**

D

DECIMAL SCALE (x) In homeopathy, the scale that measures the potency of remedies in tenths. One drop of mother tincture is mixed with nine drops of water or alcohol to make a remedy of 1 x potency. This remedy is then diluted with a further nine drops of water or alcohol to make a remedy of 2x potency. The sequence is repeated. The more the remedy is diluted, the more powerful it becomes.

DECOCTION A herbal preparation, where the plant material (usually hard or woody) is boiled in water and reduced to make a concentration extract

DECONGESTIVE An agent for the relief or reduction of congestion, e. g. mucus

DEMULCENT Agent that protects mucous membranes and allays irritation

DETOXIFICATION The removal of toxins from the body

DIAPHORETIC — see **SUDORIFIC**

DIGESTIVE Agent that promotes or aids the digestion of food

DISCHARGE An excretion or substance evacuated from the body

DIURETIC Agent that aids production of urine, promotes urination, increases flow

DYSFUNCTION Abnormal functioning of a system or organ within the body

DYSMENORRHEA Severe pains accompany monthly period

DYSPEPSIA Difficulty with digestion associated with pain, flatulence, heartburn, and nausea

DYSPNEA Labored or difficult breathing

E

EDEMA A painless swelling caused by fluid retention beneath the skin's surface

EMETIC Agent that induces vomiting

EMMENAGOGUE Agent that induces or assists menstruation

EMOLLIENT Agent that softens and soothes the skin

ENDORPHINS A group of chemicals manufactured in the brain that influence the body's response to pain

ENGORGEMENT Congestion of a part of the tissues, or fullness (as in the breasts)

ENZYME Complex proteins that are produced by the living cells and catalyze specific biochemical reaction

ESSENCE The integral part of a plant, its

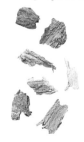

life-force, as used in flower remedies, herbalism, and aromatherapy

ESSENTIAL OIL A volatile and aromatic liquid (sometimes semisolid) which generally constitutes the odorous principles of a plant. It is obtained by a process of expression or distillation from a single botanical form or species.

ESTROGEN A hormone produced by the ovary, necessary for the development of female secondary sexual characteristics

EXPECTORANT Helps promote the removal of mucus from the respiratory system

F

FEBRIFUGE Agent that combats fever

FECES Excrement, stools

FEVER Elevation of body temperature above normal 36. 8°C (98. 4°F)

FIXATIVE A material that slows down the rate of evaporation of the more volatile components in a perfume composition

FIXED OIL The name given to a vegetable oil obtained from plants that, in contradistinction to essential oils, are fatty, dense, and non-volatile, such as olive or sweet almond oil

FUNGICIDAL Agent that prevents and combats fungal infection

G

GALACTAGOGUE Agent that increases secretion of milk

GAS EXCHANGE The exchange of waste carbon dioxide in the blood for fresh oxygen; it takes place in the alveoli of the lungs

GENERALS In homeopathy, symptoms relating to the whole person that can be expresse "I am..."; compare **PARTICULARS**

GERMICIDAL Destroys germs or micro-organisms such as bacteria

GUM "True" gum is little used in perfumery, being virtually odorless. However, the term "gum" is often applied to "resins," especially with relation to turpentines, as in the Australian "gum tree." Strictly speaking, gums are natural or synthetic water-soluble materials, such as gum arabic.

H

HALLUCINOGENIC Causes visions or delusions

HEMORRHAGE Loss of blood

HEMORRHOIDS Piles, anal varicose veins

HEMOSTATIC Arrests bleeding

HEPATIC Relating to the liver; an agent that tones the liver and aids its function.

HOLISTIC Aiming to treat the individual as an entity, incorporating body, mind, and spirit, from the Greek word holos, meaning whole

HOMEOPATHY Medical therapy devised by the 19th-century German doctor, Samuel Hahnemann, based on the premise that like cures like; sick persons are given minute doses of a remedy that will cause the symptoms of their disease, which helps the body to cure itself

HOMEOSTASIS Tendency for the internal environment of the body to remain constant in spite of varying external conditions

HORMONE A product of living cells that produces a specific effect on the activity cells remote from its point of origin

HYBRID A plant originating by fertilization of one species or subspecies by another

HYPERTENSION Raised blood pressure

HYPNOTIC Causing sleep

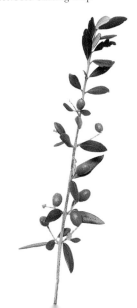

HYPOTENSION Low blood pressure, or a fall in blood pressure below the normal range

I

INCONTINENCE Partial or complete loss of control of urination

INFECTION Multiplication of pathogenic (disease-producing) micro-organisms within the body

INFLAMMATION Protective tissue response to injury or destruction of body cells characterized by heat, swelling, redness, and usually pain

INFUSION A herbal remedy prepared by steeping the plant material in water

INHALANT A remedy or drug that is breathed in through the nose or mouth

-ITIS (suffix) "Inflammation of..." for example, arthritis, inflammation of the joints

L

LAXATIVE Substance that promotes evacuation of the bowels

LEGUME A fruit consisting of one carpel, opening on one side, such as a pea

LEUCOCYTE White blood cells responsible for fighting disease

M

MACERATE Soak until soft

MATERIA MEDICA A branch of science dealing with the origins and properties of remedies; a complete description of remedies suggested in therapies such as homeopathy and herbalism

MENOPAUSE The normal cessation of menstruation, a life change for women

MENORRHAGIA An excess loss of blood occurring during menstruation

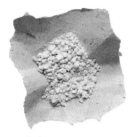

MENTALS In homeopathy, symptoms relating to the mental state, mood, and ideas

METABOLISM The complex process that is the fundamental chemical expression of life itself and the means by which food is converted to energy to maintain the body

METRORRHAGIA Bleeding that occurs in the middle of the menstrual cycle

MICROBE A minute living organism, especially pathogenic bacteria, viruses, etc.

MICTURATION Involuntary leakage of urine during coughing, laughing, or muscular effort

MODALITY In homeopathy, factor that makes symptoms better or worse

MOTHER TINCTURE In homeopathy, the source remedy, which is diluted to make the therapeutic dosages prescribed by homeopathic practitioners

MUCILAGE A substance containing gelatinous constituents that are demulcent

MUCOUS MEMBRANES Surface linings of the body, which secrete mucus

NARCOTIC Agent that induces sleep; intoxicating or poisonous in large doses

NERVINE Strengthening and toning to the nerves and nervous system

NOSODE In homeopathy, a remedy made from a diseased source, such as tuberculinum, made from tissue infected with tuberculosis

NUTRITIVE Substance that promotes nutrition

O

OLEO GUM resin A natural exudation from trees and plants that consists mainly of essential oil, gum, and resin

OLEORESIN A natural resinous exudation from plants, or an aromatic liquid preparation extracted from botanical matter using solvents. They consist almost entirely of a mixture of essential oil and resin

PANACEA A cure-all

PARASITICIDE Parasite killer

PARTICULARS In homeopathy, symptoms relating to a part of the person, that can be expressed "My..."; compare **GENERALS**

PARTURIENT Encouraging onset of labor

PECULIARS In homeopathy, strange, rare, and peculiar symptoms, which relate to the individual and are not common in illness

PEPTIC Term applied to gastric secretions and areas affected by them

PERENNIAL A plant that lives for more than two years, normally flowering every year

PERISTALSIS Rhythmic movement of the gut to push food along the intestinal tract

PHARMACOPEIA An official publication of drugs in common use, in a given country

PHLEGM Thick, shiny mucus produced in the respiratory passage

PHOTOTOXIC Substance that becomes poisonous on exposure to light

PHYTOTHERAPY The treatment of disease by plants; herbal medicine

POLYCREST A homeopathic remedy that has a broad spectrum of actions, and can therefore be used for a variety of different conditions

POMADE A prepared perfume material obtained by the enfleurage process

POTENCY "Strength" of a homeopathic remedy; the higher the number, the greater the strength and the greater the dilution

POULTICE The therapeutic application of a soft moist mass (such as fresh herbs) to the skin, to encourage local circulation and to relieve pain

PROGESTERONE A female sex hormone that prepares the uterus for the fertilized ovum and maintains pregnancy

PROPHYLACTIC Preventive of disease or infection

PROVING The process used in homeopathy for testing a remedy; it can occur when the wrong remedy is prescribed and taken over a period of time, and the symptoms of the condition it is aimed at manifest themselves

PSYCHOSOMATIC The manifestation of physical symptoms resulting from a mental state

PURGATIVE Agent stimulating evacuation of the bowels

PURULENT Containing pus

R

RECTIFICATION The process of redistillation applied to essential oils to rid them of certain constituents

REGULATOR Agent that helps balance and regulates the functions of the body

RELAXANT Substance that promotes relaxation (either muscular or psychological)

REMEDY PICTURE In homeopathy the collection of symptoms that characterize a remedy

RESIN A natural or prepared product, either solid or semi-solid in nature. Natural resins are exudations from trees, such as mastic; prepared resins are oleoresins from which essential oil has been removed

RESOLVENT An agent that disperses swelling, or effects absorption of a new growth

RESTORATIVE An agent that helps strengthen and revive the body systems

RHIZOME An underground plant stem lasting more than one season

RUBEFACIENT Substance that causes redness of the skin, possibly irritation

S

SCLEROSIS Hardening of tissue due to inflammation

SEDATIVE An agent that reduces functional activity; calming

SELF-LIMITING A condition that lasts a set length of time and usually clears of its own accord

SEPTIC Putrefying due to the presence of pathogenic (disease-producing) bacteria

SHOCK Sudden and disturbing mental or physical impression; also a state of collapse characterized by pale, cold, sweaty skin, rapid, weak, thready pulse, faintness, dizziness, and nausea

SIALOGOGUE An agent that stimulates the secretion of saliva

SOPORIFIC Agent that induces sleep

SPASM Sudden, violent involuntary muscular contraction

SPECIFIC Remedy effective for a particular ailment

STIMULANT Agent that quickens the physiological functions of the body

STOMACHIC Agent that stimulates function of the stomach

STYPTIC An astringent agent that stops or reduces external bleeding

SUCCUSSION The shaking method used in preparing homeopathic remedies

SUDORIFIC Agent that causes sweating

SYMPTOM PICTURE Homeopathic term for the overall pattern of symptoms characterizing each individual patient

SYMPTOMS Perceived changes in, or impaired function of, body or mind indicating the presence of disease or injury

T

TACHYCARDIA An unduly rapid heartbeat

TINCTURE A herbal remedy, or perfumery material prepared in an alcohol base

TISSUE SALT Inorganic compound essential to the growth and function of the body's cells

TONIC Strengthens and enlivens the whole or specific parts of the body

TOPICAL Local application of cream, ointment, tincture, or other medicine

TOPICAL IRRITANT A substance that irritates the skin

TOXIN Substance that is poisonous to the body

TRAUMA Physical injury or wound; also unpleasant and disturbing experience causing psychological upset

TRIGEMINAL NERVE Nerve that divides into three and supplies the mandibular (jaw), maxillary (cheek) and ophthalmic (eye), and forehead areas

TUBER A swollen part of an underground plant stem of one year's duration, capable of new growth

TYPE A term used by Bach and other flower remedy therapists to describe a person's general personality and approach to life

U

ULCER Slow-healing sore occurring internally or externally

UTERINE TONIC Substance that has a toning effect on the whole reproductive system

V

VASOCONSTRICTOR Agent that causes narrowing of the blood vessels

VASODILATOR Agent that dilates the blood vessels and so improves circulation

VERMIFUGE Anthelmintic remedy that eliminates worms from the body

VESICANT Causing blistering to the skin; a counter-irritant

VOLATILE Unstable, evaporates easily, as in "volatile oil"; see ESSENTIAL OIL

VULNERARY An agent that helps heal wounds and sores by external application

Healing Plant Directory

All plant names (both Latin and common) followed by a page reference feature in the book. Those names followed by "see" and a Latin name do not feature directly, but are popular alternatives by which particular plants may be known. They are included for ease of reference.

A

Aaron's rod see *Verbascum thapsus*
Achillea millefolium 132
Aconite 132
Aconitum napellus 132
Actaea racemosa 149
Adam's flanner see *Verbascum thapsus*
Aesculus x carnea 133
Aesculus hippocastanum 133
Agnus castus 215
Agrimonia eupatoria 134
Agrimony 134
Alchemilla mollis see *Alchemilla vulgaris*
Alchemilla vulgaris 134
Allium sativum 135
Aloe barbardensis see *Aloe vera*
Aloe vera 136
Althaea officinalis 136
Amantilla see *Valeriana officinalis*
American arbor vitae see *Thuja occidentalis*
Anaminta cocculus 154
Andropogon martinii see *Cymbopogon martinii*
Angelica 137
Angelica archangelica 137
Angelica sinensis 137
Anise 187
Aniseed 187
Annual knawel see *Scleranthus annuus*

Annual marjoram see *Origanum majorana*
Apple see *Malus sylvestris*
Apple geranium see *Pelargonium odoratissimum*
Arbor-vitae 208
Arbutus uva-ursi see *Arctostaphylos uva-ursi*
Archangel see *Angelica archangelica*
Arctium lappa 138
Arctium minus 138
Arctostaphylos uva-ursi 138
Arnica 139
Arnica montana 139
Aspen 36, 190
Ass ear see *Symphytum officinale*
Astragalus membranaceus 140
Astragalus root 140
Atlas cedar see *Cedrus atlantica*
Atropa belladonna 140
Auld wife's huid see *Aconitum napellus*
Avena futua 141

B

Bad man's plaything see *Achillea millefolium*
Baldmoney see *Gentiana amarella*
Barbados aloe see *Aloe vera*
Barbe-de-capuchin see *Cichorium intybus*
Basil 49, 184
Batchelor's buttons see *Tanacetum parthenium*
Bath asparagus see *Ornithogalum umbellatum*
Bay 187
Bearberry leaves 138
Bear's foot see *Aconitum napellus*
Bear's foot see *Alchemilla vulgaris*
Bear's grape see *Arctostaphylos uva-ursi*
Bee balm see *Melissa officinalis*
Beech 36, 163
Beggar's blanket see *Verbascum thapsus*
Beggar's buttons see *Arctium lappa*

Beggar's stalk see *Verbascum thapsus*
Belladonna 140
Bergamot 150
Bergamot orange see *Citrus bergamia*
Bigarade see *Citrus aurantium*
Bitter apple see *Cucumis colocynthis*
Bitter cucumber 157
Bitter orange see *Citrus aurantium*
Bitterwort see *Gentianella amarella*
Black-berried white bryony see *Bryonia alba*
Black bryony root and berries 206
Black cherry see *Atropa belladonna*
Black cohosh 149
Black elder see *Sambucus nigra*
Blackeye root see *Tamus communis*
Black haw see *Viburnum opulus*
Black sampson see *Echinacea angustifolia*
Black snake root 149
Black-tang see *Fucus vesiculosis*
Black walnut see *Juglans regia*
Blackwort see *Symphytum officinale*
Bladder fucus see *Fucus vesiculosis*
Bladderwrack 165
Blanket weed see *Verbascum thapsus*
Blessed thistle see *Silybum marianum*
Blister beetle 145
Bloodwort see *Achillea millefolium*
Blue gum see *Eucalyptus globulus*
Blue rocket see *Aconitum napellus*
Blue-sailors see *Cichorium intybus*
Boneset see *Symphytum officinale*
Bonnet bellflower see *Codonopsis pilosula*
Bore tree see *Sambucus nigra*
Boswellia carteri 141
Boswellia sacra see *Boswellia carteri*
Bottle-brush see *Equisetum arvense*
Bour tree see *Sambucus nigra*
Bramble of Mount Ida see *Rubus idaeus*
Brassica nigra 203

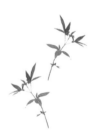

Further Reading

All books on this list have been published in the UK, unless otherwise noted

AROMATHERAPY

Aromatherapy
Christine Wildwood. Element Books, 1991

Aromatherapy for Pregnancy and Childbirth
Margaret Fawcett. Element Books, 1993

Aromatherapy from Provence
Nelly Grosjean. C. W. Daniel, 1994

Aromatherapy: Massage with Essential Oils
Christine Wildwood. Element Books, 1991

The Illustrated Encyclopaedia of Essential Oils
Julia Lawless. Element Books, UK/USA, 1995

FLOWER REMEDIES

Flower Remedies: Natural Healing with Flower Essences
Christine Wildwood. Element Books, 1991

A Guide to Bach Flower Remedies
Julian Barnard.
C. W. Daniel, 1987

GENERAL

A-Z of Natural Healthcare
Belinda Grant. Optima, 1993

All Day Energy
Kathryn Marsden. Bantam Books, 1995

The Alternative Dictionary of Symptoms and Cures
Dr. Caroline Shreeve. Century, 1987

The Alternative Health Guide
Brian Inglis & Ruth West.
Michael Joseph, 1983

The Anatomy of Change
Richard Strozzi Heckler.
Shambala, 1984

Back to Eden
Jethro Kloss. Woodbridge Press, USA, 1981

Better Health through Natural Healing
Ross Tratler. McGraw-Hill, USA, 1987

Body and Soul
Sara Martin. Arkana, 1989

Choices in Healing
Michael Lerner. MIT Press, USA/UK, 1994

The Complete Family Guide to Alternative Medicine
General Editor Richard Thomas.
Element Books, 1996

The Complete Guide to Food Allergy and Environmental Illnesses
Dr. Keith Mumby. Thorsons, 1993

The Encyclopaedia of Alternative Health Care
Kristen Olsen. Piatkus, 1989

Encyclopaedia of Natural Medicine
Brian Inglis and Ruth West. Michael Joseph, 1983

Encyclopaedia of Natural Medicine
Michael Murray and Joseph Pizzorno.
Macdonald Optima, 1990

Gentle Medicine
Angela Smyth. Thorsons, 1994

The Greening of Medicine
Patrick Pietroni. Gollancz, 1990

Guide to Complementary Medicine and Therapies
Anne Woodham. Health Education Authority, 1994

The Handbook of Complementary Medicine
Stephen Fulder. Oxford Medical Publications, 1988

Headaches
Dr. John Lockie with Karen Sullivan.
Bloomsbury, 1992

How to Live Longer and Feel Better
Linus Pauling. W. H. Freeman, USA, 1986

Life, Health and Longevity
Kenneth Seaton. Scientific Hygiene, USA, 1994

Maximum Immunity
Michael Wiener. Gateway Books, 1986

Medicine and Culture
Lynn Payer. Gollancz, 1990

Miracles Do Happen
C. Norman Shealy. Element Books, UK/USA, 1995

Reader's Digest Family Guide to Alternative Medicine
ed. Dr. Patrick Pietroni.
The Reader's Digest Association, UK/ USA/South Africa/ Aus, 1991

You Don't Have to Feel Unwell
Robin Needes. Gateway Books, 1994

HERBALISM

The Complete Illustrated Holistic Herbal
David Hoffman. Element Books, UK/USA, 1996

The Complete New Herbal
ed. Richard Mabey. Penguin Books, UK/ USA/NZ/Aus/Can, 1991

Evening Primrose
Kathryn Marsden. Vermillion, 1993
The Family Medical Herbal
Kitty Campion. Dorling Kindersley, 1988
Herbal Medicine: The Use of Herbs for Health and Healing
Vicki Pitman. Element Books, 1994
The Herbal for Mother and Child
Anne McIntyre. Element Books, 1992
Herbs for Common Ailments
Anne McIntyre. Gaia, 1992
The Herb Society's Complete Medicinal Herbal
Penelope Ody. Dorling Kindersley, 1993
The Home Herbal
Barbara Griggs. Pan Books, 1995
The Illustrated Herbal Handbook for Everyone
Juliette de Bairacli Levy. Faber & Faber, 1991

HOMEOPATHY

The Complete Family Guide to Homeopathy
Dr. Christopher Hammond. Element Books, UK/USA, 1996
Emotional Healing with Homoeopathy: A Self-Help Manual
Peter Chappell. Element Books, 1994
The Family Guide to Homoeopathy
Andrew Lockie. Hamish Hamilton, 1990
The Family Health Guide to Homoeopathy
Dr. Barry Rose. Dragon's World, 1992
Homoeopathy: The Family Handbook
British Homoeopathic Association Thorsons, 1992

How to Use Homeopathy: A Comprehensive Instruction Book
Dr. Christopher Hammond. Element Books, 1991
The New Concise Guide to Homeopathy
Nigel and Susan Garion-Hutchings. Element Books, 1993
The Women's Guide to Homoeopathy
Andrew Lockie and Nicola Geddes. Hamish Hamilton, 1992

NUTRITION AND DIET

The Amino Revolution
Robert Erdmann & Meirion Jones. Century, 1987
Anorexia and Bulimia
Julia Buckroyd. Element Books, UK/USA, 1996

Food: Your Miracle Medicine
Jean Carper. Simon & Schuster, 1993
Healing Nutrients
Patrick Quillen. Contemporary Books, USA/Beaverbooks, Can, 1987, Penguin, 1989
Nutritional Medicine
Stephen Davies and Alan Stewart. Pan Books, 1987
Prescription for Nutritional Healing
James & Phyllis Balch. Avery Press, USA, 1990
Raw Energy
Leslie & Susannah Kenton. Arrow Books, 1985
Total Body Colon Cleansing,
Brian Wright. Clearlight Books, 1995

The Vitamin Bible
Earl Mindell. Arrow, 1993
Vitamin C, The Common Cold and Flu
Linus Pauling. Berkley, USA, 1970
Vitamin C: The Master Nutrient
Sandra Goodman. Keats, USA, 1991
The Vitamin Guide: Using Vitamins for Optimum Health
Hasnain Walji. Element Books, 1992
The Wright Diet
Celia Wright. Clearlight Books, 1995

Useful Addresses

AROMATHERAPY

Europe

ACADEMY OF
  AROMATHERAPY AND MASSAGE
50 Cow Wynd, Falkirk Sterlingshire
FK1 1PU Great Britain
Tel: 44 1324 612658

INTERNATIONAL FEDERATION OF
  AROMATHERAPISTS
Stamford House 2-4 Chiswick High
Road
London W4 1TH
Great Britain
Tel: 44 181 742 2605
Fax: 44 181 742 2606

INTERNATIONAL SOCIETY OF
  PROFESSIONAL AROMATHERAPISTS
ISPA House, 82 Ashby Road Hinckley,
Leics OE10 1SN Great Britain
Tel: 44 1455 637987
Fax: 44 1455 890956

TISSERAND INSTITUTE
65 Church Road, Hove
East Sussex BN3 2BD Great Britain
Tel: 44 1273 206640
Fax: 44 1273 329811

North America

AMERICAN ALLIANCE OF AROMA THERAPY
PO Box 750428, Petaluma
California 94975-0428
USA
Tel: 1 707 778 6762
Fax: 1 707 769 0868

AMERICAN AROMATHERAPY ASSOCIATION
PO Box 3679, South Pasadena
California 91031
USA
Tel: 1 818 457 1742

NATIONAL ASSOCIATION OF HOLISTIC
  AROMATHERAPY

PO Box 17622, Boulder
Colorado 80308-0622
USA
Tel: 1 303 258 3791

BACH FLOWER REMEDIES

Australasia

MARTIN & PLEASANCE
137 Swan Street, Richmond
Victoria 3121
Australia
Tel: 61 39 427 7422

Europe

DR EDWARD BACH CENTRE
Mount Vernon, Sotwell
Wallingford, Oxon OX10 0PZ
Great Britain
Tel: 44 1491 834678
Fax: 44 1491 825022

North America

NELSON BACH USA LTD
Wilmington Technology Park 100
Research Drive Wilmington
Massachusetts 01887-4406
USA
Tel: 1 508 988 3833

DIET THERAPY

North America

AMERICAN ASSOCIATION
  OF NUTRITION CONSULTANTS
1641 East Sunset Road Apt B-117,
Las Vegas Nevada 89119
USA
Tel: 1 709 361 1132

AMERICAN DIETETICS ASSOCIATION
216 West Jackson Boulevard Apt 800,
Chicago Illinois 60606-6995
USA
Tel: 1 800 877 1600

FLOWER THERAPY

Europe

FLOWER ESSENCE FELLOWSHIP
Laurel Farm Clinic
17 Carlingcott, Peasedown St John
Bath BA2 8AN
Great Britain
Tel: 44 1761 434098
Fax: 44 1761 434905

HERBALISM

Australasia

NATIONAL HERBALISTS
  ASSOCIATION OF AUSTRALIA
Suite 305, BST House 3 Smail Street,
Broadway New South Wales 2007
Australia
Tel: 61 2 211 6437
Fax: 61 2 211 6452

Europe

SCHOOL OF HERBAL
  MEDICINE/PHYTOTHERAPY
Bucksteep Manor
Bodle Street Green
Near Hailsham, Sussex BN27 4RJ
Great Britain
Tel: 44 1323 833 812/4
Fax: 44 1323 833 869

North America

AMERICAN HERBALISTS GUILD
PO Box 1683, Soquel California 95073
USA

HOLISTIC MEDICINE

Europe

BRITISH HOLISTIC MEDICAL ASSOCIATION
Trust House Royal Shrewsbury Hospital
  South Shrewsbury, Shropshire SY3 8XF
  Great Britain
Tel: 44 1743 261155
Fax: 44 1743 353637

HOLISTIC AND CREATIVE THERAPY
ASSOCIATION
2A Burston Drive, St. Albans
Herts AL2 2HR
Great Britain
Tel: 44 1727 674567

HOLISTIC HEALTH FOUNDATION
2 De La Hay Avenue, Plymouth
Devon PL3 4HH
Great Britain
Tel: 44 1752 671 485
Fax: 44 1345 251759

North America

AMERICAN HOLISTIC HEALTH
ASSOCIATION
PO Box 17400, Anaheim California
90017-7100 USA
Tel: 1 714 779 6152/777 2917

AMERICAN HOLISTIC MEDICAL ASSOCIATION
4101 Lake Boone Trail Suite 201,
Raleigh North Carolina 27607
USA
Tel: 1 919 787 5181
Fax: 1 919 787 4916

ASSOCIATION OF HOLISTIC HEALING
CENTERS
109 Holly Crescent, Suite 201 Virginia
Beach, Virginia 23451 USA
Tel: 1 804 422 9033
Fax: 1 804 422 8132

CANADIAN HOLISTIC MEDICAL ASSOCIATION
491 Eglington Avenue West Apt 407,
Toronto Ontario M5N 1A8 Canada
Tel: 1 416 485 3071

INTERNATIONAL ASSOCIATION OF HOLISTIC
HEALTH PRACTITIONERS
5020 West Spring Mountain Road,
Las Vegas, Nevada 89102
USA
Tel: 1 702 873 4542

HOMEOPATHY

Australasia

AUSTRALIAN FEDERATION FOR
HOMEOPATHY
PO Box 806, Spit Junction New South
Wales 2088 Australia

AUSTRALIAN INSTITUTE OF HOMEOPATHY
21 Bulah Heights Berdwra Heights New
South Wales 2082 Australia

INSTITUTE OF CLASSICAL HOMEOPATHY
24 West Haven Drive, Tawa
Wellington
New Zealand

Europe

BRITISH HOMOEOPATHIC ASSOCIATION
27A Devonshire Street London WIN
1RJ Great Britain
Tel: 44 171 935 2163

CENTRE D'ETUDES
HOMEOPATHIQUES DE FRANCE
228 Boulevard Raspail
75014 Paris
France

SOCIÉTÉ MÉDICAL DE BIOTHÉRAPIE
62 rue Beaubourg, 75003 Paris France

SOCIETY OF HOMOEOPATHS
2 Artisan Road Northampton NN1 4HU
Great Britain
Tel: 44 1604 21400
Fax: 44 1604 22622

North America

AMERICAN FOUNDATION FOR HOMEOPATHY
1508 S. Garfield, Alhambra
California 91801
USA

AMERICAN INSTITUTE OF HOMEOPATHY
1585 Glencoe Street, Suite 44 Denver,
Colorado 80220-1338
USA
Tel: 1 303 321 4105

FOUNDATION FOR HOMEOPATHIC
EDUCATION AND RESEARCH
2124 Kittredge Street Berkeley,
California 94704
USA

HOMEOPATHIC COUNCIL
FOR RESEARCH AND EDUCATION
50 Park Avenue
New York 10016
USA

INTERNATIONAL FOUNDATION FOR
HOMEOPATHY
2366 Eastlake Avenue East Suite 301,
Seattle Washington 98102
USA

NATIONAL CENTER FOR HOMEOPATHY
801 North Fairfax Street Suite 306,
Alexandria Virginia 22314
USA

Index

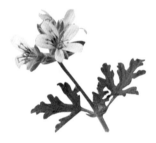

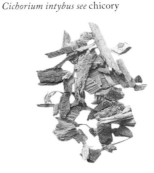

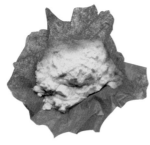

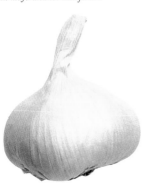

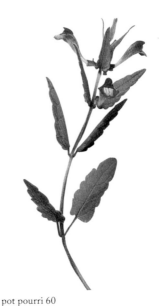

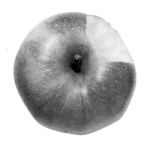

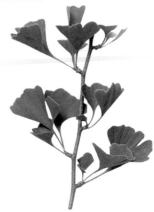

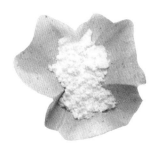

Acknowledgements

The publishers would like to thank the following for the use of pictures:

ARDEA: 24t, 152b, 166t, /sage 171t
HEATHER ANGEL: 126t, 168b
BIOFOTOS; 165b
ANTHONY BLAKE LIBRARY: 36t
BRIDGEMAN ART LIBRARY:
Bib. Nationale 34t, /Brit. Mus. 34b, /Uffizi 35t
BRIDGEWATER BOOK CO.: 14t, 14b
E. T. ARCHIVE: 35b, 44t
FLPA:
Thomas 62b, /Batten 133t, /Rose 141b,/
Hosking 150t, 157, /Merlet 169t, /Hosking 183b
BOB GIBBONS: Natural Image: 117t
HAHNEMANN HOUSE TRUST: 22t
ROBERT HARDING PICTURE LIBRARY: IPC 30b, 57t, 65b, /Liaison 92b, 230t
HOLT STUDIOS:
Cattlin 114t, /Silva 122b, /Gibbons 138b, /Gibbons 172b,/
Cattlin 175t, /Cattlin 175b, /Cherry 178t, /Cattlin 220
HUTCHISON LIBRARY: Parker 163t, /Francis 233
IMAGE BANK: Rakke 90
IMAGES COLOUR LIBRARY: 24b, 40b, 57b, 66br, 69, 229tl
NHPa: Hutchison /A. N. T 152t, /Keller /A. NT 153t
OSF: Fogden 26b, 146t, /West 114b, /Bown 155b, /159t, Davies 176t,/West 178b
PREMAPHOTOS: 134, 182t
SUPERSTOCK: 24t, 41
ELIZABETH WHITING LIBRARY: 17
ZEFA: 80

The publishers would also like to thank
MODELS: Tom Aitken, Ian Clegg, Judith Cox, Carly Evans, Janice Jones, Julia Holden, Simon Holden,
Kay Macmullan, Sally-Ann Russell, Stephen Sparshatt, and Robin Yarnton; Elphick & Son Ltd, Lewes,
East Sussex; The Pine Chest, Lewes, East Sussex; Sussex Trugs Ltd,
Herstmonceux, East Sussex.

Other Books in the Complete Illustrated Guide Series

The Complete Illustrated Guide to Massage
The Complete Illustrated Guide to Reflexology
The Complete Illustrated Guide to Palmistry
The Complete Illustrated Guide to Tai Chi
The Complete Illustrated Guide to Herbs
The Complete Illustrated Guide to Crystal Healing